*Study Guide for*

# Essentials of Pediatric Nursing

## SECOND EDITION

**TERRI KYLE, MSN, CPNP**
Director of Nursing
El Camino College
Torrance, California

**SUSAN CARMAN, MSN, MBA**
Professor of Nursing
Most recently, Edison Community College
Fort Myers, Florida

Wolters Kluwer | Lippincott Williams & Wilkins
Health

Philadelphia · Baltimore · New York · London
Buenos Aires · Hong Kong · Sydney · Tokyo

*Acquisitions Editor:* Carrie Brandon
*Product Manager:* Helene T. Caprari
*Editorial Assistant:* Jacalyn Clay
*Design Coordinator:* Holly McLaughlin
*Illustration Coordinator:* Brett MacNaughton
*Manufacturing Coordinator:* Karin Duffield
*Prepress Vendor:* Aptara, Inc.

Second edition

Printed in China

ISBN: 978-1-60547-630-8

Care has been taken to confirm the accuracy of the information presented and to describe generally accepted practices. However, the authors, editors, and publisher are not responsible for errors or omissions or for any consequences from application of the information in this book and make no warranty, expressed or implied, with respect to the currency, completeness, or accuracy of the contents of the publication. Application of this information in a particular situation remains the professional responsibility of the practitioner; the clinical treatments described and recommended may not be considered absolute and universal recommendations.

The authors, editors, and publisher have exerted every effort to ensure that drug selection and dosage set forth in this text are in accordance with the current recommendations and practice at the time of publication. However, in view of ongoing research, changes in government regulations, and the constant flow of information relating to drug therapy and drug reactions, the reader is urged to check the package insert for each drug for any change in indications and dosage and for added warnings and precautions. This is particularly important when the recommended agent is a new or infrequently employed drug.

Some drugs and medical devices presented in this publication have Food and Drug Administration (FDA) clearance for limited use in restricted research settings. It is the responsibility of the health care provider to ascertain the FDA status of each drug or device planned for use in his or her clinical practice.

LWW.com

# Preface

This Study Guide was developed by Kim Cooper and Kelly Gosnell, to accompany the second edition of *Essentials of Pediatric Nursing* by Terri Kyle and Susan Carman. The Study Guide is designed to help you practice and retain the knowledge you have gained from the textbook, and it is structured to integrate that knowledge and give you a basis for applying it in your nursing practice. The following types of exercises are provided in each chapter of the Study Guide.

## SECTION I: ASSESSING YOUR UNDERSTANDING

The first section of each Study Guide chapter concentrates on the basic information of the textbook chapter and helps you to remember key concepts, vocabulary, and principles.

- *Fill in the Blanks*
  Fill in the blank exercises test important chapter information, encouraging you to recall key points.

- *Labeling*
  Labeling exercises are used where you need to remember certain visual representations of the concepts presented in the textbook.

- *Matching*
  Matching questions test your knowledge of the definition of key terms.

- *Sequencing*
  Sequencing exercises ask you to remember particular sequences or orders, for instance, testing processes and prioritizing nursing actions.

- *Short Answers*
  Short answer questions will cover facts, concepts, procedures, and principles of the chapter. These questions ask you to recall information as well as demonstrate your comprehension of the information.

## SECTION II: APPLYING YOUR KNOWLEDGE

The second section of each Study Guide chapter consists of case-study-based exercises that ask you to begin to apply the knowledge you have gained from the textbook chapter and reinforced in the first section of the Study Guide chapter. A case study scenario based on the chapter's content is presented, and then you are asked to answer some questions, in writing, related to the case study. The questions cover the following areas:
- Assessment
- Planning Nursing Care
- Communication
- Reflection

## SECTION III: PRACTICING FOR NCLEX

The third and final section of the Study Guide chapters helps you practice NCLEX-style questions while further reinforcing the knowledge you have been gaining and testing for yourself through the textbook chapter and the first two sections of the Study Guide chapter. In keeping with the NCLEX, the questions presented are multiple choice and scenario based, asking you to reflect, consider, and apply what you know and to choose the best answer out of those offered.

## ANSWER KEYS

The answers for all of the exercises and questions in the Study Guide are provided at the back of the book, so you can assess your own learning as you complete each chapter.

We hope you will find this Study Guide to be helpful and enjoyable, and we wish you every success in your studies toward becoming a nurse.

**The Publishers**

# Contents

# CHAPTER 1

# Introduction to Child Health and Pediatric Nursing

## Learning Objectives

- Compare the past definitions of health and illness to the current definitions.
- Identify the key milestones in the history of child health.
- Discuss different methods of measuring child health.
- Discuss the philosophy of pediatric nursing care.
- Identify the major roles and functions of pediatric nursing, including the scope of practice and the professional standards for pediatric nurses.
- Explain the components of the nursing process as they relate to nursing practice for children and their families.
- Identify ethical concepts related to providing nursing care to children and their families.
- Describe legal issues related to caring for children and their families.

## SECTION I: ASSESSING YOUR UNDERSTANDING

### Activity A  FILL IN THE BLANKS

1. More children and adolescents die from _Unintentional_ injuries than any other cause.

2. The current health care delivery system, based on diagnostic-related groups, improve access to preventative care, but limit access to _Specialty_ care.

3. With the emphasis on reducing costs, _anticipatory_ guidance and education by pediatric nurses has become ever more important.

4. The comparatively high rate of infant _Mortality_ is believed to be related to the high incidence of low-birth-weight infants being born.

5. Children's medical records are only shared with legal parents, _gaurdians_, or others with written authorization by the parents.

### Activity B  MATCHING

*Match the types of nursing skills in Column A with their description in Column B.*

| Column A | Column B |
|---|---|
| _D_ 1. Pediatric nurse practitioner | a. Supervises a group of patients |
| _E_ 2. Family nurse practitioner | b. Consults in an area of expertise |
| _C_ 3. Neonatal nurse practitioner | c. Specialty within a specialty |
| _B_ 4. Clinical nurse specialist | d. Certified specialist |
| _A_ 5. Case manager | e. Provides health care across the life span |

**Column A**

___ **1.** Febrile seizures

___ **2.** Reye's syndrome

___ **3.** Craniosynostosis

___ **4.** Aseptic meningitis

___ **5.** Positional plagiocephaly

**Column B**

**a.** Treat aggressively with intravenous antibiotics initially

**b.** Position the infant so that the flatten area is up

**c.** Surgical correction to allow brain growth

**d.** Rectal diazepam

**e.** Maintain cerebral perfusion, manage intracranial pressure, manage hydration, and safety measures

**Activity C** SEQUENCING

*Place the following federal programs in the proper order of their enactment.*

**1.** Aid to dependent families and children

**2.** Child Health Assessment Program

**3.** Children's Bureau

**4.** Medicaid coverage for poor children

**5.** Special education in public schools

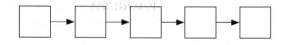

**Activity D** SHORT ANSWERS

**1.** What are the three levels of care provided by pediatric nurses?

_____

_____

_____

**2.** Describe the components of case management.

_____

_____

_____

**3.** Name the six standards of care formulated by the American Nurses Association (ANA) and the Society of Pediatric Nurses (SPN). What is the purpose of these standards?

_____

_____

_____

**4.** What is the purpose of the government's *Healthy People* agenda?

_____

_____

_____

**5.** What does the term "child mortality rates" refer to? What are the rates for each of the age groups?

_____

_____

_____

# SECTION II: APPLYING YOUR KNOWLEDGE

## Activity E CASE STUDY

Remember Isabelle Romano, the 6-year-old female with a history of cerebral palsy, introduced in chapter 1. She was born at 28 weeks and is currently admitted to the hospital due to difficulty breathing secondary to pneumonia. Her parents are very active in her care. Isabelle lives at home with her parents and two brothers, Sergio and Tito.

1. Discuss the barriers to health care that the Romano family may encounter.

2. Discuss your various roles as the nurse caring for Isabelle.

# SECTION III: PRACTICING FOR NCLEX

## Activity F NCLEX-STYLE QUESTIONS

*Answer the following questions.*

1. The nurse is promoting health while caring for a 6-year-old girl who has a cold. Which of the following interventions best supports Healthy People 2010 goals?
   a. Explaining good diet in child's terms
   b. Promoting frequent hand washing
   c. Recommending a helmet for biking
   d. Telling the mother how to treat head lice

2. The nurse is caring for a 14-year-old boy with a debilitating illness who wants to attend school. Which of the following interventions addresses the child's physical health but not his quality of life?
   a. Helping the child modify trendy clothing to his needs
   b. Consulting with the school nurse at the child's school

   c. Assessing the child's daily oxygen supplement needs
   d. Adapting technologies for use outside of the home

3. The nurse is talking with the mother of a 2-year-old girl during a scheduled visit. Which of the following teaching subjects least supports the emphasis on preventive care?
   a. Reminding that child will imitate parents
   b. Explaining how to toddler proof the house
   c. Describing self-care for brushing teeth
   d. Explaining how to teach self hand washing

4. The nurse is caring for a 7-year-old boy with cystic fibrosis whose parents are intensely interested in all aspects of the child's condition and care. Which of the following interventions is least important for empowering these health care consumers?
   a. Teaching the parents how to perform chest physiotherapy
   b. Educating the parents about the lung transplant list
   c. Keeping the family apprised of all developments in care
   d. Locating the best deal on a high frequency chest compression vest

5. The nurse is updating the records of a 10-year-old girl who had her appendix removed. Which of the following actions could jeopardize the privacy of the child's medical records?
   a. Changing identification and passwords monthly
   b. Letting another nurse use the nurse's log-in session
   c. Closing files before stepping away from computer
   d. Printing out confidential information for transmittal

6. The nurse is assessing a 9-year-old boy during a back-to-school check up. Which of the following findings is a factor for childhood injury?

   a. Records show child weighed 2,450 g at birth.

   b. Mother reports she has abused alcohol and drugs.

   c. The parents adopted the boy from Guatemala.

   d. Mother reports the child is hostile to other children.

7. The school nurse is caring for several children who witnessed an 8-year-old girl get hit by car on the way to school. Which of the following interventions is least important to the nursing plan of care for these children?

   a. Determining that the children were traumatized by what they saw

   b. Arranging for counseling for the children who saw the accident

   c. Including friends of the injured child to receive counseling too

   d. Making phone calls to the parents of the children counseled

8. The nurse is assessing a 9-year-old girl with pneumonia. Which of the following findings is a factor for this child's morbidity?

   a. Records show the child has asthma

   b. The mother says she is single parent

   c. The mother was 16 when she delivered this child

   d. The mother's boyfriend abused the child

9. The nurse is caring for 16-year-old boy with injuries from a car accident. Which of the following activities is least likely to be part of the nurse's role as case manager?

   a. Facilitating the doctor's diagnosis and treatment plan

   b. Prescribing services needed to improve the outcome

   c. Helping the child and family access the services needed

   d. Evaluating the child's progress toward recovery

10. The nurse is promoting good health to a 15-year-old girl during an annual visit. Which of the following health promotions is most important for this child?

    a. Assessing for signs of depression or anxiety

    b. Discussing ways to plan and enjoy a healthy diet

    c. Recommending the child get a vaccination for flu

    d. Promoting safe sex to avoid pregnancy and disease

11. The nurse is preparing a program for adolescents concerning health promotion. Based upon the leading cause of mortality for this age group, the best focus for the program will be

    a. Communicable disease prevention

    b. Safety and reduction of risks

    c. Tobacco use

    d. Nutritional counseling

12. During a well child visit, a mother laughingly reports that her 10-year-old child's teacher has recommended a mental health evaluation for the child. What response by the nurse is most appropriate?

    a. Your child is too young to be concerned with mental health problems.

    b. Mental health issues in children are pretty rare.

    c. Does anyone in your family have mental health problems?

    d. What types of issues is the teacher concerned about?

13. A nurse is considering employment in a practice that promotes family-centered care. When considering this position, the nurse recognizes that this philosophy

    a. Will embrace teaching the parents to manage the health care needs of their child.

    b. Will promote the involvement of the child and parents as members of the health care team.

    c. Will focus primarily on the use of herbal remedies to manage health concerns.

    d. Will consider the wishes of the child as the leading force in planning care.

14. The nursery nurse is preparing a consent form for the circumcision of a newborn baby. The mother of the child is 16 years of age. The baby's father is not participating in the care. When planning to complete the surgical consent, the action by the nurse is most appropriate?

a. Ask the grandmother of the newborn to sign the surgical consent.

b. Determine if the baby's father is older than 18 years, and if so ask for him to sign.

c. Recommend that the court appoint a guardian for the baby.

d. Ask for the baby's mother to sign the surgical consent.

15. The parents of a 12-year-old child preparing to undergo surgery explain to the nurse that their religious beliefs do not allow for blood transfusions. What initial action by the nurse is most appropriate?

a. Explain to the parents that the surgeon will make the final decision in the event a blood transfusion is needed by the child.

b. Ask the child what their preference will be.

c. Contact the hospital attorney.

d. Document the parents' requests.

# CHAPTER 2

# Factors Influencing Child Health

## Learning Objectives

- Discuss genetic influences on child health.
- Compare and contrast the factors associated with health status and lifestyle that affect a child's health.
- Explain the concept of resiliency as it relates to children and their health status.
- Discuss health care and its effect on child health.
- Delineate the structures, functions, and roles of families and their influence on children and their health.
- Differentiate discipline from punishment.
- Discuss culture and ethnicity in relation to child health.
- Discuss community and its effects on a child's health.
- Discuss the sources of violence and how exposure to violence affects children.
- Describe the impact of poverty and homelessness on the health of children.

## SECTION I: ASSESSING YOUR UNDERSTANDING

### Activity A  FILL IN THE BLANKS

1. The process of increasing desirable behavior and decreasing or eliminating undesirable behaviors is a process known as _____.

2. Children's temperaments are categorized into three major groups. The largest group of children (40%) is classified as _____ children.

3. The ability to apply knowledge about a child's culture to adapt their health care accordingly is known as cultural _____.

4. When children have been exposed to violence at home and do not appear to suffer negative consequences, they are demonstrating _____.

5. In 2003, _____ was the third leading cause of death in young people, ranging in age from 10 to 24 years.

**Activity B** MATCHING

*Match the cultural group in Column A with the proper belief or practice impacting children's health in Column B.*

**Column A**

_____ **1.** Asian American

_____ **2.** African American

_____ **3.** Arab American

_____ **4.** Native American

**Column B**

a. Women as the verbal decision makers; celebrations to mark the stages of growth and development; health as harmony with nature; illness due to disharmony, evil spirits

b. Use of complementary modalities with Western health care practices; view of life as a cycle with everything connected to health

c. Illness as due to inadequate diet, shifts in hot and cold, exposure of stomach while sleeping, emotional or spiritual distress and "evil eye"; view of pain as unpleasant requiring immediate relief

d. Health as God's will maintainable with a balance of hot and cold food intake; freedom from pain indicative of good health; pain tolerated stoically due to belief that it is God's will

e. Pain and suffering inevitable; relief achieved through prayers and laying on of hands; food as a symbol of health and wealth

**Activity C** SEQUENCING

*Write in order the stages of Duvall's developmental theory.*

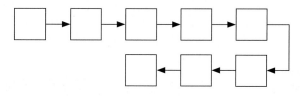

**Activity D** SHORT ANSWERS

1. When using positive reinforcement discipline strategies, name three characteristics of feedback that are pivotal to success.

_____

_____

_____

2. Identify three protective factors that boost resilience in children.

_____

_____

_____

3. List three major religions that include "last rites" or special burial customs at the time of death.

_____

_____

_____

# SECTION II: APPLYING YOUR KNOWLEDGE

## Activity E CASE STUDY

Joel Loveland, 8 years old, is brought to the clinic for his annual exam. During the health history you learn that Joel's parents have been divorced for several years and his mother recently remarried a man who has two children from a previous marriage. Joel's mother states, "Joel's step father is a wonderful man but we have different discipline beliefs. He firmly believes the child should obey the family rules without questioning them and he does not see anything wrong with a spanking now and then."

1. How would you address the mother's concerns?

   _____

   _____

   _____

2. Later during your assessment, the mother expresses concerns of how the divorce and now remarriage may affect Joel. How would you respond?

   _____

   _____

   _____

# SECTION III: PRACTICING FOR NCLEX

## Activity F NCLEX-STYLE QUESTIONS

*Answer the following questions.*

1. A 10-year-old girl is living with her grandparents. Which nursing intervention is most important with this family structure?
   a. Teaching the couple basic child care skills
   b. Determining who the decision maker is
   c. Assessing the child for emotional problems
   d. Helping to access the need for financial aid

2. The nurse is assessing a woman who is pregnant. Her health history reveals she has three young adult children. Which nursing intervention would be most appropriate according to Duvall's developmental theory?
   a. Assessing the parent's coping abilities
   b. Providing developmental anticipatory guidance
   c. Promoting the importance of vaccinations
   d. Describing nutritional value of breastfeeding

3. The nurse is caring for a 7-year-old child who is being treated for multiple fractures after being involved in an automobile accident. The nurse observes that the father frequently takes on the role of nurturer in the family. When planning care, which nursing intervention would most involve the father?
   a. Assuring medications are received on time
   b. Staying with the child at the hospital
   c. Meeting with the discharge planner to discuss plans after discharge
   d. Bathing the child

4. Nurse is providing education concerning discipline to the parents of a 2-year-old girl. Which of the nurse's comments follows the strategies for good discipline?
   a. "Always have the father do the disciplining."
   b. "Tell what will result in her being sent to her room."
   c. "Tell her adults can do as they please, children can't."
   d. "You can modify the discipline when she is sick."

5. The nurse is caring for an Arab American child. The nurse's observations reveal the family follows traditional Arab American cultural values. Which approach would be most successful?
   a. Inquiring about folk remedies used
   b. Coordinating care through the mother
   c. Dealing exclusively with the father
   d. Promoting preventative health care

6. Bookish parents have a child with a 3-year-old boy with a difficult temperament. Which guidance will be most successful for the nurse to use?

    a. "Give him time out for running in the house."

    b. "Encourage him to do quiet activities."

    c. "Provide a place for him to roughhouse."

    d. "Spank him for throwing a tantrum."

7. The mother of two school age children is getting divorced. Which would be the best advice for the nurse to give?

    a. "It's best to treat your children like adults."

    b. "Make your side of the disagreement clear."

    c. "Move out when the children are in school."

    d. "Discuss how things will work after the divorce."

8. The nurse is caring for a single mother and her two preschool age children. Which is the priority intervention?

    a. Maintaining the vaccination schedule

    b. Assessing the mother's psychological status

    c. Referring the mother to Parents Without Partners

    d. Asking the children about their concerns and fears

9. The nurse is assessing for violence in the home. Which response by the mother represents the greatest risk to the child?

    a. The mother says she dreads going home

    b. The mother's partner calls the child names

    c. The boyfriend is very strict with the child

    d. The boyfriend may leave for days at a time

10. Nurse is teaching techniques for effective discipline to the parents of a 9-year-old girl. Which of the following topics is an example of extinction discipline?

    a. Going out for ice cream

    b. Going home early from shopping

    c. Letting her go to a friend's house

    d. Praising her for polite behavior

11. The nurse is discussing the impact of smoking with the mother of a toddler. Which of the following statements by the mother indicates an adequate understanding of the impact of her smoking?

    a. "Smoking will not harm my son as long as I am in another room."

    b. "Smoking outside will protect my child from harm.

    c. "Even the clothing I wear when smoking can pose a danger to my son."

    d. "Exposure to cigarette smoke will be of the greatest danger to my son when he is school aged."

12. A woman has presented to the clinic with her sick school aged child. The child's mother reports she rarely has enough money to meet the health care needs of her chronically ill child. What information should be provided to the woman?

    a. Medicaid is a federal program that is designed to meet the specific needs of children.

    b. Medicaid is a state assistance program that will provide health care for all children under the age of 13.

    c. Medicare is available to help with the health care needs of indigent children.

    d. Low-income parents and their children may qualify for Medicaid.

13. The nurse is caring for a 12-year-old African American female. The child is in pain as a result of a back injury. The nurse correctly recognizes which of the following beliefs regarding pain to be most consistent with the child's culture?

    a. Pain is a part of life and must be endured to increase strength.

    b. Pain may be relieved through prayer and laying on of hands.

    c. Pain is best treated by establishing balance within all other areas of life.

    d. Pain results when there has been negative behavior.

14. The nurse is preparing to discuss preparations for discharge and follow-up care of an Arab American child. The nurse correctly recognizes:

    a. Items requiring written consent will likely be managed by the child's father.

    b. The mother will make the majority of health care decisions.

    c. The viewpoints of the child will be taken into consideration when making health care decisions.

    d. The family will gather and make health care decisions as a group.

15. Traditionally, hot and cold are viewed as potential causes of disease by which of the following groups?

    a. African Americans

    b. Arab Americans

    c. Native Americans

    d. Hispanic Americans

# CHAPTER 3

# Growth and Development of the Newborn and Infant

## Learning Objectives

- Identify normal developmental changes occurring in the newborn and infant.
- Identify the gross and fine motor milestones of the newborn and infant.
- Express an understanding of language development in the first year of life.
- Describe nutritional requirements of the newborn and infant.
- Develop a nutritional plan for the first year of life.
- Identify common issues related to growth and development in infancy.
- Demonstrate knowledge of appropriate anticipatory guidance for common developmental issues.

## SECTION I: ASSESSING YOUR UNDERSTANDING

### Activity A  FILL IN THE BLANKS

1. Inconsolable crying, known as _____, lasts longer than 3 hours.

2. The education of parents about what to expect in the next phase of development is referred to as _____ guidance.

3. Milk production is stimulated by _____, a hormone secreted by the anterior pituitary.

4. The thin, yellowish fluid called _____ is produced by the breasts for the first 2 to 4 days after birth.

5. Stranger anxiety is an indicator that the infant is recognizing himself as _____ from others.

6. The sequential process by which infants and children gain various skills and function is referred to as _____.

7. The anterior fontanel normally remains open until _____ months of life.

## Activity B LABELING

*Label the tooth and age of eruption on the figure provided.*

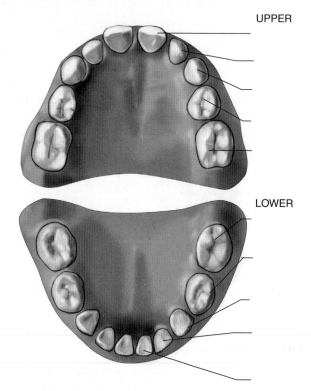

UPPER

LOWER

## Activity C MATCHING

*Match the infant age in Column A with the proper motor skill in Column B.*

**Column A**

_____ **1.** 1-month old

_____ **2.** 2-month old

_____ **3.** 3-month old

_____ **4.** 4-month old

_____ **5.** 5-month old

_____ **6.** 6-month old

**Column B**

**a.** Raises head and chest

**b.** Hold open hand to face

**c.** Tripod sits

**d.** Grasps rattle or toy

**e.** Rolls from prone to supine

**f.** Lifts head while prone

*Match the reflex in Column A with the description in Column B.*

**Column A**

_____ **1.** Asymmetric tonic neck

_____ **2.** Babinski

_____ **3.** Moro

_____ **4.** Parachute

_____ **5.** Root

**Column B**

**a.** Fanning and hyper-extension

**b.** Fencing position

**c.** Prepare to "catch themselves"

**d.** Hands form "C"

**e.** Searches with the mouth

## Activity D SEQUENCING

*List the motor skills of the infant in order of occurrence.*

**1.** Crawls on hands and knees

**2.** Pokes with index finger

**3.** Puts objects in container

**4.** Sits unsupported

**5.** Transfers object from one hand to the other

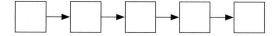

## Activity E SHORT ANSWER

*Briefly answer the following.*

**1.** What are the nursing interventions that will help achieve the Healthy People 2020 objective of increasing the proportion of mothers who breastfeed?

_____

_____

_____

**2.** In what incidences is breastfeeding contraindicated?

_____

_____

_____

3. When providing education to a new parent about how to tell if her infant is hungry, what behavioral cues should be discussed as early cues of hunger?

_____

_____

_____

4. The nurse is reviewing the adjusted age of an infant. What is the adjusted age and how is it calculated?

_____

_____

_____

5. Identify four primitive reflexes present at birth.

_____

_____

_____

6. What changes normally take place in the cardiovascular system during the first year of life?

_____

_____

_____

# SECTION II: APPLYING YOUR KNOWLEDGE

**Activity F** CASE STUDY

Remember Allison Johnson, the 6-month old from Chapter 4, who was brought to the clinic by her mother and father for her 6-month check-up. As new parents, Allison's mother and father had many questions and concerns.

1. Allison's parents ask "What can we do to encourage Allison's development?".

_____

_____

_____

2. Allison's dad states in college he took a psychology class and remembers there are different development theories. He asks how those relate to Allison right now.

_____

_____

_____

3. During your assessment, Allison's parents ask what findings would concern you. Discuss specific developmental warning signs you are assessing.

_____

_____

_____

# SECTION III: PRACTICING FOR NCLEX

**Activity G** NCLEX-STYLE QUESTIONS

*Answer the following questions.*

1. The nurse is examining a 6-month-old girl who was born 8 weeks early. Which of the following findings is cause for concern?
   a. The child measures 21 inches in length
   b. The child exhibits palmar grasp reflex
   c. Head size increased 5 inches since birth
   d. The child weighs 10 pounds 2 ounces

2. The nurse is caring for the family of a 2-month-old boy with colic. The mother reports feeling very stressed by the baby's constant crying. Which of the following interventions would provide the most help in the short term?
   a. Urging the baby's mother to take time for herself away from the child
   b. Educating the parents about when colic stops
   c. Assessing the parents' care and feeding skills
   d. Watching how the parents respond to the child

3. The mother of 1-week-old baby boy voices concerns about her baby's weight loss since birth. At birth the baby weighed 7 pounds; the baby currently weighs 6 pounds 1 ounce. What response by the nurse is most appropriate?

   a. "All babies lose a substantial amount of weight after birth."

   b. "Your baby has lost too much weight and may need to be hospitalized."

   c. "Your baby's weight loss is well within the expected range."

   d. "Your baby has lost a bit more than the normal amount."

4. The nurse is teaching the parents of a 6-month-old boy about proper child dental care. Which of the following actions will the nurse indicate as the most likely to cause dental caries?

   a. Not cleaning a neonate's gums when he is done eating

   b. Putting the child to bed with a bottle of milk or juice

   c. Using a cloth instead of a brush for cleaning teeth

   d. Failure to clean the teeth with fluoridated toothpaste

5. The nurse is assessing the sleeping practices of the parents of a 4-month-old girl who wakes repeatedly during the night. Which of the following parent comments might reveal a cause for the night waking?

   a. They sing to her before she goes to sleep

   b. They put her to bed when she falls asleep

   c. If she is safe, they lie her down and leave

   d. The child has a regular, scheduled bedtime

6. The nurse is educating the mother of a 6-month-old boy about the symptoms for teething. Which of the following symptoms would the nurse identify?

   a. The child may run a mild fever or vomit

   b. The child avoids hard foods for soft ones

   c. The child increases biting and sucking

   d. The child has frequent loose stools

7. The nurse is teaching healthy eating habits to the parents of a 7-month-old girl. Which of the following recommendations is the most valuable advice?

   a. Let the child eat only the foods she prefers

   b. Actively urge the child to eat new foods

   c. Provide small portions that must be eaten

   d. Keep serving new foods several times

8. The nurse is providing helpful feeding tips to the mother of a 2-week-old boy. Which of the following recommendations will best help the child feed effectively?

   a. Maintaining a feed-on-demand approach

   b. Applying warm compresses to the breast

   c. Encouraging the infant to latch on properly

   d. Maintaining adequate diet and fluid intake

9. The nurse is providing anticipatory guidance to the mother of a 1-week-old girl. Which of the following is reason for the mother to contact her care provider?

   a. The dried umbilical cord stump falls off

   b. Rectal temperature is greater than 100.4°F

   c. The child is eating but still losing weight

   d. The child wets her diaper 8 times per day

10. The nurse is observing a 6-month-old boy for developmental progress. Which of the following milestones would be typical for him?

    a. Shifts a toy to his left hand and reaches for another

    b. Picks up an object using his thumb and finger tips

    c. Puts down a little ball to pick up a stuffed toy

    d. Enjoys hitting a plastic bowl with a large spoon

11. The nurse is assessing an infant at his 6 month well baby check-up. The nurse notes that at birth the baby weighed 8 pounds and was 20 inches in length. Which of the following findings is most consistent with the normal infant growth and development?

   a. The baby weighs 21 pounds and is 30 inches in length.

   b. The baby weighs 16 pounds and is 26 inches in length.

   c. The baby weighs 15 pounds and is 24 inches in length.

   d. The baby weighs 24 pounds and is 26 inches in length.

12. A 1-month-old infant's mother voices concern about her baby's respirations. She states they are rapid and irregular. What information should be provided by the nurse?

   a. The normal respiratory rate for an infant at this age is between 20 and 30 breaths per minute.

   b. The respirations of a 1-month-old infant are normally irregular and periodically pause.

   c. An infant at this age should have regular respirations.

   d. The physician should be notified about the irregularity of the infant's respirations.

13. The nurse is assessing the oral cavity of a 4-month-old infant. Which of the following findings are consistent with a child of this age?

   a. The infant has 1 to 3 natal teeth.

   b. The infant has no teeth.

   c. The infant has 1 to 2 lower teeth.

   d. The infant has 1 upper tooth.

14. The nurse is educating the mother of a newborn baby about feeding practices. The nurse correctly advises the mother:

   a. The best feeding schedule offers food every 4 to 6 hours.

   b. Most newborns need to eat about 4 times per day.

   c. The newborn's stomach can hold between one-half to 1 ounce.

   d. Demand scheduled feeding is associated with increased difficulty getting the baby to sleep through the night.

# CHAPTER 4

# Growth and Development of the Toddler

## Learning Objectives

- Explain normal physiologic, psychosocial, and cognitive changes occurring in the toddler.
- Identify the gross and fine motor milestones of the toddler.
- Demonstrate an understanding of language development in the toddler years.
- Discuss sensory development of the toddler.
- Demonstrate an understanding of emotional/social development and moral/spiritual development during toddlerhood.
- Implement a nursing care plan to address common issues related to growth and development in toddlerhood.
- Encourage growth and learning through play.
- Develop a teaching plan for safety promotion in the toddler period.
- Demonstrate an understanding of toddler needs related to sleep and rest, as well as dental health.
- Develop a nutritional plan for the toddler based on average nutritional requirements.
- Provide appropriate anticipatory guidance for common developmental issues that arise in the toddler period.
- Demonstrate an understanding of appropriate methods of discipline for use during the toddler years.

- Identify the role of the parent in the toddler's life and determine ways to support, encourage, and educate the parents about toddler growth, development, and concerns during this period.

## SECTION I: ASSESSING YOUR UNDERSTANDING

### Activity A   FILL IN THE BLANKS

1. When _____ of the spinal cord is achieved around age 2 years, the toddler is capable of exercising voluntary control over the sphincters.

2. The leading cause of unintentional injury and death in children in this country is due to _____.

3. The ability to understand what is being said or asked is called _____ language.

4. The _____ remains short in both the male and female toddler, making them more susceptible to urinary tract infections compared to adults.

5. During the _____ stage of development, according to Piaget, children begin to become more sophisticated with symbolic thought.

## Activity B MATCHING

*Match the word in Column A with the correct description in Column B.*

**Column A**

_____ **1.** Echolalia

_____ **2.** Regression

_____ **3.** Individuation

_____ **4.** Ritualism

_____ **5.** Egocentrism

_____ **6.** Telegraphic speech

**Column B**

**a.** Self-interest due to an inability to focus on another's perspective

**b.** Familiar routine that provides structure and security for the toddler

**c.** Speech that uses essential words only

**d.** Repetition of words and phrases without understanding

**e.** Internalizing a sense of self and one's environment

**f.** Returning to a prior developmental stage

*Match the nutrients in Column A with the appropriate food source in Column B.*

**Column A**

_____ **1.** Dietary fiber

_____ **2.** Folate

_____ **3.** Vitamin A

_____ **4.** Vitamin C

_____ **5.** Calcium

**Column B**

**a.** Avocados, broccoli, green peas, dark greens

**b.** Apricots, cantaloupe, carrots, sweet potatoes

**c.** Applesauce, carrots, corn, green beans

**d.** Dairy products, broccoli, tofu, legumes

**e.** Broccoli, oranges, strawberries, tomatoes

## Activity C SEQUENCING

*Place the following descriptions of expressive language in the order the toddler will display them:*

**1.** Uses primarily descriptive words (hungry, hot)

**2.** Talks about something that happened in the past

**3.** Babbles in what sounds like sentences

**4.** Uses a finger to point to things

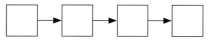

## Activity D SHORT ANSWERS

*Briefly answer the following.*

**1.** Discuss ways to prevent temper tantrums in toddlers.

_____

_____

_____

**2.** Describe appropriate discipline for a toddler.

_____

_____

_____

**3.** Explain the care for the toddler's teeth and gums. How does the care change after the child reaches the age of 2?

_____

_____

_____

**4.** Discuss the changes in the genitourinary system in the toddler that allow for readiness for toilet training.

_____

_____

_____

**5.** Toddlers generally have a swayback appearance. What is the underlying cause of this manifestation?

_____

_____

_____

# SECTION II: APPLYING YOUR KNOWLEDGE

## Activity E  CASE STUDY

Jose Gonzales is a 2-year-old boy brought to the clinic by his mother and father for his 2-year-old check-up. The following questions refer to him.

1. Jose's parents state "We speak Spanish at home to Jose and are working to make him bilingual." What do you need to consider when assessing language development in Jose?

   _____

   _____

   _____

2. Jose's mother asks what they can do to encourage Jose's language development.

   _____

   _____

   _____

3. Jose's father states that Jose's favorite word is "No." He asks if this is normal at this age. How would you respond? (include a discussion on Erikson stage of development and suggestions for dealing with this)

   _____

   _____

   _____

# SECTION III: PRACTICING FOR NCLEX

## Activity F  NCLEX-STYLE QUESTIONS

*Answer the following questions.*

1. The parents of an overweight 2-year-old boy admit that their child is a bit "chubby," but argue that he is a picky eater who will eat only junk food. Which is the best response by the nurse to facilitate a healthier diet?

   a. "You may have to serve a new food 10 or more times."

   b. "Serve only healthy foods. He'll eat when he's hungry."

   c. "Give him more healthy choices with less junk food available."

   d. "Calorie requirements for toddlers are less than infants."

2. The nurse is observing a 36-month-old boy during a well visit. Which motor skill has he most recently acquired?

   a. The child is able to undress himself

   b. He is able to push a toy lawnmower

   c. The child is able to kick a ball

   d. The child can pull a toy while walking

3. The nurse is providing anticipatory guidance to the parents of an 18-month-old girl. Which recommendation will be most helpful to the parents?

   a. Giving the child time out for 1 ½ minutes

   b. Ignoring bad behavior and praising good

   c. Slapping her hand using one or two fingers

   d. Describing proper behavior when she misbehaves

4. The nurse is teaching a first-time mother with a 14-month-old boy about child safety. Which is the most effective overall safety information to provide guidance for the mother?

   a. "Place a gate at the top of stairways."

   b. "Never let him out of your sight."

   c. "Put chemicals in a locked cabinet."

   d. "Don't smoke in the house or car."

5. The parents of a 2-year-old girl are concerned with her behavior. For which behavior would the nurse share their concern?

   a. The child refuses to share her toys with her sister

   b. She frequently babbles to herself when playing

   c. The child likes to change toys frequently

   d. She plays by herself even when other children are present

6. The nurse is discussing sensory development with the mother of a 2-year-old boy. Which parental comment suggests the child may have a sensory problem?

   a. "He wasn't bothered by the paint smell."

   b. "He was licking up the dishwashing soap."

   c. "He doesn't respond if I wave to him."

   d. "I dropped a pan behind him and he cried."

7. The nurse is assessing the language development of a 3-year-old girl. Which finding would suggest a problem?

   a. The child can make simple conversation

   b. She tells the nurse she saw Na-Na today

   c. The child speaks in 2- to 3-word sentences

   d. She can tell the nurse what her name is

8. The nurse is observing a 3-year-old boy in a daycare center. Which behavior might suggest an emotional problem?

   a. The child has persistent separation anxiety

   b. He goes from calm to tantrum suddenly

   c. The child sucks his thumb periodically

   d. He is unable to share toys with others

9. The nurse is teaching a mother of a 1-year-old girl about weaning her from the bottle and breast. Which recommendation would be part of the nurse's plan?

   a. Wean from breast by 18 months of age at the latest

   b. Give the child an iron-fortified cereal

   c. Switch the child to a no-spill sippy cup

   d. Wean from the bottle at 15 months of age

10. The parents of a 3-year-old boy have asked the nurse for advice about a preschool for their child. Which suggestion is most important for the nurse to make?

    a. "Look for a preschool that is clean and has a loving staff."

    b. "Check to make sure your child can attend with the sniffles."

    c. "Make sure that you can easily get an appointment to visit."

    d. "The staff should be trained in early childhood development."

11. The nurse is assessing a 2-year-old boy during a well child visit. The nurse correctly identifies the child's current stage of Erickson's growth and development as:

    a. Trust versus mistrust

    b. Autonomy versus shame and doubt

    c. Initiative versus guilt

    d. Industry versus inferiority

12. The nurse is assessing a 3-year-old child. The nurse notes the child is able to understand that objects hidden from sight still exist. The nurse correctly documents the child is displaying:

    a. Tertiary circular reactions

    b. Mental combinations

    c. Preoperational thinking

    d. Concrete thinking

**13.** The nurse is discussing the activities of a 20-month-old child with his mother. The mother reports the children of her friends seem to have more advanced speech abilities than her child. After assessing the child, which of the following findings is cause for follow up?

   **a.** Inability to point to named body parts

   **b.** Inability to talk with the nurse about something that happened a few days ago

   **c.** Points to pictures in books when asked

   **d.** Understands approximately 75 to 100 words

**14.** The mother of an 18-month-old girl voices concerns about her child's social skills. She reports that the child does not play well with others and seems to ignore other children who are playing at the same time. What response by the nurse is indicated?

   **a.** "It is normal for children to engage in play alongside other children at this age."

   **b.** "Has your child displayed any aggressive tendencies toward other children?"

   **c.** "Perhaps you should consider a preschool to promote more socialization opportunities."

   **d.** "Does your child have opportunities to socialize much with other children?"

# CHAPTER 5

# Growth and Development of the Preschooler

## Learning Objectives

- Identify normal physiologic, cognitive, and psychosocial changes occurring in the preschool-aged child.
- Express an understanding of language development in the preschool years.
- Implement a nursing care plan that addresses common concerns or delays in the preschooler's development.
- Integrate knowledge of preschool growth and development with nursing care and health promotion of the preschool-aged child.
- Develop a nutrition plan for the preschool-aged child.
- Identify common issues related to growth and development during the preschool years.
- Demonstrate knowledge of appropriate anticipatory guidance for common developmental issues that arise in the preschool period.

## SECTION I: ASSESSING YOUR UNDERSTANDING

### Activity A  FILL IN THE BLANKS

1. The over-consumption of cow's milk may result in a deficiency of _____ due to the calcium blocking its absorption.

2. Communication in preschool children is _____ in nature, as they are not yet capable of abstract thought.

3. Preschool age children are more susceptible to bladder infections than are adults due to the length of the _____.

4. During a night _____ a child will scream and thrash but not awaken.

5. A nutrient _____ diet along with physical activity is the foundation for obesity prevention in the preschool child.

**Activity B** MATCHING

*Match the theorist and stage in Column A with the proper activities/behaviors in Column B*

**Column A**

_____ **1.** Erikson – Initiative versus guilt

_____ **2.** Piaget – Preconceptual

_____ **3.** Piaget – Intuitive

_____ **4.** Kohlberg – Punishment–obedience orientation

_____ **5.** Kohlberg – Preconventional morality

_____ **6.** Freud – Phallic stage

**Column B**

**a.** Displays animism

**b.** Able to classify and relate objects

**c.** Children may learn inappropriate behavior if the parent does not intervene to teach the behavior is wrong

**d.** Likes to please parents

**e.** Super-ego is developing and the conscience is emerging

**f.** Determines good and bad dependent upon associated punishment

**Activity C** SEQUENCING

*Place the following motor skills in the order of acquisition.*

**1.** Swings and climbs well

**2.** Copies circles and traces squares

**3.** Throws ball overhand

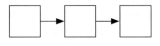

**Activity D** SHORT ANSWERS

*Briefly answer the following.*

**1.** Describe the cognitive abilities of a child in the intuitive phase.

_____

_____

_____

**2.** Explain the difference between nightmares and night terrors.

_____

_____

_____

**3.** Name three ways to promote healthy teeth and gums in preschoolers.

_____

_____

_____

**4.** What strategies should be used by the parents of a preschool-aged child who has lied?

_____

_____

_____

**5.** What is the primary social task of the preschool-aged child?

_____

_____

_____

# SECTION II: APPLYING YOUR KNOWLEDGE

### Activity E CASE STUDY

Remember Nila Patel, the 4-year-old from Chapter 5, who was brought to the clinic by her parents for her school check-up.

1. Nila's mother states that "Nila loves to play make believe. She is constantly playing in a fantasy world. I am not sure if this is healthy behavior." How would you address Mrs. Patel's concerns?

   _____

   _____

   _____

2. Nila's parents express concerns about the transition to Kindergarten. What guidance can you give them regarding this?

   _____

   _____

   _____

3. During your assessment, Nila's mother asks what findings would concern you. Discuss specific developmental warning signs you are assessing for.

   _____

   _____

   _____

# SECTION III: PRACTICING FOR NCLEX

### Activity F NCLEX-STYLE QUESTIONS

*Answer the following questions.*

1. The nurse is conducting a well child assessment of a 4-year-old. Which of the following assessment findings would warrant further investigation?

   a. Presence of 20 deciduous teeth

   b. Presence of 10 deciduous teeth

   c. Absence of dental caries

   d. Presence of 19 deciduous teeth

2. The nurse is conducting a health screening of a 5-year-old boy as required for kindergarten. The boy is fearful about going to a new school. The mother asks for the nurse's advice. Which is the best response by the nurse?

   a. "Kindergarten is a big step for a child. Be patient with him."

   b. "Talk to your son's new teacher and schedule a tour with him."

   c. "Be aware that he may have difficulty adjusting being away from home 5 days a week."

   d. "Remind him that kindergarten will be a lot of fun and he'll make new friends."

3. The nurse is conducting a well child examination of a 4-year-old and is assessing the child's height. The nurse would expect that the child's height would have increased by which of the following since last year's examination?

   a. ½ to 1 inch

   b. 1 to 2 inches

   c. 2 ½ to 3 inches

   d. 3 ½ to 4 inches

4. A nurse is providing a routine wellness examination for a 5-year-old boy. Which of the following responses by the parents indicates a need for an additional referral or follow-up?

   a. "He can count to 30 but gets confused after that."

   b. "We often have to translate his speech to others."

   c. "He is always talking and telling detailed stories."

   d. "He knows his name and address."

5. The parents of a 4-year-old girl tell the nurse that their daughter is having frequent nightmares. Which of the following statements would indicate that the girl is having night terrors instead of nightmares?

   a. "She screams and thrashes when we try to touch her."

   b. "She is scared after she wakes up."

   c. "She comes and wakes us up after she awakens."

   d. "She has a hard time going back to sleep."

6. The nurse is providing teaching to the mother of a 4-year-old girl about bike safety. Which of the following statements indicates a need for further teaching?

   a. "The balls of her feet should reach both pedals while sitting."

   b. "Pedal back brakes are better for her age group."

   c. "She should always ride on the sidewalk."

   d. "She can ride on the street if I am riding with her."

7. The nurse is conducting a health screening for a 3-year-old boy as required by his new preschool. Which of the following statements by the parents would warrant further discussion and intervention?

   a. "The school has a looser environment which is a good match for his temperament."

   b. "The school requires processed foods and high sugar foods be avoided."

   c. "The school is quite structured and advocates corporal punishment."

   d. "There is a very low student teacher ratio and they do a lot of hands on projects."

8. A nurse is caring for a 4-year-old girl. The parents indicate that their daughter often reports that objects in the house are her friends. They are concerned because the girl says that the grandfather clock in the hallway smiles and sings to her. How should the nurse respond?

   a. "Your daughter is demonstrating animism which is common."

   b. "Attributing life-like qualities to inanimate objects is quite normal at this age."

   c. "Do you think your daughter is hallucinating?

   d. "Is there a family history of mental illness?"

9. The nurse is providing teaching about child safety to the parents of a 4-year-old girl. Which of the following statements by the parents would indicate a need for further teaching?

   a. "She should use a helmet when riding her bike."

   b. "She still needs a booster seat in the car."

   c. "We need to know the basics of CPR and first aid."

   d. "We need to continually remind her about safety rules."

10. The nurse is providing teaching about proper dental care for the parents of a 5-year-old girl. Which of the following responses indicates a need for further teaching?

    a. "Too much fluoride can contribute to fluorosis."

    b. "We should use only a pea-sized amount of toothpaste."

    c. "She needs to floss her teeth before brushing."

    d. "She should see a dentist every 6 months."

11. The father of a preschool boy reports concerns about the short stature of his son. The nurse reviews the child's history and notes the child is 4 years old and is presently 41 inches tall and has grown 2.5 inches in the past year. What response by the nurse is most appropriate?

    a. "Is there a reason you are concerned about your child's height?"

    b. "Your son is slightly below the normal height for his age group but may still grow to be a normal height in the coming year."

c. "Your son is slightly below the normal height for his age but he had demonstrated a normal growth rate this year."

d. "Both your son's height and rate of growth are within normal limits for his age."

12. The mother of a 4-year-old girl reports her daughter has episodes of wetting her pants. The nurse questions the mother about the frequency. The nurse determines these episodes occur about once every 1 to 2 weeks. What response by the nurse is indicated?

a. "You should consider restricting your daughter's fluid intake."

b. "Discipline should be applied after these times."

c. "At this age it is helpful to remind children to go to the bathroom."

d. "The frequency of these wetting episodes may be consistent with a low-grade urinary tract infection."

13. The nurse is caring for a 4-year-old child hospitalized in traction. The child talks about an invisible friend to the nurse. What action by the nurse is indicated?

a. The nurse should document the reports of hallucinations by the child.

b. The nurse should explain to the child that there are no friends present.

c. The nurse should discourage the child from talking about the imaginary friend.

d. The nurse should recognize this behavior as normal for the child's developmental age and do nothing.

14. The mother of a 4-year-old boy reports her son has voiced curiosity about her breasts. She asks the nurse what she should do. What is the best information that the nurse can give to the parent?

a. Advise the parent that sexual curiosity is unusual at this age.

b. Encourage the parent to provide a detailed discussion about human sexuality with the child.

c. Encourage the parent to determine what the child's specific questions are and answer them briefly.

d. Advise the parent to explain to the child that he is too young to discuss such things.

15. The mother of a 3-year-old child reports her son is afraid of dark. She asks the nurse for help. Which of the following is the best advice the nurse can offer?

a. Encourage the parent to allow a small night light.

b. Encourage the parent to consider allowing the child to sleep with her until he feels more able to sleep alone.

c. Encourage the mother to allow a night light until the child falls asleep and then recommend she turn it off.

d. Encourage the parent to avoid the use of night lights as they interfere with restful sleep in children.

# Growth and Development of the School-Age Child

## Learning Objectives

- Identify normal physiologic, cognitive, and moral changes occurring in the school-age child.
- Describe the role of peers and schools in the development and socialization of the school-age child.
- Identify the developmental milestones of the school-age child.
- Identify the role of the nurse in promoting safety for the school-age child.
- Demonstrate knowledge of the nutritional requirements of the school-age child.
- Identify common developmental concerns in the school-age child.
- Demonstrate knowledge of the appropriate nursing guidance for common developmental concerns.

## SECTION I: ASSESSING YOUR UNDERSTANDING

### Activity A  FILL IN THE BLANKS

1. An 8-year-old who is the size of an 11-year-old will think and act like a(n) _____ year-old.

2. The Academy of Pediatrics recommends _____ hours or less of television viewing per day.

3. Brain growth is complete by the time the _____ birthday is celebrated.

4. Between the ages of 10 and 12 (the pubescent years for girls), _____ levels remain high, but are more controlled and focused than previously.

5. Motor vehicle accidents are a common cause of _____ in the school-aged child.

6. Most young children are not capable of handling _____ or making decisions on their own before 11 or 12 years of age.

7. Ways to develop self-worth is termed _____.

8. During school children are influenced by _____ and teachers.

9. Compared with the earlier years, caloric needs of the school-age child are _____.

10. The bladder capacity for a 10-year-old would be _____ ounces.

## Activity B MATCHING

*Match the terms with the descriptions.*

**Column A**

_____ **1.** Inferiority

_____ **2.** Burxism

_____ **3.** Malocclusion

_____ **4.** Caries

_____ **5.** Secondary sexual characteristics

_____ **6.** Principle of conservation

**Column B**

**a.** Gritting or grinding of teeth

**b.** Tooth decay

**c.** Feelings of inability or not measuring up to the abilities of others

**d.** Matter does not change when forms change

**e.** Improper teeth alignment

**f.** Changes in breast development and genitalia during late school age or early adolescent

*Match the systems with the capacities.*

**Column A**

_____ **1.** Lymph system

_____ **2.** Heart

_____ **3.** Bones

**Column B**

**a.** Mineralization not complete until maturity

**b.** Smaller in size, in relation to the rest of the body, than any other developmental stage

**c.** Continues to grow until the child is 9 years old

*Match the theorists with characteristics of their theories for the school-age child.*

**Column A**

_____ **1.** Kohlberg

_____ **2.** Feud

_____ **3.** Piaget

_____ **4.** Erikson

**Column B**

**a.** Industry versus inferiority

**b.** Conventional: "good child, bad child"

**c.** Latency

**d.** Concrete operational

## Activity C SEQUENCING

*Place the following developmental milestones in the proper sequence.*

**1.** Brain growth is complete

**2.** Fine motor skills develop

**3.** Frontal sinuses development is complete

**4.** Gross motor skills develop

**5.** Lymphatic tissue growth is complete

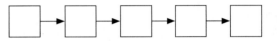

## Activity D SHORT ANSWERS

*Briefly answer the following.*

**1.** Describe the development of children's gross motor skills as they correspond to age groups.

_____

_____

_____

**2.** Describe the child who is labeled "slow to warm."

_____

_____

_____

**3.** Define the nurse's role in school-age children's growth and development.

_____

_____

_____

**4.** Detail the sleep requirements for school-age children.

_____

_____

_____

**5.** Discuss the importance of body image on the school-aged child.

_____

_____

_____

# SECTION II: APPLYING YOUR KNOWLEDGE

## Activity E  CASE STUDY

*Olivia Anderson, 9 years old, is brought to the clinic by her mother for her annual check-up.*

1. During your assessment you note the interaction between the mother and the daughter. While asking Olivia about her friends at school, the mother responds "Olivia does not have many friends. I have told her if she would just care more about her appearance, other children will want to spend time with her."

   How would you respond to the mother?

   _____

   _____

   _____

2. Olivia's mother expresses concerns regarding discipline and how best to approach this.

   How would you respond?

   _____

   _____

   _____

3. During your assessment, you discover that Olivia spends most of her time watching television and playing video games. What guidance can you give to Olivia and her mother regarding this?

   _____

   _____

   _____

# SECTION III: PRACTICING FOR NCLEX

## Activity F  NCLEX-STYLE QUESTIONS

*Answer the following questions.*

1. The nurse is about to see a 9-year-old girl for a well child check-up. Knowing that the child is in Piaget's period of concrete operational thought, which of the following characteristics will the child display?

   a. The child can consider an action and its consequences

   b. The child views the world in terms of her own experience

   c. The child makes generalized assumptions about groups of things

   d. The child knows lying is bad because she gets sent to her room for it.

2. The nurse is educating the parents of a 6-year-old boy how to manage the child's introduction into elementary school. The child has an easy temperament. Which of the following would the nurse most likely suggest?

   a. Comforting the child when he is frustrated

   b. Helping the child deal with minor stresses

   c. Schedule several visits to the school before classes start

   d. Being firm with the anticipated episodes of moodiness and irritability

3. The mother of a 7-year-old girl is asking the nurse's advice about getting her daughter a 2-wheel bike. Which of the following responses by the nurse is most important?

   a. "Teach her where she'll land on the grass if she falls."

   b. "Be sure to get the proper size bike."

   c. "She won't need a helmet if she has training wheels."

   d. "Learning to ride the bike will improve her coordination."

4. The school nurse is assessing the nutritional status of an overweight 12-year-old girl. Which of the following questions would be appropriate for the nurse to ask?

   a. Does your family have rules about foods and how they are prepared?

   b. What does your family do for exercise?

   c. How often does everyone in your family eat together?

   d. Have you gained weight recently?

5. The nurse has taken a health history and performed a physical exam for a 12-year-old boy. Which of the following findings will most likely be made?

   a. The child's body fat has decreased since last year

   b. The child has different diet preferences than his parents

   c. The child has a leaner body mass than a girl at this age

   d. The child described a somewhat reduced appetite

6. The nurse is teaching parents of an 11-year-old girl how to deal with the issues relating to peer pressure to use tobacco and alcohol. Which of the following suggestions provides the best course of action for the parents?

   a. Avoiding smoking in the house or in front of the child

   b. Hiding alcohol out of the child's reach

   c. Forbidding the child to have friends that smoke or drink

   d. Discuss tobacco and alcohol use with the child

7. The nurse is assessing the nutritional needs of an 8-year-old girl who weighs 65 pounds. Which of the following amounts would provide the proper daily caloric intake for this child?

   a. 1,895 calories per day

   b. 2,065 calories per day

   c. 2,245 calories per day

   d. 2,385 calories per day

8. The nurse is talking with the parents of an 8-year-old boy who has been cheating at school. Which of the following comments should be the primary message for the nurse to present?

   a. "The punishment should be severe and long lasting."

   b. "Make sure that your behavior around your son is exemplary."

   c. "Resolve this by providing an opportunity for him to cheat and then dealing with it."

   d. "You may be putting too much pressure on him to succeed."

9. A 9-year-old boy has arrived for a health maintenance visit. Which of the following milestones of physical growth would the nurse expect to observe?

   a. Brain growth is complete and the shape of the head is longer

   b. Lymphatic tissue growth is complete providing greater resistance to infections

   c. Frontal sinuses are developed while tonsils have decreased in size

   d. All deciduous teeth are replaced by 32 permanent teeth

10. The nurse is educating the parents of a 10-year-old girl in ways to help their child avoid tobacco. Which of the following suggestions would be part of the nurse's advice?

    a. "Keep your cigarettes where she can't get to them."

    b. "Always go outside when you have a cigarette."

    c. "Tell her only losers smoke and chew tobacco."

    d. "As parents, you need to be good role models."

11. The parents of a 7-year-old girl report concerns about her seemingly low self-esteem. The parents question how self-esteem is developed in a young girl. What response by the nurse is most appropriate?

    a. "The peers of a child at this age are the greatest influence on self-esteem."

    b. "Several interrelated factors are to blame for low self-esteem."

    c. "Your daughter's self-esteem is influenced by feedback from people they view as authorities at this age."

    d. "A child's self-esteem is greatly inborn and environmental influences guide it."

12. The parents of an 8-year-old boy report their son is being bullied and teased by a group of boys in the neighborhood. What information can be accurately provided by the nurse?

    a. "Perhaps teaching your son self-defense courses will help him to have a greater sense of control and safety."

    b. "Bullying can have lifelong effects on the self-esteem of a child."

    c. "Fortunately the scars of being picked on will fade as your son grows up."

    d. "Your son is at high risk for bullying other children as a result of this situation."

13. During a well child check at the ambulatory clinic, the mother of a 10-year-old boy reports concerns about her son's frequent discussions about death and dying. Based upon knowledge of this age grout the nurse understands which of the following?

    a. Discussions about death and dying are not normal for this age group.

    b. Preoccupations about death and dying may hint at a psychological disorder.

    c. Preoccupation with thoughts related to death and dying in this age group are consistent with the later development of depression.

    d. Preoccupation with death and dying is common in the school-aged child.

14. The parents of a 9-year-old boy report they have been homeschooling their son and now plan to enroll him in the local public school. They voice concerns about the influence of the other children on their son's values. What information can be provided to the parents by the nurse?

    a. "At your son's age, values are most influenced by peers."

    b. "The values of the family will likely prevail for your son."

    c. "Values are largely inborn and will be impacted only in a limited way by environmental influences."

    d. "Teacher will begin to have the largest influence on a child's values at this age."

15. The nurse is caring for a hospitalized 5-year-old child. The child's mother has reported her child is becoming very "clingy." What advice can be provided to the parent by the nurse? Select all that apply.

    a. "Regression is normal during hospitalization."

    b. "Be careful not to coddle the child or it will result in regressive behaviors."

    c. "These behaviors are the result of a loss of self-control and are likely temporary."

    d. "Allowing the child to have some input in the care may be helpful in managing these behaviors."

# Growth and Development of the Adolescent

- Identify normal physiologic changes, including puberty, occurring in the adolescent.
- Discuss psychosocial, cognitive, and moral changes occurring in the adolescent.
- Identify changes in relationships with peers, family, teachers, and community during adolescence.
- Describe interventions to promote safety during adolescence.
- Demonstrate knowledge of the nutritional requirements of the adolescent.
- Demonstrate knowledge of the development of sexuality and its influence on dating during adolescence.
- Identify common developmental concerns of the adolescent.
- Demonstrate knowledge of the appropriate nursing guidance for common developmental concerns.

## SECTION I: ASSESSING YOUR UNDERSTANDING

### Activity A FILL IN THE BLANKS

1. Risk-taking behaviors of adolescents are those that could lead to physical or _____ injury.

2. Second only to growth during _____, adolescence provides the most rapid and dramatic changes in size and proportions.

3. Adolescents proceed from thinking in concrete terms to thinking in _____ terms.

4. Families who listen and continue to demonstrate affection for and acceptance of their adolescent have a more _____ outcome.

5. The prevalence of obesity is highest in _____ and African American teens between the ages of 12 and 19.

6. The family can experience a _____ if an adolescent's striving for independence is met with stricter parental limits.

7. According to Erikson, it is during adolescence that teenagers achieve a sense of _____.

8. The _____ of the skeletal system is completed earlier in girls than in boys.

9. During middle adolescence gross motor skills such as speed, accuracy, and _____ improve.

10. It is important for the nurse to take into consideration the effects culture, ethnicity, and _____ have on adolescents.

## Activity B MATCHING

*Match the illicit drug in Column A with the proper descriptive word or phrase in Column B.*

| Column A | Column B |
|---|---|
| \_\_\_\_ **1.** Amphetamines | **a.** Pressured speech and anorexia |
| \_\_\_\_ **2.** Barbiturates | **b.** Drowsiness, constricted pupils |
| \_\_\_\_ **3.** Cocaine | **c.** Depression in children |
| \_\_\_\_ **4.** Hallucinogens | **d.** Violence, irrational behavior |
| \_\_\_\_ **5.** Opiates | **e.** Hypertension, distorted perceptions |
| \_\_\_\_ **6.** Phencyclidine hydrochloride (PCP) | **f.** Hyperactivity in children |

*Match the type of contraceptive with the correct description.*

| Column A | Column B |
|---|---|
| \_\_\_\_ **1.** Condom | **a.** Requires fitting and education |
| \_\_\_\_ **2.** Depo-Provera | **b.** Effective if used with a barrier method |
| \_\_\_\_ **3.** Diaphragm | **c.** Injectable, administered every 3 months |
| \_\_\_\_ **4.** Emergency contraceptive pills | **d.** Not appropriate for routine use |
| \_\_\_\_ **5.** Oral contraception | **e.** Inexpensive, protects against disease |
| \_\_\_\_ **6.** Spermicides | **f.** Highly effective, expensive |

*Match the nutrient in Column A with the daily requirement in Column B.*

| Column A | Column B |
|---|---|
| \_\_\_\_ **1.** Calcium (boys and girls) | **a.** 12 mg/day |
| | **b.** 45 to 59 g/day |
| \_\_\_\_ **2.** Iron (boys) | **c.** 1,200 to 1,500 mg /day |
| \_\_\_\_ **3.** Iron (girls) | |
| \_\_\_\_ **4.** Protein (boys) | **d.** 15 mg/day |
| \_\_\_\_ **5.** Protein (girls) | **e.** 46 g/day |

## Activity C SEQUENCING

*Beginning with early adolescence and ending with late adolescence, place the following physiological changes in sequential order.*

**1.** Voice changes

**2.** Eruption of last four molars

**3.** Head, neck, hands, and feet reach adult proportions

**4.** Increase in shoulder, chest, and hip breadth

**5.** First menstrual period (average = 12.8 years)

**6.** Increase in percentage of body fat

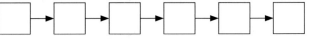

## Activity D SHORT ANSWERS

*Briefly answer the following.*

**1.** List eight reasons why adolescents become pregnant.

_____

_____

_____

**2.** Describe the adolescent's achievement of his or her identity, including how previous developmental stages and culture play a role.

_____

_____

_____

**3.** Explain how the school experience comprises an integral component of the adolescent's preparation for the future.

_____

_____

_____

**4.** Explain the importance of sexuality discussions between parents and teens.

_____

_____

_____

5. Discuss the physical growth and development of the teenager. What factors influence the growth of teens? How has growth of teens changed over the past few decades?

_____

_____

_____

6. Discuss the cognitive development/capabilities of the teenaged child.

_____

_____

_____

# SECTION II: APPLYING YOUR KNOWLEDGE

## Activity E CASE STUDY

_Cho Chung, a 15-year-old, is brought to the clinic by her mother for her annual school check-up._

1. During your assessment, Cho states she wants to get her belly button pierced but her parents refuse. She states, "They just don't understand that there is really no risk. I have at least 10 friends who have one, and none of them have had any problems." How would you address this?

_____

_____

_____

2. During your assessment, you find out Cho has recently become sexually active. How would you address sexually transmitted infections and teen pregnancy during Cho's visit?

_____

_____

_____

3. After the exam, Cho's mother expresses concerns about communicating with her daughter. How would you respond?

_____

_____

_____

# SECTION III: PRACTICING FOR NCLEX

## Activity F NCLEX-STYLE QUESTIONS

_Answer the following questions._

1. The nurse knows that the 13-year-old girl in the exam room is in the process of developing her own set of values. Which of the following activities will this child be experiencing according to Kohlberg's theory?
   a. Wishing her parents were more understanding
   b. Assuming everyone is interested in her favorite pop star
   c. Wondering what is the meaning of life
   d. Comparing morals with those of peers

2. The nurse is promoting safe sex to a 14-year-old boy who is frequently dating. Which of the following points is most likely to be made during the talk?
   a. "Adolescents account for 25% of sexually transmitted infection (STI) cases."
   b. "Contraception is a shared responsibility."
   c. "Be careful or you'll wind up being a teenage dad."
   d. "Girls are more susceptible to STIs than boys."

3. The school nurse is providing nutritional guidance during a 9th grade health class. Which of the following foods would be recommended as a good source for calcium?
   a. Strawberries, watermelon, and raisins
   b. Beans, poultry, and fish
   c. Peanut butter, tomato juice, and whole grain bread
   d. Cheese, yogurt, and white beans

4. The nurse is talking to a 13-year-old boy about choosing friends. Which of the following functions do peer groups provide that can have a negative result?
   a. Following role models
   b. Sharing problems
   c. Negotiating differences
   d. Developing loyalties

5. The school nurse is assessing a 16-year-old girl who was removed from class because of disruptive behavior. She arrived in the nurse's office with dilated pupils and talking rapidly. Which of the following drugs might she be using?

   a. Opiates

   b. Barbiturates

   c. Amphetamines

   d. Marijuana

6. The nurse is providing anticipatory guidance for violence prevention to a group of parents with adolescent children. Which of the following actions would be most effective in preventing suicide?

   a. Watching for aggressive behavior or racist remarks

   b. Checking for signs of depression or lack of friends

   c. Becoming acquainted with the teen's friends

   d. Monitoring video games, TV shows, and music

7. A 16-year-old girl has arrived for her sports physical with a new piercing in her navel. What is the best approach for the nurse to use?

   a. "Be sure to clean the navel several times a day."

   b. "I hope for your sake the needle was clean."

   c. "This is a risk for hepatitis, tetanus, and AIDS."

   d. "This is a wound and can become infected."

8. Throughout a health surveillance visit, a 12-year-old boy complains to the nurse about his parents intruding on his personal space, but then says he is looking forward to the family vacation. Which of the following characteristics also suggests the boy has entered adolescence?

   a. Growing interest in attracting girls' attention

   b. Feels secure with his body image

   c. Experiences frequent mood changes

   d. Understands that actions have consequences

9. The nurse is performing a physical assessment on an 11-year-old girl during a health surveillance visit. Which of the following findings would suggest the child has reached adolescence?

   a. A significant muscle mass increase

   b. Eruption of last four molars

   c. Increased shoulder, chest and hip widths

   d. The child has higher blood pressure

10. The nurse is promoting nutrition to a teen who is going through a growth spurt. Knowing that the teen has a need for increased amounts of zinc, calcium, and iron, which of the following foods would be recommended for its high iron content?

    a. Fat-free milk

    b. Whole grain bread

    c. Organic carrots

    d. Fresh orange juice

11. The nurse is collecting data from a 15-year-old boy who is being seen at the ambulatory care clinic for immunizations. During the initial assessment, he voices concerns about being a few inches shorter than his peers. What response by the nurse is indicated?

    a. "Being short is nothing to be ashamed of."

    b. "I am sure you are not the shortest guy in your class."

    c. "Boys your age will often continue growing a few more years."

    d. "Are the other men in your family short?"

12. The nurse is meeting with a 16-year-old female child who reports being physically active on the track and basketball teams at school. The child reports a weight loss of 7 pounds since she began training for the track season. When reviewing her caloric needs the nurse recognizes the diet should include how many calories?

    a. 1,800 calories per day

    b. 2,000 calories per day

    c. 2,200 calories per day

    d. 2,400 calories per day

13. Which of the following behaviors by an 18-year-old is consistent with successful progression through the stages of Piaget's theory of development?

    a. There is a strong sense of understanding of internal identity.

    b. The individual reflects a strong moral code.

    c. The individual is able to use critical thought processes to handle a problem.

    d. The individual is able to be a part of a large group of peers while maintaining a sense of self.

14. The nurse is counseling an overweight, sedentary 15-year-old female child. The nurse is assisting her to make appropriate menu choices. Which of the following indicates the child understands the appropriate dietary selections to make?

    a. "I avoid all fat intake."

    b. "Because of my age, my dairy intake is unlimited."

    c. "I need to have 2 servings of fruit each day."

    d. "To lose weight my protein intake should be limited to 2 to 4 servings per day."

15. The nurse is performing an assessment on a 12-year-old male child. Which of the following findings is consistent with the child's age?

    a. Absence of pubic hair

    b. Presence of curling pubic hair

    c. Coarse pubic hair

    d. Presence of sparse pubic hair

# Atraumatic and Family-Centered Care of Children

- Describe the major principles and concepts of atraumatic care.
- Incorporate atraumatic care to prevent and minimize physical stress for children and families.
- Discuss the major components and concepts of family-centered care.
- Utilize excellent therapeutic communication skills when interacting with children and their families.
- Use culturally competent communication when working with children and their families.
- Describe the process of health teaching as it relates to children and their families.

## SECTION I: ASSESSING YOUR UNDERSTANDING

### Activity A  FILL IN THE BLANKS

1. Therapeutic care that decreases or eliminates the psychological and physical distress experienced by children and their families when receiving health care is referred to as _____ care.

2. Communication that is goal-directed, focused, and purposeful is considered _____ communication.

3. Things such as eye contact and body position are part of _____ communication.

4. A _____ nurse practitioner helps ensure that children and families receive atraumatic care.

5. Clarifying the parent's feelings by paraphrasing parts of a conversation is utilization of _____ communication.

6. Paying attention to what the child and parents are saying by nodding one's head and making eye contact is considered _____ listening.

7. When communicating with a family that speaks a different language than the nurse or with a child that is deaf may require the use of a reliable _____.

## Activity B MATCHING

*Match the development level in Column A with the communication technique in Column B appropriate for the developmental age.*

**Column A**

_____ **1.** Adolescents

_____ **2.** Infants

_____ **3.** Preschoolers

_____ **4.** School-age children

_____ **5.** Toddlers

**Column B**

**a.** Use a soothing voice

**b.** Prepare child just before procedure

**c.** Use diagrams and illustrations

**d.** Use storytelling and play

**e.** Define medical words as necessary

## Activity C SEQUENCING

*Place the following methods of learning in order from lowest percent of information remembered to the highest percent remembered after 2 weeks:*

**1.** Actively discussing

**2.** Hearing

**3.** Performing an activity

**4.** Reading

**5.** Watching a demonstration

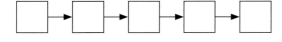

## Activity D SHORT ANSWERS

*Briefly answer the following.*

**1.** Discuss how therapeutic hugging is beneficial during certain procedures?

_____

_____

_____

**2.** Describe four ways to evaluate the success of child and family education.

_____

_____

_____

**3.** What incidents would alert the nurse that a family may be suffering from health literacy difficulties?

_____

_____

_____

**4.** Name six suggestions to enhance learning if literacy problems exist.

_____

_____

_____

**5.** How can the nurse help prevent or minimize child and family separation during a child's hospitalization?

_____

_____

_____

# SECTION II: APPLYING YOUR KNOWLEDGE

## Activity E CASE STUDY

Emma is a 4-year-old female admitted to your pediatric unit secondary to a suspected head injury from a fall. She was playing at a playground with her babysitter and fell from the top of the slide. Emma also has a laceration to her arm that will require stitches. She is scheduled for a CT scan. Her parents are with her and are very supportive and display no difficulties with health literacy.

1. How would you explain a head CT to Emma?

   _____

   _____

   _____

2. What technique should be used to restrain Emma while she receives her stitches?

   _____

   _____

   _____

# SECTION III: PRACTICING FOR NCLEX

## Activity F NCLEX-STYLE QUESTIONS

*Answer the following questions.*

1. The nurse is assessing the learning needs of the parents of 5-year-old girl who is scheduled for surgery. Which of the following nonverbal cues shows them that the nurse is interested in what the family members are saying?
   a. Sitting straight with feet flat on the floor
   b. Looking at child when the father is talking
   c. Nodding head while the mother speaks
   d. Standing several steps away from parents

2. The nurse is caring for a 3-year-old boy who must have a lumbar puncture. Which of the following actions would provide the greatest contribution toward atraumatic care?
   a. Having a child life nurse practitioner play with the child
   b. Explaining the lumbar puncture procedure
   c. Letting the child take his teddy bear with him
   d. Keeping the parents calm in front of the child

3. The nurse is caring for a 14-year-old boy, and his parents, who has just been diagnosed with a malignant tumor on his liver. Which of the following interventions is most important to this child and family?
   a. Arranging an additional meeting with the nurse practitioner
   b. Discussing treatment options with the child and parents
   c. Involving the child and family in decision making
   d. Describing postoperative home care for the child

4. The nurse is educating a 15-year-old girl with Grave's disease and her family about the disease and its treatment. Which of the following methods of evaluating learning is least effective?
   a. Having the child and family demonstrate skills
   b. Asking closed-ended questions for specific facts
   c. Requesting the parent to teach the child skills
   d. Setting up a scenario for them to talk through

5. The nurse is caring for a 14-year-old girl with terminal cancer and her family. Which of the following interventions would best provide therapeutic communication?
   a. Recognizing the parents' desire to use all options
   b. Supporting the child's desires for treatment
   c. Presenting options for treatment
   d. Informing the child in terms she can understand

6. The nurse is caring for a 6-year-old boy and his parents. The child will need chemotherapy for which informed consent is necessary. Which of the following is the most important nursing intervention?

   a. Teaching the parents about optional treatments

   b. Explaining the procedure and possible side effects

   c. Asking questions to determine the parents' understanding

   d. Witnessing the signing of the consent form

7. The nurse is caring for a 3-year-old girl with a ruptured appendix. Her parents have strong religious beliefs against certain types of medical treatment. Which of the following interventions best ensures that the child receives appropriate care?

   a. Recognizing the parents' religious beliefs

   b. Communicating using appropriate terms

   c. Educating the parents about the surgery and prognosis

   d. Assuring the parents that the surgeon is competent

8. The nurse is assessing the teaching needs of the parents of an 8-year-old boy with leukemia. Which of the following assessments would disclose a possible health literacy issue?

   a. The parents missed the last scheduled appointment

   b. The entire family is fluently bi-lingual

   c. The parents are taking notes on answers to their questions

   d. The mother seems to ask most of the questions regarding care

9. The nurse is teaching a 7-year-old girl about the tonsillectomy she will have. Which of the following techniques would be appropriate for this child? (Select all that apply)

   a. Allowing the child to do as much self care as possible

   b. Explaining the procedure that will happen later in the day

   c. Offering choices of drinks and gelatin after the procedure

   d. Explaining that anesthesia is a lot like falling asleep

   e. Use plays or puppets to help explain the procedure

10. The nurse is educating the family of a 2-year-old Chinese boy with bronchiolitis about the disorder and its treatment. Which of the following actions, involving an interpreter, can jeopardize the family's trust?

    a. Allowing too little appointment time for the translation

    b. Using a person who is not a professional interpreter

    c. Asking the interpreter questions not meant for the family

    d. Using an older sibling to communicate with the parents

11. The child life nurse practitioner has been assigned to assist the hospitalized child and the child's parents. Which of the following are appropriate interventions for the child life nurse practitioner to perform? Select all that apply.

    a. The child life nurse practitioner talks to the family about a diagnostic test that the child is scheduled for later in the day

    b. The child life nurse practitioner gives the child an influenza vaccination

    c. The child life nurse practitioner starts the child's intravenous line

    d. The child life nurse practitioner shows the child where the pediatric play room is located

    e. The child life nurse practitioner speaks to the physician as the child's advocate

12. The child and her mother are receiving discharge instructions from the nurse. Which of the following statements by the child's mother are "red flags" that the mother may have poor literacy skills? Select all that apply.

    a. "I forgot my glasses today and can't seem to read this form."

    b. "I'm going to take a few notes while you're teaching us."

    c. "The receptionist told me that we missed another appointment."

    d. "I guess I just forgot to give her the medication the way you told me to."

    e. "I'm going to take these instructions home to read them."

13. The nurse is preparing to educate the child about a procedure that the child is scheduled for tomorrow morning. Which of the following techniques used by the nurse indicate the need for further education about communicating with a child? Select all that apply.

    a. The nurse stands at the foot of the child's bed while teaching the child.

    b. The nurse uses terms that the child will likely understand.

    c. The nurse speaks quickly.

    d. The nurse requests that the parents leave the room while the nurse educates the child.

    e. The nurse is patient with the child and looks for nonverbal cues.

14. The nurse is educating a young child about what to expect during an upcoming procedure. Which of the following statements by the nurse are appropriate to use? Select all that apply.

    a. "This little tube will go in your nose and down into your belly."

    b. "I'm going to give you this shot and it will put you to sleep."

    c. "You'll end up in 'ICU' where you'll wake up with some electrodes on your thorax."

    d. "When they come to get you, you'll get on a special rolling bed."

    e. "They're going to give you some special medicine to help the doctor see what's happening inside your belly."

15. The child has been admitted to a pediatric unit in a hospital. Which of the following nursing interventions indicate that atraumatic care principles are being used? Select all that apply.

    a. The nurse requests that parent assist the nurse by "holding the child down."

    b. The nurse applies a numbing cream prior to starting the child's intravenous line.

    c. The nurse asks the child if he would like to take a bath before or after he takes his medication.

    d. The nurse encourages the family to bring in the child's favorite stuffed animal from home.

    e. The nurse shows the parent how to unfold the chair in the child's room into a bed.

# CHAPTER 9

# Health Supervision

## Learning Objectives

- Describe the principles of health supervision.
- Identify challenges to health supervision for children with chronic illnesses.
- List the three components of a health supervision visit.
- Use instruments appropriately for developmental surveillance and screening of children.
- Demonstrate knowledge of the principles of immunization.
- Identify barriers to immunization.
- Identify the key components of health promotion.
- Describe the role of anticipatory guidance in health promotion.

## SECTION I: ASSESSING YOUR UNDERSTANDING

### Activity A  FILL IN THE BLANKS

1. Because of the impact that hearing loss can have on _____, it is crucial that even slight hearing loss be identified by age 3 months.

2. Screening for iron deficiency at 6 months of age is important because the _____ iron stores of full-term infants are almost depleted.

3. If a client's family has difficulty accessing health care facilities, health promotion activities may be carried out in _____ settings such as schools and churches.

4. Health supervision has three components: screening, _____, and health promotion.

5. When obtaining an immunization history, asking _____ and where the last immunization was received provides more information than asking if immunizations are current.

6. The purpose of hyperlipidemia screening is to reduce the incidence of adult _____ disease.

7. The Weber test screens for hearing by assessing sound conducted via _____.

8. Vaccinations may be postponed if the child has a severe illness with high fever or _____, or has recently received blood products.

9. For children less than 3 years of age, vision screening based on the child's ability to _____ and follow objects.

10. _____ immunity is acquired when a person's own immune system generates the immune response.

## Activity B  MATCHING

*Match the age and developmental warning sign in Column A with the possible developmental concern in Column B.*

**Column A**

___ **1.** Rolls over before 3 months

___ **2.** Persistent head lag after 4 months

___ **3.** Not smiling at 6 months

___ **4.** Not babbling at 6 months

___ **5.** Not walking by 18 months

___ **6.** Hand dominance present before 18 months

**Column B**

**a.** Hemiplegia in opposite upper extremity

**b.** Hypertonia

**c.** Visual defect of attachment issue

**d.** Gross motor delay

**e.** Hypotonia

**f.** Hearing deficit

*Match the developmental screening tool in Column A with the descriptive phrase in Column B.*

**Column A**

___ **1.** Ages and Stages Questionnaire (ASQ)

___ **2.** Child Development Inventory (CDI)

___ **3.** Denver II

___ **4.** Goodenough Harris Drawing Test

___ **5.** Parent's Evaluation of Developmental Status (PEDS)

**Column B**

**a.** Simple questions about infant, toddler, or preschooler behaviors

**b.** Uses props provided in kit such as a baby doll, ball, and crayons to assess personal–social, fine motor–adaptive, language and gross motor skills

**c.** Assesses communication, gross and fine motor, personal–social, and problems-solving skills

**d.** Screens for developmental, behavioral, and family issues. Tool is available in Spanish.

**e.** Nonverbal screen for mental ability

*Match the vision screening tool in Column A with the descriptive phrase in Column B.*

**Column A**

___ **1.** Color Vision Testing Made Easy (CVTME)

___ **2.** Ishihara

___ **3.** LEA symbols or Allen figures

___ **4.** Snellen letters or numbers

___ **5.** Tumbling E

**Column B**

**a.** Uses pictures instead of the alphabet

**b.** Shapes embedded in dots

**c.** Used to assess the preschooler by asking him to point the direction the letter is pointing

**d.** Numbers hidden in dots

**e.** Used in children who know the alphabet

## Activity C  SEQUENCING

*Beginning with an infant who is between birth and 3 months, and progressing in age, place the following developmental warning signs in sequential order.*

**1.** Head lag disappears

**2.** Uses spoon or crayon

**3.** Uses imitative play

**4.** Rolls over

**5.** Says first word

**6.** Primitive reflex disappears

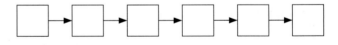

## Activity D  SHORT ANSWERS

*Briefly answer the following.*

**1.** Describe the proper technique for doing the Weber test, including what should be heard and where.

_____

_____

_____

2. What conditions seen in parents or grandparents who are less than 55 years of age would suggest screening for hyperlipidemia in the children?

_____

_____

_____

3. Describe the process of screening for hearing loss in older children, beginning with a history from the primary caregivers.

_____

_____

_____

4. Describe the potential impact of iron deficiency in children. During what periods of time is a child at the greatest risk for the development of the condition?

_____

_____

_____

5. Discuss the recommendations for screening children for hypertension. What factors increase the risk for the development of this condition?

_____

_____

_____

# SECTION II: APPLYING YOUR KNOWLEDGE

## Activity E  CASE STUDY 1

Jasmine Chase, a 15-year-old female, is seen in your clinic for her annual exam. During this health supervision visit, Jasmine expresses concerns about her weight. She states she has been attempting to diet and has reduced her number of meals a day by skipping breakfast. She also decided to give up meat, fish, and poultry, and eats mostly salads for lunch and dinner.

1. During the health interview and exam, what information do you want to elicit?

_____

_____

_____

2. What screening test may be warranted for Jasmine and why?

_____

_____

_____

3. During today's exam, you determine Jasmine's height is 5 feet and her weight is 150 pounds. What can you do to help promote a healthy weight for Jasmine?

_____

_____

_____

**CASE STUDY 2**

Claire Rosemount is a 5-year-old female who was recently diagnosed with Type I diabetes mellitus. Your clinic has been her medical home since birth. Health supervision of a child with a chronic illness can be challenging.

1. What can nurses do to meet these challenges and ensure proper care for Claire and other children with chronic illnesses?

_____

_____

_____

# SECTION III: PRACTICING FOR NCLEX

## Activity F  NCLEX-STYLE QUESTIONS

*Answer the following questions.*

1. During the health history of a 2-month-old infant, the nurse identified a risk factor for developmental delay and is preparing to screen the child's development. Which of the following risks did the nurse find?
   a. The child had neonatal conjunctivitis
   b. The parents are both in college
   c. The child was born at 36 weeks
   d. The child has small eyes and chin

2. The nurse is promoting achieving the benefits of a healthy weight to an overweight 12-year-old child and her parents. Which of the following approaches is best?

   a. Showing the family the appropriate weight for the child

   b. Asking what activities she enjoys such as dance or sports

   c. Suggesting that the child join a little league softball team

   d. Pointing out fattening foods and excesses in their diet

3. The nurse is discussing Varicella immunization with a mother who is reluctant about vaccinating her 13-month-old because she feels it is "not necessary." Which of the following comments will be most persuasive for immunization?

   a. "Mild reactions occur in 5% to 10% of children."

   b. "Varicella is a highly contagious herpes virus."

   c. "Children not immunized are at risk if exposed to the disease."

   d. "Risk of Varicella is greater than the risk of vaccine."

4. The nurse is doing a health history for a 14-year-old boy during a health supervision visit. The boy says he has outgrown his clothes recently. Which of the following conditions needs to be checked for based on this information?

   a. Developmental problems

   b. Hyperlipidemia

   c. Iron deficiency anemia

   d. Systemic hypertension

5. A mother and her 2-week-old infant have arrived for a health supervision visit. Which of the following activities will the nurse perform?

   a. Assess the child for an upper respiratory infection

   b. Take a health history for a minor injury

   c. Administer a Varicella injection

   d. Warn against putting the baby to bed with a bottle

6. During a physical assessment of a 6-year-old child, the nurse observes the child has lost a tooth and uses the opportunity to promote oral health care. Which of the following comments would be included in this discussion?

   a. "Oral health can affect general health."

   b. "Fluoridated water has significantly reduced cavities."

   c. "Try to keep the child's hands out of the mouth."

   d. "Limit the amount of soft drinks in the child's diet."

7. The mother of a 5-year-old with eczema is getting a check-up for her child before school starts. Which of the following will the nurse do during the visit?

   a. Change the bandage on a cut on the child's hand

   b. Assess how the family is coping with the chronic illness

   c. Discuss systemic corticosteroid therapy

   d. Assess the child's fluid volume

8. The nurse is performing a vision screening for 6-year-old child. Which of the following screening charts would be best for determining the child's ability to discriminate color?

   a. Snellen

   b. Ishihara

   c. Allen figures

   d. CVTME

9. The nurse is anticipating that health supervision for a 5-year-old child will be challenging. Which of the following indicators supports this concern?

   a. Grandparents play a significant role in the family

   b. The child has a number of chores and responsibilities

   c. The mother dotes on the child

   d. The home is in a high-crime neighborhood

10. During the health history, the parent of a 10-year-old child mentions the child seems to have trouble hearing. Which of the following tests is the nurse likely to use?

    a. Rinne test

    b. Whisper test

    c. Evoked otoacoustic emissions test

    d. Auditory brain stem response test

11. The nurse is collecting data from the mother of a 3-year-old child. Which of the following reports will warrant further follow-up?

    a. The child cannot stack five blocks

    b. The child cannot grasp a crayon with the thumb and fingers

    c. The child cannot copy a circle

    d. The child is not able to throw a ball overhand

12. The student nurse is preparing to assist the registered nurse to perform the Denver II screening test. Which of the items will the student nurse correctly plan to use with the assessment? Select all that apply.

    a. Ball

    b. Four plastic rings

    c. Doll

    d. Crayon

    e. Crackers

13. The mother of a 2-year-old child questions when she will need to initially have her child's vision screened. What information should be provided by the nurse?

    a. Vision screening begins at 2 years of age

    b. Vision screening begins at 2 ½ years of age

    c. Vision screening begins at 3 years of age

    d. Vision screening begins just prior to kindergarten

14. The nurse is counseling a child about the health benefits associated with breastfeeding. Which of the following statements by the child indicates understanding?

    a. "Breastfeeding my baby passes on a type of active immunity."

    b. "Breastfeeding my baby passes on passive immunity."

    c. "Breastfeeding my baby provides lifelong immunity against certain diseases."

    d. "Breastfeeding my baby will help to stimulate my baby's immune system to activate."

15. Which of the following children poses the greatest risk for elevated lead levels?

    a. A Caucasian child who is 2 years of age

    b. An African American child who is 18 months of age

    c. A Caucasian child who is 10 years of age

    d. An Asian child who is 2 years of age

# Health Assessment of Children

# SECTION I: ASSESSING YOUR UNDERSTANDING

## Activity A  FILL IN THE BLANKS

1. _____ is an acronym that means pupils are equal, round, reactive to light and accommodation.

2. _____ is the measure of body weight relative to height.

3. The _____ is the area on an infant's head that is not protected by skull bone.

4. Auscultation is listening with a _____.

5. When assessing the thorax and lungs, an inspiratory high pitched sound is referred to as audible _____.

6. During assessment of the newborn the nurse notes small white papules on the infant's forehead, chin, nose, and cheeks. The nurse is correct in documenting this finding as

   _____.

7. Following inspection, _____ of the abdomen should be performed next during assessment of the abdomen.

## Activity B  LABELING

*Consider the following figure.*

*Identify the point of maximal intensity (PMI) or apical impulse, for birth to 4 years, age 4 to 6 years, and 7 years and older.*

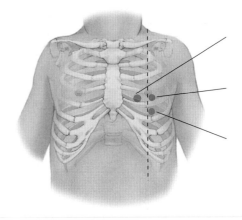

**Activity C** **MATCHING**

*Match the term in Column A with the proper definition in Column B.*

**Column A**

_____ **1.** Acrocyanosis

_____ **2.** Cerumen

_____ **3.** Lanugo

_____ **4.** Stadiometer

_____ **5.** Accommodation

**Column B**

**a.** Soft downy hair found on the newborn's body

**b.** Ability of the eyes to focus at different distances

**c.** Transient blueness in the hands and feet

**d.** Instrument to measure standing height

**e.** Waxy substance normally found lubricating and protecting the external ear canal

**Activity D** **SEQUENCING**

*Place the following questions in the health interview of an adolescent in the proper sequence in the boxes provided below:*

**1.** Are you sexually active?

**2.** What is your name?

**3.** What can I help you with today?

**4.** Do you have any allergies?

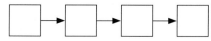

**Activity E** **SHORT ANSWERS**

*Briefly answer the following.*

**1.** Briefly describe the six grades of heart murmurs in children.

_____

_____

_____

**2.** Differentiate between ecchymosis, petechiae, and purpura.

_____

_____

_____

**3.** Briefly describe the expected appearance of the healthy ear canal and tympanic membrane.

_____

_____

_____

**4.** How does the heart rate vary according to a child's age?

_____

_____

_____

**5.** What are some possible reasons for inaccurate pulse oximetry readings?

_____

_____

_____

**6.** Identify four risk factors that would indicate the need to assess the blood pressure of a child under the age of 3 years.

_____

_____

_____

# SECTION II: APPLYING YOUR KNOWLEDGE

## Activity F  CASE STUDY

As the nurse on a pediatric unit you are assigned to care for three children. You receive the following information on each child in report. Based on this information, rank in order of priority when to assess each child. Provide rationale for your answers.

1. A 5-year-old hospitalized with an acute asthma attack. Vital signs are: heart rate 124, respiratory rate 28 to 30, blood pressure 93/48, and axillary temperature of 98.6F.

   _____

   _____

   _____

2. A 3-month-old hospitalized for rule out sepsis secondary to fever. Vital signs are: heart rate 165, respiratory rate 34, blood pressure 108/64, and rectal temperature of 102.5F taken immediately before report. No intervention was initiated.

   _____

   _____

   _____

3. A 7-month-old hospitalized with pneumonia. Vital signs are: heart rate of 165 with brief episodes of dropping into the 60's during the previous shift, respiratory rate of 78, blood pressure 112/72, and axillary temperature of 99.5F.

   _____

   _____

   _____

# SECTION III: PRACTICING FOR NCLEX

## Activity G  NCLEX-STYLE QUESTIONS

*Answer the following questions.*

1. The nurse is examining the genitals of a healthy newborn girl. The nurse would expect to observe which of the following normal findings?
   a. Swollen labia minora
   b. Lesions on the external genitalia
   c. Labial adhesions
   d. Swollen labia majora

2. The nurse is caring for a 13-year-old girl. As part of a routine health assessment the nurse needs to address areas relating to sexuality and substance abuse. Which of the following should the nurse say first to encourage communication?
   a. Do you smoke cigarettes or marijuana?
   b. I promise not to tell your mother any of your responses.
   c. Tell me about some of your current activities at school.
   d. Are you considering sexual activity?

3. The nurse is caring for a 10-year-old girl and is trying to obtain clues about the child's state of physical, emotional, and moral development. Which of the following questions would most likely elicit the desired information?
   a. "Do you like your school and your teacher?"
   b. "Would you say that you are a good student?"
   c. "Tell me about your favorite activity at school?"
   d. "Do you have a lot of friends at school?"

4. A nurse is caring for a very shy 4-year-old girl. During the course of a well child assessment the nurse must take the girl's blood pressure. Which of the following is the best approach?

   a. "May I take your blood pressure?"

   b. "Your sister did a great job when I took hers"

   c. "Help me take your dolls blood pressure"

   d. "Will you let me put this cuff on your arm?"

5. The nurse is preparing to see a 14-month-old child and needs to establish the chief complaint or purpose of the visit. Which of the following would be the best approach with the parents?

   a. "What is your chief complaint?"

   b. "What can I help you with today?"

   c. "Is your child feeling sick?"

   d. "Has your child been exposed to infectious agents?"

6. A nurse is conducting a physical examination of an uncooperative preschooler. In order to encourage deep breathing during lung auscultation what could the nurse say?

   a. "You must breathe deeply so I can hear your lungs"

   b. "You may not leave until I listen to your breathing"

   c. "Do you think you can blow out my light bulb on this pen?"

   d. "Do you want your mother to listen to your lungs?"

7. The nurse is conducting a physical examination of a healthy 6-year-old. Which of the following would the nurse do first?

   a. Observe the skin for its overall color and characteristics.

   b. Tap with the knee with a reflex hammer to check for deep tendon reflexes.

   c. Palpate the skin for texture and hydration status.

   d. Auscultate the heart, lungs, and the abdomen.

8. A nurse is assessing an infant's reflexes. The nurse places his or her thumb to the ball of the infant's foot to elicit which reflex?

   a. Parachute

   b. Plantar grasp

   c. Babinski

   d. Palmar grasp

9. The emergency department nurse is caring for a child who is showing signs of anaphylaxis. The nurse evaluates how comprehensive the history of the child should be and determines that which action takes priority?

   a. Taking a problem-focused history

   b. Obtaining a complete and detailed history

   c. Stabilizing the child's physical status

   d. Getting the child's history from other providers

10. The nurse is conducting a physical examination of a 5-year-old girl. The nurse asks the girl to stand still with her eyes closed and arms down by her side. The girl immediately begins to lean. This tells the nurse which information?

    a. The child has poor coordination and poor balance

    b. The child warrants further testing for cerebellar dysfunction

    c. The child has a negative Romberg test; no further testing is necessary

    d. The child has a possible inner ear infection

11. The nurse needs to calculate the child's body mass index (BMI). The child's weight is 42 kg and is 142 cm tall. Calculate the child's BMI using the metric method, round answer to the nearest whole number.

12. The experienced nurse is assessing the child's lungs. Rank the following steps in the proper order of assessment:

a. The nurse percusses over the child's lungs.

b. The nurse visually inspects the child's thorax.

c. The nurse palpates the child's thorax.

d. The nurse auscultates the child's lungs.

# Caring for Children in Diverse Settings

- Identify the major stressors of illness and hospitalization for children.
- Identify the reactions and responses of children and their families during illness and hospitalization.
- Explain the factors that influence the reactions and responses of children and their families during illness and hospitalization.
- Describe the nursing care that minimizes stressors for children who are ill or hospitalized.
- Discuss the major components of admission for children to the hospital.
- Discuss appropriate safety measures to use when caring for children of all ages.
- Review nursing responsibilities related to child discharge from the hospital.
- Describe the various roles of community and home care nurses.
- Discuss the variety of settings in which community-based care occurs.
- Discuss the advantages and disadvantages of home health care.

## SECTION I: ASSESSING YOUR UNDERSTANDING

### Activity A FILL IN THE BLANKS

1. Therapeutic _____ is the use of a holding position that promotes close physical contact between the child and a parent or caregiver that is used when the child needs to remain still for procedures such as IV insertion.

2. Restraints should be checked every _____ minutes following initial placement, then every hour for proper placement.

3. A good time to assess the skin is during _____ time.

4. Forcing a child to _____ can exacerbate any nausea or vomiting.

5. _____ play allows a child to express his or her feelings and fears, as well as providing a means to promote energy expenditure.

6. Nurses in the school setting develop _____ to plan how the school staff will collaborate with the student and family in meeting the needs of students with complex health care issues.

7. _____ nurses focus on health supervision services and connecting children to needed community resources.

## Activity B MATCHING

*Match the term in Column A with the proper definition in Column B.*

**Column A**

____ **1.** Denial

____ **2.** Regression

____ **3.** Sensory overload

____ **4.** Separation anxiety

____ **5.** Sensory deprivation

**Column B**

**a.** Increased stimulation for the child

**b.** Defense mechanism used by children to avoid unpleasant realities

**c.** Distress related to being removed from primary caregivers and familiar surroundings

**d.** Lack of stimulation

**e.** Defense mechanism used by children to avoid dealing with conflict by returning to a previous stage that may be more comfortable to the child

## Activity C SEQUENCING

*Place the three stages of separation anxiety in the proper sequence.*

**1.** Despair

**2.** Denial

**3.** Protest

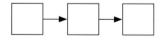

## Activity D SHORT ANSWERS

*Briefly answer the following.*

**1.** How can the nurse address and minimize separation anxiety in the hospitalized child?

_____

_____

_____

**2.** When does discharge planning begin? Why?

_____

_____

_____

**3.** What are some common behaviors or methods children use for coping with hospitalization?

_____

_____

_____

**4.** What are the most common reasons for children to be hospitalized?

_____

_____

_____

**5.** What are some ways the home care nurse can establish a trusting relationship with the child and caregivers?

_____

_____

_____

# SECTION II: APPLYING YOUR KNOWLEDGE

## Activity E CASE STUDY

A variety of reactions and responses are seen as a result of the stressors children experience in relation to hospitalization. Nurses often spend more time with children and their families compared to other physicians during hospitalization. Therefore, it is essential that nurses establish strategies to care and intervene in order to help children cope with their experience. Nurses must examine effects of hospitalization within the child's developmental stage and understand the reactions and responses of the child and family to hospitalization.

While working on the pediatric unit, your child care assignment involves children of differing developmental ages. Read the below reactions and identify interventions and rationales for each of the following children in your care.

1. Leslie Lucas, a 6-month-old female with a club foot repair, is hospitalized post-surgery. She has been irritable and difficult to console.

   _____

   _____

   _____

2. Eli Castle, an 18-month-old male admitted with pneumonia, has not slept more than 1 hour without waking.

   _____

   _____

   _____

3. Amelia Lionhart, a 4-year-old female admitted with dehydration, repeatedly wakes up crying after having nightmares.

   _____

   _____

   _____

4. Jamal Anderson, a 10-year-old male, hospitalized secondary to asthma, has eaten very little from his meal trays for the past few days.

   _____

   _____

   _____

5. Cheryl Erikson, a 16-year-old female with lymphoma, expresses a desire to be left alone in her darkened room.

   _____

   _____

   _____

# SECTION III: PRACTICING FOR NCLEX

## Activity F NCLEX-STYLE QUESTIONS

*Answer the following questions.*

1. The nurse is caring for an 18-month-old boy hospitalized with a gastrointestinal disorder. The nurse knows that the child is at risk for separation anxiety. The nurse understands to watch carefully for which of the following behaviors, indicating that the first phase of separation anxiety is occurring?

   a. Crying and acting out

   b. Embracing others who attempt to comfort him

   c. Disinterest in play and food

   d. Exhibiting apathy and withdrawing from others

2. The nurse is caring for a preschooler who is hospitalized with a suspected blood disorder and receives an order to draw a blood sample. Which of the following would be the best way to approach the child for this procedure?

   a. "I need to take some blood."

   b. "We need to put a little hole in your arm."

   c. "I need to remove a little blood."

   d. "Why don't you sit on your mom's lap?"

3. The nurse is caring for a child hospitalized with complications from asthma. Which of the following statements by the parents indicates a need for careful observation of the child's anxiety level?

   a. "My mother passed away here after surgery."

   b. "Our twins were born here 18 months ago."

   c. "My son was born at this hospital."

   d. "We attended a 'living with asthma' class here."

4. A nurse is caring for a 6-year-old boy hospitalized due to an infection requiring intravenous antibiotic therapy. The child's motor activity is restricted and he is acting out, yelling, kicking, and screaming. Which of the following responses by the nurse would help promote positive coping?

   a. "Your medicine is the only way you will get better."

   b. "Let me explain why you need to sit still."

   c. "Would you like to read or play video games?"

   d. "Do I need to call your parents?"

5. A nurse is telling the parents how to help their 10-year-old daughter deal with an extended hospital stay due to surgery, followed by traction. Which of the following responses indicates a need for further teaching?

   a. "I should not tell her how long she will be here."

   b. "She will watch our reactions carefully."

   c. "We must prepare her in advance."

   d. "She will be sensitive to our concerns."

6. A nurse is preparing to admit a child for a tonsillectomy. How should the nurse establish rapport?

   a. "Let's take a look at your tonsils."

   b. "Do you understand why you are here?"

   c. "Are you scared about having your tonsils out?"

   d. "Tell me about your cute stuffed dog you have."

7. The nurse is preparing to admit a 4-year-old who will be having tympanostomy tubes placed in both ears. Which of the following strategies would most likely reduce the child's fears of the procedure?

   a. "The doctor is going to insert tympanostomy tubes in your ears"

   b. "Don't worry, you will be asleep the whole time"

   c. "Let me show you how tiny these tubes are"

   d. "Let me show you the operating room"

8. A nurse is developing a preoperative plan of care for a 2-year-old. The nurse understands to pay particular attention to which of the child's age-related fears?

   a. Separation from friends

   b. Separation from parents

   c. Loss of control

   d. Loss of independence

9. The nurse is providing teaching for the parents of a 7-year-old boy, scheduled for surgery, to help prepare the child for hospitalization. Which of the following statements by the parents indicates a need for further teaching?

   a. "We should talk about going to the hospital and what it will be like coming home"

   b. "We should visit the hospital and go through the preadmission tour in advance"

   c. "It is best to wait and let her bring up the surgery or any questions she has"

   d. "It is a good idea to read stories about experiences with hospitals or surgery"

10. The nurse is caring for a 7-year-old boy in a body cast. He is shy and seems fearful of the numerous personnel in and out of his room. How can the nurse help reduce his fear?

   a. Remind the boy he will be out of the hospital and going home soon.

   b. Encourage the boy's parents to stay with him at all times to reduce his fears.

   c. Write the name of his nurse on a board and identify all staff on each shift, every day.

   d. Tell him not to worry; explain that everyone is here to care for him.

11. The nurse is providing care for a hospitalized child. Rank the following phases in the order of occurrence based on the nurse's statements.

    a. "Let's sit over here and play a game of 'Go Fish'."

    b. "You handled that procedure so well! Would you like me to get Mr. Snuggles for you?"

    c. "Would you like your medicine before or after your mom helps take a bath?"

    d. "Hi, my name is Cindy and I'm going to be your nurse for today."

12. The nurse has applied a restraint to the child's right wrist to prevent the child from pulling out an intravenous line. Which of the following assessment findings are important to note to ensure that there is proper circulation to the child's right arm?

    a. Capillary refill is less than 2 seconds in upper extremities bilaterally

    b. Fingers are pink and warm bilaterally

    c. Lungs are clear throughout

    d. Radial pulses are easily palpable bilaterally

    e. Bowel sounds present in all four quadrants

13. The student nurse is assisting the more experienced pediatric nurse. Which of the following statements by the student indicate further education is required?

    a. "Could you give the nauseated child some medicine before it is time for him to start thinking about ordering lunch?"

    b. "I'm going to redress the child's IV site while she is in the playroom."

    c. "I took our new teenaged child down to show him the playroom."

    d. "It would be easy to perform a straight catheterization while the baby is in his crib."

    e. "I told the child's mom to go ahead and bring in his blanket and stuffed animal."

14. The nurse is documenting the child's intake. The child ate four cups of ice during this shift. How many cups of fluid did the child ingest?

    a. 4 cups of fluid

    b. 1 cup of fluid

    c. ½ cup of fluid

    d. 2 cups of fluid

# Caring for the Special Needs Child

- Analyze the impact that being a child with special needs has on the child and family.
- Identify anticipated times when the child and family will require additional support.
- Describe ways that nurses assist children with special needs and their families to obtain optimal functioning.
- Discuss early intervention and public school education for the special needs child.
- Plan for transition of the special needs child from the inpatient facility to the home, and from pediatric to adult medical care.
- Discuss key elements related to pediatric end-of-life care.
- Differentiate developmental responses to death and appropriate interventions.

## SECTION I: ASSESSING YOUR UNDERSTANDING

### Activity A  FILL IN THE BLANKS

1. The Individuals with Disabilities Education Act (IDEA) of 2004 mandates government-funded care coordination and special education for children up to _____ years of age.

2. _____ care provides an opportunity for families to take a break from the daily intensive care giving responsibilities.

3. When working with a dying child, always focus on the _____ as the unit of care.

4. _____ remains the leading cause of death from disease in all children over the age of 1 year.

5. A _____ consent is necessary for organ donation, so the family must be appropriately informed and educated.

6. _____ care provides the best quality of life possible at the end of life while alleviating physical, psychological, emotional, and spiritual suffering.

7. During the last stages of a terminal illness, _____ care allows for family-centered care in the child's home or appropriate facility.

## Activity B MATCHING

*Match the child's stage in Column A with their needs as they go through the dying process in Column B.*

**Column A**

_____ **1.** Toddler (1 to 3 years)

_____ **2.** 3 to 5 years

_____ **3.** 5 to 10 years

_____ **4.** 10 to 14 years

_____ **5.** 14 to 18 years

**Column B**

a. Need to know death is not a punishment; need to know that although they will be missed, the family will function without them

b. Specific honest details; old enough to help in some decision making

c. Reinforcement of self-esteem; privacy and time alone, time with peers; participation in decision making

d. Support through honest, detailed explanations; wants to feel truly involved and listened to

e. Need familiarity, routine, favorite toys and physical comfort

## Activity C SEQUENCING

*Place the Adolescent Health Transition Project (AHTP) recommendations schedule for transitioning child care to adult care for the child with special health care needs in the proper sequence.*

**1.** Explore health care financing for young adults. If needed, notify the local division of vocational rehabilitation by the autumn before the teen is to graduate from high school of the impending transition. Initiate guardianship procedures if appropriate.

**2.** Ensure that a transition plan is initiated and that the individualized education plan (IEP) reflects post-high school plans.

**3.** Ensure that the young adult has registered with the Division of Developmental Disabilities for adult services if applicable.

**4.** Notify the teen that all rights transfer to him or her at the age of majority. Check the teen's eligibility for SSI the month the child turns 18. Determine if the child is eligible for SSI work incentives.

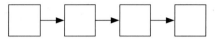

## Activity D SHORT ANSWERS

*Briefly answer the following.*

**1.** Name four different complementary therapies that might be adopted for treatment of children with chronic illness.

_____

_____

_____

**2.** Explain dietary requirements and how they are best met for formerly premature infants who need to "catch-up" on weight.

_____

_____

_____

**3.** How should the nurse explain DNR orders (do not resuscitate) to a family when they are trying to make this decision regarding a terminally ill child?

_____

_____

_____

**4.** List the principles that the Last Acts Palliative Care Task Force has established regarding the care of children with a terminal illness.

_____

_____

_____

**5.** Since the body requires less nutrition during the dying process, what are some important care measures to keep in mind for the dying child?

_____

_____

_____

# SECTION II: APPLYING YOUR KNOWLEDGE

## Activity E  CASE STUDY

1. Preet Singh is a 2-year-old boy born at 27 weeks gestation and has a history of hydrocephalus and developmental delay. What role can the nurse play in assisting the family to obtain optimal functioning?

_____

_____

_____

2. Georgia Lansing, a 7-year-old girl, has been diagnosed with lymphoma. She recently had a relapse and has not responded to treatment. The family has decided on palliative care. Discuss ways the nurse can support the dying child and family.

   Include the type of support and education that the dying child needs according to the developmental stage.

_____

_____

_____

# SECTION III: PRACTICING FOR NCLEX

## Activity F  NCLEX-STYLE QUESTIONS

*Answer the following questions.*

1. The nurse is caring for the family of a medically fragile 2-year-old girl. Which activity is most effective in building a therapeutic relationship?
   a. Helping access an early intervention program.
   b. Teaching physiotherapy techniques.
   c. Listening to parents' triumphs and failures.
   d. Getting free samples of the child's medications.

2. A 14-year-old boy is aware that he is dying. Which action best meets the child's need for self-esteem and sense of worth?
   a. Providing full participation in decision making.
   b. Initiating conversations about his feelings.
   c. Giving direct, honest answers to his questions.
   d. Listening to his fears and concerns about dying.

3. A 10-year-old girl with bone cancer is near death. Which action would best minimize her 8-year-old sister's anxiety?
   a. Correcting her when she says her sister won't die.
   b. Telling her that her sister won't need food any more.
   c. Discouraging the child's questions about death.
   d. Explaining how the morphine drip works.

4. A 15-year-old boy with special needs is attending high school. Which nursing intervention will be most beneficial to his education?
   a. Collaborating with the school nurse about his care.
   b. Serving on his individualized education plan (IEP) committee.
   c. Advocating for financial aid for a motorized wheelchair.
   d. Assessing how attending school will affect his health.

5. A 6-month-old girl is significantly underweight. Which assessment finding will point to an inorganic cause of failure to thrive?
   a. Examining to see if the infant refuses the nipple.
   b. Observing to see if the child avoids eye contact.
   c. Asking the mother if the birth was premature.
   d. Checking the health history for risk factors.

6. The nurse is caring for the family of a 9-year-old boy with cerebral palsy. Which intervention will best improve communication between the nurse and the family?

   a. Giving direct, understandable answers.

   b. Sharing cell phone numbers with the parents.

   c. Using reflective listening techniques.

   d. Saying the same thing in different ways.

7. It is difficult for the father of a technologically dependent 7-year-old girl to leave his work. Which nursing intervention would best involve him in family-centered care?

   a. Leave a voice mail for the father at work.

   b. Email a status report to the father's office.

   c. Urge the father to come to the hospital at lunch.

   d. Schedule education sessions in the evening.

8. The nurse is caring for the family of a medically fragile child in the hospital. Which intervention is most important to the parents?

   a. Educating the parents about the course of treatment.

   b. Evaluating the emotional strength of the parents.

   c. Preparing a list of supplies the family will need.

   d. Assessing the adequacy of the home environment.

9. The nurse at a hospice care facility is caring for a 12-year-old girl. Which intervention best meets the needs of this child?

   a. Assuring her the illness is not her fault.

   b. Urging her to invite her friends to visit.

   c. Acting as the child's personal confidant.

   d. Explaining her condition to her in detail.

10. The nurse is caring for a 15-year-old boy with cystic fibrosis. Which intervention will help avert risky behavior?

    a. Assessing for signs of depression.

    b. Encouraging participation in activities.

    c. Monitoring compliance with treatment.

    d. Urging that he join a support group.

11. The infant was born prematurely. Which of the following assessment findings may indicate that the child is suffering from a medical condition associated with being born prematurely?

    a. The child's parents stated that the child began losing baby teeth earlier than their other children.

    b. The child's hearing is not within normal limits and the child requires a hearing aid.

    c. The child eyes deviate inward.

    d. The child is noted to be above the 95th percentile for height and at the 85th percentile for weight.

    e. The child started speaking multi-word sentences at 18 months old.

12. The infant was born at 32 weeks gestation and is now 9 months old. What is the infant's corrected age?

13. The child has been hospitalized for failure to thrive. The child weighs 23.2 kg. The child is to receive 120 kilocalories per kg of weight per day. How many kilocalories should the child eat each day?

14. Rank the following psychosocial development stages in the proper order of occurrence.

    a. Initiative

    b. Autonomy

    c. Industry

    d. Trust

**15.** The child has been diagnosed with vulnerable child syndrome. Which of the following statements by the child's parent is associated with the presence of this syndrome?

    **a.** "I discipline all of three of my kids very fairly."

    **b.** "He was always a sweet and happy baby."

    **c.** "For the first few weeks of his life, he was so yellow I was afraid he would glow."

    **d.** "When she was a toddler she developed meningitis and the doctors told me they didn't think she'd make it."

    **e.** "She was born with a cleft lip and palate. I was so afraid she wasn't getting enough formula."

# CHAPTER 13

# Key Pediatric Nursing Interventions

## Learning Objectives

- Describe the "eight rights" of pediatric medication administration.
- Explain the physiologic differences in children affecting a medication's pharmacodynamic and pharmacokinetic properties.
- Accurately determine recommended pediatric medication doses.
- Demonstrate the proper technique for administering medication to children via the oral, rectal, ophthalmic, otic, intravenous, intramuscular, and subcutaneous routes.
- Integrate the concepts of atraumatic care in medication administration for children.
- Identify the preferred sites for peripheral and central intravenous medication administration.
- Describe nursing management related to maintenance of intravenous infusions in children, as well as prevention of complications.
- Explain nursing care related to enteral tube feedings.
- Describe nursing management of the child receiving total parenteral nutrition.

## SECTION I: ASSESSING YOUR UNDERSTANDING

### Activity A  FILL IN THE BLANKS

1. A port-a-cath is a type of _____ central venous access device.

2. _____ is the behavior of a medication at the cellular level.

3. Encouraging the child to count aloud or asking a child to blow bubbles during a medical procedure is a method to create a _____.

4. When inserting a rectal suppository for any child under the age of 3, the nurse should use the _____ finger.

5. _____ typically occurs with too rapid cessation of TPN (total parenteral nutrition).

6. _____ tubes are inserted through the nose and terminate in the stomach and are used for short-term enteral feeding.

7. Administration of medication into the eyes is referred to as the _____ route.

## Activity B   LABELING

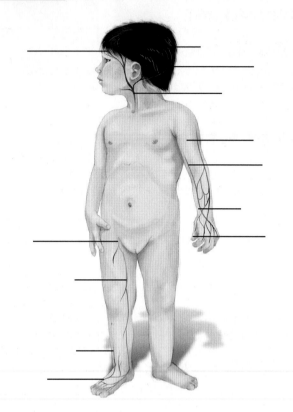

*Provide labels for the preferred peripheral sites for IV insertion.*

a. Dorsal arch
b. Great saphenous
c. Basilic
d. Superficial temporal
e. Femoral
f. Cephalic
g. Frontal
h. Dorsal arch
i. External jugular
j. Occipital
k. Digital
l. Small saphenous

## Activity C   MATCHING

*Match the term in Column A with the proper definition in Column B.*

**Column A**

_____ **1.** Gavage feedings

_____ **2.** Enteral nutrition

_____ **3.** Bolus feeding

_____ **4.** Parenteral nutrition

_____ **5.** Residual

**Column B**

a. Nutrition delivered directly into the intestinal tract

b. Administration of a specified feeding solution at specific intervals, usually over a short period of time

c. Intravenous delivery of nutritional substances

d. The amounts of contents remaining in the stomach indicating gastric emptying time

e. Feeding administered via a tube into the stomach or intestines

## Activity D   SEQUENCING

*Place the steps of administering a gavage enteral feeding in the proper sequence.*

1. Measure the amount of gastric residual.

2. Flush the tube with water and administer the feeding.

3. Check tube for placement.

4. Flush the tube with water.

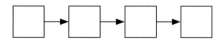

## Activity E  SHORT ANSWERS

*Briefly answer the following.*

1. What is the rationale for performing all invasive procedures outside of the child's hospital room?

_____

_____

_____

2. There are eight rights of pediatric medication administration. How can the nurse ensure that the medication is being administered to the right child?

_____

_____

_____

3. What are the key measures to reduce the risk of complications related to the use of central venous access devices and total parenteral nutrition?

_____

_____

_____

4. What are the eight rights of medication administration for children?

_____

_____

_____

5. Briefly explain the methods for verifying proper feeding tube placement.

_____

_____

_____

# SECTION II: APPLYING YOUR KNOWLEDGE

## Activity F  CASE STUDY

Jennifer Michels, a 7-month-old, has a rectal temperature of 102.5 F. As the nurse caring for her, you are preparing to administer oral acetaminophen per the physicians order. Jennifer's weight is 15 lbs.

1. Discuss the steps you will take for administering a PRN dose of oral acetaminophen for Jennifer. Include rationale for your actions.

_____

_____

_____

2. The physician ordered 70 mg po every 4 hours for fever or discomfort. Calculate the correct dose for Jennifer's weight based on recommended dosing for acetaminophen of 10 to 15 mg/kg every 4 to 6 hours. Is the physician's order a safe and therapeutic dose?

_____

_____

_____

3. Obtain the amount to be drawn up using a concentration of acetaminophen infant drops 80 mg/0.8 ml.

_____

_____

_____

# SECTION III: PRACTICING FOR NCLEX

## Activity G NCLEX-STYLE QUESTIONS

*Answer the following questions.*

1. The nurse is caring for a 4-year-old who requires a venipuncture. Which of the following explanations to prepare the child for the procedure is most appropriate?

    a. "The doctor will look at your blood to see why you are sick."

    b. "The doctor wants to see if you have strep throat."

    c. "The doctor needs to take your blood to see why you are sick."

    d. "The doctor needs to culture your blood to see if you have strep."

2. The nurse is caring for a child with an intravenous device in his hand. Which of the following signs would alert the nurse that infiltration is occurring?

    a. Warmth, redness

    b. Cool, puffy skin

    c. Induration

    d. Tender skin

3. The nurse is preparing to administer a medication via a syringe pump as ordered for a 2-month-old girl. What is the priority nursing action?

    a. Gather the medication

    b. Verify the medication order

    c. Gather the necessary equipment and supplies

    d. Wash hands and put on gloves

4. A nurse is teaching the parents of a 5-year-old boy who requires daily oral medication how to administer it. Which of the following responses indicates a need for further teaching?

    a. "I should never refer to the medicine as candy."

    b. "We should never bribe our child to take the medicine."

    c. "He needs to take his medicine or he will lose a privilege."

    d. "We checked that the medicine can be mixed with yogurt or applesauce."

5. A nurse is preparing to administer an ordered IM injection to an infant. The nurse knows that the most appropriate injection site for this child is the:

    a. Deltoid

    b. Ventrogluteal

    c. Dorsogluteal

    d. Vastus lateralis

6. The nurse is preparing to remove an IV device from the arm of a 6-year-old girl. Which of the following is the best approach to minimize fear and anxiety?

    a. "This won't be painful; you'll just feel a tug and a pinch."

    b. "The first step is for you to help me remove this dressing from your IV."

    c. "Be sure to keep your hands clear of the scissors so I don't cut you."

    d. "Please be a big girl and don't cry when I remove this."

7. The nurse is teaching the parents of a 5-month-old how to administer an oral antibiotic. Which of the following responses indicates a need for further teaching?

    a. "We can mix the antibiotics into his formula or food."

    b. "We can follow his medicine with some applesauce or yogurt."

    c. "We can place the medicine along the inside of his cheek."

    d. "We should not forcibly squirt the medication in the back of his throat."

8. A nurse is caring for a child who requires intravenous maintenance fluid. The child weighs 30 kg. The nurse calculates the child's daily maintenance fluid requirement to be:

    a. 1,500 mL

    b. 1,600 mL

    c. 1,700 mL

    d. 1,800 mL

9. The nurse is assessing the aspirate of a gavage feeding tube to confirm placement. Which of the following assessment findings indicates intestinal placement?

    a. Clear aspirate

    b. Yellow aspirate

    c. Tan aspirate

    d. Green aspirate

10. The nurse is preparing to administer medication to a 10-year-old who weighs 70 pounds. The prescribed single dose is 3 to 4 mg/kg per day. Which of the following is the appropriate dose range for this child?

    a. 96 to 128 mg

    b. 105 to 140 mg

    c. 210 to 280 mg

    d. 420 to 560 mg

11. The child weighs 47 pounds. How many kilograms does the child weigh? Round the answer to the nearest tenth.

12. The child weighs 27 kg. Using the following formula, calculate how many milliliters of intravenous fluids should be administered to the child in a 24 hour period.

Formula:

    100 milliliters per kilogram of body weight for the first 10 kilograms
    50 milliliters per kilogram of body weight for the next 10 kilograms
    20 milliliters per kilogram of body weight for the remainder of body weight in kilograms

13. The adolescent weighs 113 pounds. The nurse closely monitors the child's urine output. How many milliliters of urine is the least amount that the adolescent should make during an 8-hour shift? Round to the nearest whole number.

14. The nurse is calculating the urinary output for the infant. The infant's diaper weighed 40 grams prior to placing the diaper on the infant. After removal of the wet diaper, the diaper weighed 75 grams. How many milliliters of urine can the nurse document as urinary output?

15. Age affects how the medication is distributed throughout the body. Which of the following are factors that affect how medication distribution is altered in infants and young children? Select all that apply.

    a. Infants and young children have an increased percentage of water in their bodies

    b. Infants and young children have an increased percentage of body fat

    c. Infants and young children have an increased number of plasma proteins available for binding to drugs

    d. The blood–brain barrier in infants and young children does not easily allow permeation by many medications

    e. The livers in infants and young children are immature

# CHAPTER 14

# Pain Management in Children

## Learning Objectives

- Identify the major physiologic events associated with the perception of pain.
- Discuss the factors that influence the pain response.
- Identify the developmental considerations of the effects and management of pain in the infant, toddler, preschooler, school-age child, and adolescent.
- Explain the principles of pain assessment as they relate to children.
- Understand the use of the various pain rating scales and physiologic monitoring for children.
- Establish a nursing care plan for children related to management of pain, including pharmacologic and nonpharmacologic techniques and strategies.

## SECTION I: ASSESSING YOUR UNDERSTANDING

### Activity A FILL IN THE BLANKS

1. Two of the most commonly used agents for conscious sedation are _____ and fentanyl.

2. EMLA should be applied _____ minutes before a superficial procedure such as a heel stick or venipuncture.

3. Conscious sedation is a medically controlled state of _____ consciousness.

4. _____ is considered the "gold standard" for all opioid agonists and is the drug to which all other opioids are compared.

5. Patient controlled analgesia is usually reserved for use by children _____ years of age and older.

6. The point at which an individual feels the lowest intensity of the painful stimulus is referred to as the _____.

7. _____ is the pain rating scale that is used for children that uses photographs of facial expressions.

### Activity B MATCHING

*Match the term in Column A with the proper definition in Column B.*

| Column A | Column B |
|---|---|
| ___ 1. Somatic pain | a. Process of nociceptor activation |
| ___ 2. Transduction | b. Pain due to the activation of the A delta fibers and C fibers by noxious stimulant |
| ___ 3. Nociceptive pain | c. Situated within the spinal canal, on or outside the dura mater |
| ___ 4. Neuromodulators | d. Pain that develops in the tissues |
| ___ 5. Epidural | e. Substances that modify the perception of pain |

*Match the medication in Column A with its action in Column B.*

**Column A**

\_\_\_\_ **1.** Morphine

\_\_\_\_ **2.** Pentazocine

\_\_\_\_ **3.** Ibuprofen

\_\_\_\_ **4.** Acetaminophen

**Column B**

**a.** Inhibition of prostaglandin synthesis

**b.** Opioid agonist acting primarily at μ receptor sites

**c.** Direct action of hypothalamic heat regulating center

**d.** Antagonist at μ receptor sites agonist at κ receptor sites

---

**Activity C** SEQUENCING

*Place the physiologic events that lead to the sensation of pain in the proper sequence.*

**1.** Modulation

**2.** Transmission

**3.** Transduction

**4.** Perception

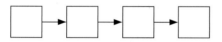

---

**Activity D** SHORT ANSWERS

*Briefly answer the following.*

**1.** What is the difference between superficial somatic pain and deep somatic pain?

_____

_____

_____

**2.** What are the three general principles that guide pain management in children?

_____

_____

_____

**3.** Which of the factors that influence a child's perception of pain can be changed?

_____

_____

_____

**4.** What is conscious sedation? What are the advantages of conscious sedation? What agents may be used to achieve conscious sedation?

_____

_____

_____

**5.** Discuss the administration of epidural anesthesia.

_____

_____

_____

---

# SECTION II: APPLYING YOUR KNOWLEDGE

**Activity E** CASE STUDY

Owen Nelson, 6 months old, is admitted to your unit post club foot repair. His parents are at the bedside and concerned about Owen's comfort. They state "We have heard that infants do not feel pain like adults do but we want to make sure Owen is not in pain. How do we do this?"

**1.** How would you address Owen's parents concerns?

_____

_____

_____

**2.** During your assessment you find that Owen is lying in his crib with his legs elevated, his face is relaxed, he appears restless but moves easily, cries occasionally but is consoled by his mother's or father's touch and voice. Using the appropriate pain assessment tool for Owen's age and development, assess Owen's pain level based on the above information. What further assessment information may be helpful in determining if Owen is in pain?

_____

_____

_____

3. Based on your above assessment, you intervene by providing pain medication to Owen per the physician's order to. What nonpharmacological interventions can you discuss with the parents to help decrease Owen's discomfort?

_____

_____

_____

# SECTION III: PRACTICING FOR NCLEX

**Activity F** **NCLEX-STYLE QUESTIONS**

*Answer the following questions.*

1. The nurse is providing postsurgical care for a 5-year-old. The nurse knows to avoid which of the following questions when assessing the child's pain level?
   a. Would you say that the pain you are feeling is sharp or dull?
   b. Would you point to the cartoon face that best describes your pain?
   c. Would you point to the spot where your pain is?
   d. Would you please show me with photograph and number best describes your hurt?

2. The nurse is assisting with the administration of parenteral opioids for a child for an initial dose. What action should the nurse take first?
   a. Ensure naloxone is readily available
   b. Assess for any adverse reaction
   c. Assess the status of bowel sounds
   d. Premedicate with acetaminophen

3. The nurse is caring for a child who has received postoperative epidural analgesia. What is the priority nursing assessment?
   a. Urinary retention
   b. Pruritus
   c. Nausea and vomiting
   d. Respiratory depression

4. A nurse is applying EMLA as ordered. The nurse understands that EMLA is contraindicated in which of the following situations?
   a. Infants less than 6 weeks of age
   b. Children with darker skin
   c. Infants less than 12 months receiving methemoglobin-inducing agents
   d. Children undergoing venous cannulation or intramuscular injections

5. A nurse is caring for a 4-year-old child who is exhibiting extreme anxiety and behavior upset prior to receiving stitches for a deep chin laceration. Which of the following is the priority nursing intervention?
   a. Ensuring that emergency equipment is readily available
   b. Serving as an advocate for the family to ensure appropriate pharmacologic agents are chosen
   c. Conducting an initial assessment of pain to serve as a baseline from which options for relief can be chosen
   d. Ensuring the lighting is adequate for the procedure but not so bright to cause discomfort

6. A nurse is interviewing the mother of a sleeping 10-year-old girl in order to assess the level of the child's postoperative pain. Which of the following comments would trigger additional questions and necessitate further teaching?
   a. "She is asleep, so she must not be in pain."
   b. "She has never had surgery before."
   c. "She is very articulate and will tell you how she feels."
   d. "She has a very easy going temperament."

7. The nurse is providing teaching the parents of a 9-year-old boy with episodes of chronic pain how to help him manage his pain nonpharmacologically. Which of the following statements indicates a need for further teaching?
   a. "We should perform the techniques along with him."
   b. "We should start the method as soon as he feels pain."
   c. "We need to identify the ways in which he shows pain."
   d. "We should select a method that he likes the best."

8. A nurse is assessing the pain level of an infant. Which of the following findings is not a typical physiologic indicator of pain?

   a. Decreased oxygen saturation

   b. Decreased heart rate

   c. Palmar sweating

   d. Plantar sweating

9. The nurse is preparing to assess the postsurgical pain level of a 6-year-old. The child has appeared unwilling or unable to accurately report his pain level. Which of the following assessment tools would be most appropriate for this child?

   a. FACES Pain Rating Scale

   b. FLACC Behavioral scale

   c. Oucher Pain rating

   d. Visual Analog and Numerical scales

10. The nurse is preparing to assess the pain of a developmentally and cognitively delayed 8-year-old. Which of the pain rating scales should the nurse choose?

   a. FACES pain rating scale

   b. Word Graphic Rating Scale

   c. Adolescent Pediatric Pain Tool

   d. Visual Analog and Numerical Scales

11. The nurse is caring for a patient who is 30 weeks gestation. The patient is preparing to undergo an invasive procedure on her unborn baby. The patient discusses the likelihood that her fetus will experience pain. Which of the following statements indicates an understanding of the influences of stimuli on the unborn fetus?

   a. "Unborn babies do not feel painful sensations."

   b. "Since my child is a boy the amount of pain that he can experience is lessened."

   c. "Painful stimuli can be felt by the fetus only in the hours prior to delivery."

   d. "The physiological maturity needed for the fetus to sense pain is present by about 23 weeks gestation."

12. A pregnant teen voices concerns related to potential paralysis about the plans for an epidural anesthetic to be administered. What information can be provided to the teen?

   a. "Paralysis is not a serious concern for the procedure."

   b. "The spinal cord will not be damaged by the insertion of the epidural catheter."

   c. "The spinal cord ends above the area where the epidural is inserted."

   d. "The risk of paralysis is limited because your physician is skilled in the administration of epidurals."

13. The nurse is assigned to care for a 14-year-old child who is hospitalized in traction for serious leg fractures after an automobile accident. The parents ask the nurse to avoid administering analgesics to their child to help prevent him from becoming addicted. What response by the nurse is indicated?

   a. "We can talk with the physician to see about reducing the amount of medications given to reduce the potential for addiction."

   b. "If there is no history of drug abuse in the family there should be no increased risk for the development of addiction."

   c. "Administering medications to manage complaints of pain is not going to cause addition."

   d. "Your child is too young to experience drug addiction."

14. The nurse is caring for a 5-year-old child who underwent a painful surgical procedure earlier in the day. The nurse notes the child has not reported pain to any of the nursing staff. What action by the nurse is indicated?

   a. Contact the physician to report the child's condition.

   b. Administer prophylactic analgesics.

   c. Observe for behavioral cues consistent with pain.

   d. Encourage the child to report pain.

15. The nurse is preparing to administer a dose of Toradol (ketorolac) to a 15-year-old child. The nurse should do which of the following to reduce the potential for gastrointestinal upset?

   a. Administer the medication before meals.

   b. Administer the medication with milk

   c. Administer the medication with meals

   d. Administer the medication with a citrus beverage

# CHAPTER 15

# Nursing Care of the Child with an Infectious or Communicable Disorder

## Learning Objectives

- Discuss anatomic and physiologic differences in children versus adults in relation to the infectious process.
- Identify nursing interventions related to common laboratory and diagnostic tests used in the diagnosis and management of infectious conditions.
- Identify appropriate nursing assessments and interventions related to medications and treatments for childhood infectious and communicable disorders.
- Distinguish various infectious illnesses occurring in childhood.
- Devise an individualized nursing care plan for the child with an infectious or communicable disorder.
- Develop child/family teaching plans for the child with an infectious or communicable disorder.

## SECTION I: ASSESSING YOUR UNDERSTANDING

### Activity A FILL IN THE BLANKS

1. The trigger of prostaglandins to increase the body's temperature set point is caused by _pyrogens_.

2. Monocytes use _phagocytosis_ as a means to eliminate pathogens.

3. B cells use _antibodies_ to attack specific foreign substances.

4. Fever can increase the production of _neutrophils_ and slow the growth of bacteria and viruses.

5. Acetaminophen and _ibuprofen_, administered at the appropriate dose and interval, are safe and effective for reducing fever in children.

## Activity B MATCHING

*Match the infection chain link in Column A with the proper word or phrase in Column B.*

**Column A**

_b_ **1.** Infectious agent
_e_ **2.** Mode of transmission
_f_ **3.** Portal of entry
_c_ **4.** Portal of exit
_d_ **5.** Reservoir
_a_ **6.** Susceptible host

**Column B**

a. Child
b. Rickettsiae
c. Gastrointestinal tract
d. Animal
e. Fomite
f. Respiratory tract

*Match the vector-borne illness in Column A with Column B.*

**Column A**

_b_ **1.** Endemic typhus
_c_ **2.** Pediculosis pubis
_a_ **3.** Rickettsialpox
_e_ **4.** Roundworm
_d_ **5.** Scabies

**Column B**

a. Mouse mite bite
b. Rat flea feces
c. Sexual contact
d. Close, prolonged contact
e. Ingested fecal matter

## Activity C SEQUENCING

*Place the following stages of an infectious disease in the proper order:*

**1.** Convalescence
**2.** Illness
**3.** Incubation
**4.** Prodromal

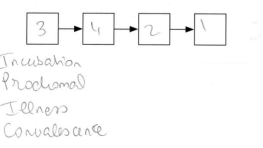

3 → 4 → 2 → 1

Incubation
Prodromal
Illness
Convalescence

## Activity D SHORT ANSWERS

*Briefly answer the following.*

**1.** Name five risk factors for sepsis that are related to pregnancy and labor.

Strep B / STD / invasive procedures / PROM

**2.** Describe the nursing management of mumps.

Respiratory isolation / support knobles / no contagious after 9 days / if orchitis present

**3.** Explain postexposure prophylaxis after an animal bite.

passive and active prophylaxis

**4.** Explain the role of fever in the child with an infection.

↑ neutrophile production + ↑ T cell multi

**5.** Explain sepsis. What is septic shock?

hypotension / low blood flow / multi system

{Endemic Typhus → Rat flea feces
{Pediculosis pubis → Sexual contact
{Rickettsialpox → Mouse mite bite
{Round worm → Ingested fecal matter

# SECTION II: APPLYING YOUR KNOWLEDGE

**Activity E** CASE STUDY

Jennifer Mikelson, a 16-year-old female, is seen in your clinic. She presents with complaints of abnormal vaginal discharge and pain with urination. Jennifer is visibly upset and not very willing to answer questions at this time. She states "can't you just give me some medicine to take."

1. How would you proceed with your assessment?

_____

_____

_____

2. Jennifer is diagnosed with Chlamydia. What home care instructions and education should you provide?

_____

_____

_____

3. By the end of the assessment Jennifer is opening up. She states she recently began having sexual relations with her boyfriend. He does not like condoms so the majority of the sexual interactions have been unprotected. How would you respond?

_____

_____

_____

# SECTION III: PRACTICING FOR NCLEX

**Activity F** NCLEX-STYLE QUESTIONS

*Answer the following questions.*

1. A 10-year-old girl with long hair is brought to the emergency room because she began acting irritable, complained of headache, and is very sleepy. What question would be most appropriate to ask the parents?
   a. "Has she done this before?"
   b. "How long has she been acting like this?"
   c. "What were you doing prior to her beginning to feel sick?"
   d. "What medications is she currently taking?"

2. A 6-year-old boy is suspected of having late-stage Lyme disease. Which of the following assessments would produce findings supporting this concern?
   a. Inspection for erythema migrans
   b. Asking the child if his knees hurt
   c. Observation of facial palsy
   d. Examination for conjunctivitis

3. The nurse is preparing to administer acetaminophen to a 4-year-old girl to provide comfort to the child. Which of the following precautions is very specific with antipyretics?
   a. Check for medicine allergies
   b. Take entire course of medication
   c. Ensure proper dose and interval
   d. Warn of possible drowsiness

4. A 10-year-old boy has an unknown infection and will need a urine for culture and sensitivity. To assure that the sensitivity results is accurate, which of the of the following steps is most important?
   a. Ensure that the specimen is obtained from proper area
   b. May need to collect three specimens on three different days
   c. Use aseptic technique when getting the specimen
   d. Obtain specimen before antibiotics are given

5. The nurse at an outpatient facility is obtaining a blood specimen from a 9-year-old girl. Which of the following techniques would most likely be used?
   a. Puncturing a vein on the dorsal side of the hand
   b. Administration of sucrose prior to beginning
   c. Accessing an indwelling venous access device
   d. Using an automatic lancet device on the heel

6. Which child needs to be seen immediately in the physician's office?

   a. A 10-month-old with a fever and petechiae who is grunting

   b. A 2-month-old with a slight fever and irritability after getting immunizations the previous day

   c. A 4-month-old with a cough, elevated temperature and wetting eight diapers every 24 hours

   d. An 8-month-old who is restless, irritable, and afebrile

7. The nurse is administering a chicken pox vaccination to a 12-month-old girl. Which of the following is a unique concern with Varicella?

   a. This disease can reactivate years later causing shingles

   b. Vitamin A is indicated for children younger than 2 years

   c. Dehydration is caused by mouth lesions

   d. Avoid exposure to pregnant women

8. The pediatric nurse knows that there are a number of anatomic and physiologic differences between children and adults. Which of the following statements about the immune systems of infants and young children is true?

   a. Children have an immature immune response

   b. Cellular immunity is not functional in children

   c. Children have an increased inflammatory response

   d. Passive immunity overlaps immunizations

9. The nurse is taking a health history for an 8-year-old boy who is hospitalized. Which of the following is a risk factor for sepsis in a hospitalized child?

   a. A maternal infection or fever

   b. Use of immunosuppression drugs

   c. Lack of juvenile immunizations

   d. Resuscitation or invasive procedures

10. The nurse is caring for a 5-year-old girl with scarlet fever. Which of the following interventions will most likely be part of her care?

    a. Exercising both standard and droplet precautions

    b. Palpating for and noting enlarged lymph nodes

    c. Monitoring for changes in respiratory status

    d. Teaching proper administration of Penicillin V

11. The nurse is caring for a 10-year-old child with a skin rash. The nurse should include which of the following interventions to manage the associated pruritis?

    a. Encourage warm baths

    b. Apply hot compresses

    c. Press the pruritic area

    d. Rub powder on the pruritic area

12. The student nurse is discussing the plan of care for a child admitted to the hospital for treatment of an infection. Which of the following actions should be taken first?

    a. Obtain blood cultures

    b. Initiate antibiotic therapy

    c. Obtain urine specimen for analysis

    d. Initiate intravenous therapy

13. The nurse is reviewing the assessment data from a 4-year-old admitted to the hospital for management of early onset sepsis. Which of the following findings are supportive of the diagnosis?

    a. The child complains about having to stay in bed

    b. The child's tympanic temperature is 98.8 F

    c. The child is hypotensive *late sign*

    d. The child is irritable

14. The nurse is preparing to perform a finger stick on a child. Which of the following actions indicates the need for further instruction?

    a. The nurse cleans the finger with an alcohol-based solution prior to the finger stick.

    b. The nurse presses the collection tube against the skin of the finger during specimen collection.

    c. The nurse uses the outer side of the finger for performing the stick.

    d. The nurse wears gloves during the collection of the specimen.

15. The nurse is providing education to the parents of a 5-year with a fever. Which of the following statements indicates the need for further instruction? Select all that apply.

a. "Fever has many therapeutic properties."

b. "I can administer two baby aspirin tablets to my child every 4 to 6 hours for the fever."

c. "Sponging my child with cold water can be a soothing way to manage the fever."

d. "I should use a cooling fan in my child's room to keep the fever down."

e. "Ibuprofen has been shown to be more beneficial than Tylenol when managing a fever."

# CHAPTER 16

# Nursing Care of the Child with a Neurologic Disorder

## Learning Objectives

- Compare how the anatomy and physiology of the neurologic system in children differs from adults.
- Identify various factors associated with neurologic disease in infants and children.
- Discuss common laboratory and other diagnostic tests useful in the diagnosis of neurologic conditions.
- Discuss common medications and other treatments used for treatment and palliation of neurologic conditions.
- Recognize risk factors associated with various neurologic disorders.
- Distinguish among different neurologic illnesses based on the signs and symptoms associated with them.
- Discuss nursing interventions commonly used for neurologic illnesses.
- Devise an individualized nursing care plan for the child with a neurologic disorder.
- Develop child and family teaching plans for the child with a neurologic disorder.
- Describe the psychosocial impact of chronic neurologic disorders on children.

## SECTION I: ASSESSING YOUR UNDERSTANDING

### Activity A FILL IN THE BLANKS

1. The _Kernig's_ sign is an indication of meningitis.

2. Lack of response to _painful_ stimuli can indicate a life-threatening condition.

3. Variation in head _circumference_ percentiles over time may indicate abnormal brain or skull growth.

4. Changes in _gait_, muscle tone, or strength may indicate certain neurologic problems.

5. The _Doll's eye_ maneuver can be helpful in assessing cranial nerves III, IV, and VI in an infant, uncooperative child, or comatose child.

6. When assessing sensory function in an infant, limit the examination to _touch_ or pain.

7. _Intracranial_ pressure is inversely related to level of consciousness.

8. During auscultation, a loud or localized _bruit_ indicates the need for immediate further investigation.

## Activity B  LABELING

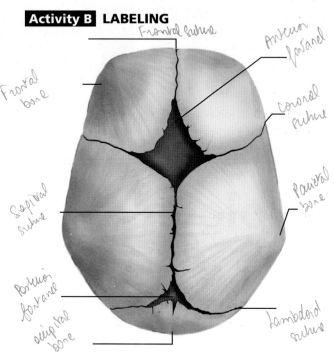

*Handwritten labels:*
- Frontal suture
- Anterior fontanel
- Coronal suture
- Frontal bone
- Sagittal suture
- Parietal bone
- Posterior fontanel
- Occipital bone
- Lambdoid suture

*Label the skull structures in the infant.*

Parietal bone
Occipital bone
Sagittal suture
Lambdoid suture
Frontal bone
Anterior fontanel
Coronal suture
Frontal suture
Posterior fontanel

## Activity C  MATCHING

*Match the term in Column A with the proper definition in Column B.*

**Column A**

___d___ 1. Febrile seizures
___e___ 2. Reye's syndrome
___c___ 3. Craniosynostosis
___a___ 4. Aseptic meningitis
___b___ 5. Positional plagiocephaly

**Column B**

a. Treat aggressively with intravenous antibiotics initially
b. Position the infant so that the flatten area is up
c. Surgical correction to allow brain growth
d. Rectal diazepam
e. Maintain cerebral perfusion, manage ICP, manage hydration, and safety measures

## Activity D  SEQUENCING

*Place the following levels of consciousness in the proper order from lowest to highest using the boxes provided below:*

1. Coma
2. Confusion
3. Full consciousness
4. Obtunded
5. Stupor

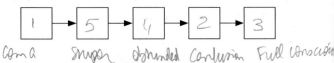

| 1 | → | 5 | → | 4 | → | 2 | → | 3 |

*Coma     Stupor     Obtunded     Confusion     Full conscious*

## Activity E  SHORT ANSWERS

*Briefly answer the following.*

1. Describe how to test for Kernig's sign, what indicates a positive sign, and what disorder is indicated.

   *Irritation meninges / meningitis*
   *flexing hip / knee then extending knee*

2. Describe the opisthotonic position, what age a child would assume this position, and what neurologic disorder is implicated.

   *hyperextended position of infant to*
   *relieve discomfort due to β meningitis*

3. What are the proper positions for a lumbar puncture for an infant and child?

   *upright c head / lened*

4. What is the purpose of a ventriculoperitoneal (VP) shunt, what causes it to malfunction, and what are the symptoms the malfunction produces?

   *relieve CSF in hydrocephalus and*
   *maint an proper intracranial pressure*

5. In regards to the Glasgow Coma Scale, what are the three major areas of assessment, and what does a low score indicate?

   *Level of consciousness less*

   *eye opening / verbal response / motor response*

# SECTION II: APPLYING YOUR KNOWLEDGE

## Activity F  CASE STUDY

Jessica Clark, 5 years old, is admitted to the neurologic unit at a pediatric hospital after having a seizure at school. Her mother reports that Jessica has a history of seizures and is taking phenobarbital to control them. The mother states, "Ever since Jessica started school this year, it has been more difficult to get her to take her medicine."

1. What diagnostic and laboratory tests can you anticipate?

2. Minutes after leaving the room, the mother calls you back because Jessica is having another seizure. Identify nursing interventions related to the care of this child during and immediately following a seizure. List in order of priority.

3. What teaching will the nurse do with this child's family? Include a discussion on ways to increase compliance with the seizure medication.

# SECTION III: PRACTICING FOR NCLEX

## Activity G  NCLEX-STYLE QUESTIONS

*Answer the following questions.*

1. The nurse is providing education to the parents of a 3-year-old girl with hydrocephalus who has just had an external ventricular drainage system placed. Which of the following questions would best begin the teaching session?
   a. "What questions or concerns do you have about this device?"
   b. "Do you understand why you clamp the drain before she sits up?"
   c. "What do you know about her autoregulation mechanism failing?"
   d. "Why do you always keep her head raised 30 degrees?"

2. During physical assessment of a 2-month-old infant, the nurse suspects the child may have a lesion on the brain stem. Which of the following signs or symptoms was observed?
   a. Only one eye is dilated and reactive
   b. A sudden increase in head circumference *Hydrocephalus*
   c. Horizontal nystagmus *Brain stem*
   d. The posterior fontanel is closed

3. After a difficult birth, the nurse observes that a newborn has swelling on part of his head. Which of the following signs suggests cephalohematoma?
   a. Swelling does not cross the midline or suture lines
   b. The swelling crosses the midline of the infant's scalp
   c. The infant had a low birth weight when born at 37 weeks
   d. The infant has facial abnormalities

4. The nurse is caring for an 8-year-old girl who was in a car accident. Which of the following symptoms would suggest the child has a cerebral contusion?

   a. She has trouble focusing when reading
   b. She has difficulty concentrating
   c. She has had some vomiting *subdural hematoma*
   d. She is bleeding from the ear *basilar skull Fx*

5. The nurse caring for an infant with craniosynostosis, specifically positional plagiocephaly, would prioritize which of the following activities? *position flatten area up*

   a. Moving the infant's head every 2 hours
   b. Measuring the intake and output every shift
   c. Massaging the scalp gently very 4 hours
   d. Giving the infant small feedings whenever he is fussy

6. Premature infants have more fragile capillaries in the periventricular area than term infants. Which of the following problems does this put them at risk for?

   a. Moderate closed-head injury
   b. Early closure of the fontanels
   c. Congenital hydrocephalus
   d. Intracranial hemorrhaging

7. The nurse is caring for a near-term pregnant woman who has not taken prenatal vitamins or folic acid supplements. Which of the following congenital defects is most likely to occur based on the mother's prenatal history?

   a. Neonatal conjunctivitis
   b. Facial deformities
   c. A neural tube defect
   d. Incomplete myelinization

8. The nurse is caring for a 3-year-old boy who is experiencing seizure activity. Which of the following diagnostic tests will determine the seizure area in the brain?

   a. Cerebral angiography
   b. Lumbar puncture
   c. Video electroencephalogram
   d. Computed tomography

9. A pregnant patient asks if there is any danger to the development of her fetus in the first few weeks of her pregnancy. The nurse would be correct in responding:

   a. "As long as you were taking good care of your health before becoming pregnant, your fetus should be fine during the first few weeks of pregnancy."
   b. "Bones begin to harden in the first 5 to 6 weeks of pregnancy so vitamin D consumption is particularly important."
   c. "During the first 3 to 4 weeks of pregnancy brain and spinal cord development occur and are affected by nutrition, drugs, infection, or trauma."
   d. "The respiratory system matures during this time so good prenatal care during the first weeks of pregnancy is very important."

10. The nurse has developed a nursing plan for the care of a 6-year-old girl with congenital hydrocephalus whose shunt has become infected. The most important discharge teaching point for this family is:

    a. Maintaining effective cerebral perfusion
    b. Educating the parents how to properly give antibiotics
    c. Establishing seizure precautions for the child
    d. Encouraging development of motor skills

11. The young child has been diagnosed with bacterial meningitis. Which of the following nursing interventions are appropriate?

    a. Initiate droplet isolation
    b. Identify close contacts of the child who will require postexposure prophylactic medication
    c. Administer antibiotics as ordered
    d. Monitor the child for signs and symptoms associated with decreased intracranial pressure
    e. Initiate seizure precautions

12. The meningococcal vaccine should be offered to high-risk populations. Which of the following people who have never been vaccinated have an increased risk of becoming infected with meningococcal meningitis?

   a. An 18-year-old student who is preparing for college in the fall and has signed up to live in a dormitory with two other suite mates

   b. A child who is 12 years old

   c. A 5-year-old child who routinely travels in the summer with her parents on mission trips to Haiti

   d. A child who was diagnosed with diabetes mellitus when he was 7 years old

   e. A child who is 8 years old

13. An 11-year-old child was recently diagnosed with chickenpox. His parents gave him aspirin for a fever and the child is now hospitalized. Which of the following nursing interventions are commonly associated with the management of Reye's syndrome?

   a. Request order for an antiemetic

   b. Assess intake and output every shift

   c. Assess child's skin for the development of distinctive rash every 4 hours

   d. Request order for anticonvulsant

   e. Monitor the child's laboratory values related to pancreatic function

14. The young child was involved in a motor vehicle accident and was admitted to the pediatric intensive care unit with changes in level of consciousness and a high-pitched cry. Which of the following are late signs of increased intracranial pressure?

   a. The child states that he feels a little "dizzy."

   b. The child's toes are pointed downward, his head and neck are arched backwards, and his arms and legs are extended. *decerebrate*

   c. The sclera of the eyes is visible above the iris.

   d. The child's heart rate is 56 beats per minute. *Bradycardia*

   e. The child's pupils are fixed and dilated.

*ICP*

*Early sign*
- dizzy
- sclera eye visible above the iris

*Late sign*
- bradycardia
- pupils fixed dilated
- decerebrate posturing

# Nursing Care of the Child with a Disorder of the Eyes or Ears

- Differentiate between the anatomic and physiologic differences of the eyes and ears in children as compared with adults.
- Identify various factors associated with disorders of the eyes and ears in infants and children.
- Discuss common laboratory and other diagnostic tests useful in the diagnosis of disorders of the eyes and ears.
- Discuss common medications and other treatments used for treatment and palliation of conditions affecting the eyes and ears.
- Recognize risk factors associated with various disorders of the eyes and ears.
- Distinguish between different disorders of the eyes and ears based on the signs and symptoms associated with them.
- Discuss nursing interventions commonly used in regard to disorders of the eyes and ears.
- Devise an individualized nursing care plan for the child with a sensory impairment or other disorder of the eyes or ears.
- Develop patient/family teaching plans for the child with a disorder of the eyes or ears.
- Describe the psychosocial impact of sensory impairments on children.

## SECTION I: ASSESSING YOUR UNDERSTANDING

**Activity A** FILL IN THE BLANKS

1. According to *Healthy People 2020* recommendations, visual acuity testing should begin at _____ 3 _____ years of age.

2. Short length and _horizontal_ position of eustachian tubes leads to greater susceptibility of acute otitis media in children less than 2 years of age.

3. Systemic _Antibiotics_ are used to treat periorbital cellulitis.

4. Permanent visual _Deterioration_ can be averted with early identification and treatment of amblyopia.

5. Vision or hearing impairment impedes _Developmental_ progress.

6. The spherical shape of the newborn's lens does not allow for _Distance_ accommodation.

## Activity B MATCHING

*Match the term in Column A with the proper definition in Column B.*

**Column A**

b **1.** Contusion

d **2.** Corneal abrasion

a **3.** Eyelid injury

e **4.** Foreign body

c **5.** Scleral hemorrhage

**Column B**

**a.** Vision is usually unaffected

**b.** Discoloration and edema of eyelid

**c.** Erythema that resolves gradually without intervention

**d.** May require ointment to sooth injury or antibiotic ointment

**e.** Requires careful removal only by a health care professional

## Activity C SEQUENCING

*Place the following vision and hearing milestones in the proper order:*

**1.** Binocular vision

**2.** Eye color

**3.** Functional hearing

**4.** Visual acuity of 20/20

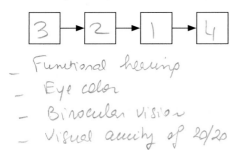

3 → 2 → 1 → 4

- Functional hearing
- Eye color
- Binocular vision
- Visual acuity of 20/20

## Activity D SHORT ANSWERS

*Briefly answer the following.*

**1.** List at least five signs and symptoms of children with hearing loss at (a) infant, (b) young child, and (c) older child stages.

_____

_____

_____

**2.** Describe how to interact with a visually impaired child, especially the use of one's voice and ways to act as the child's eyes.

_____

_____

_____

**3.** List at least three signs and symptoms that would lead the nurse to suspect a child is visually impaired at (a) infant, (b) young child, or (c) older child stages.

_____

_____

_____

**4.** List at least five factors that increase the risk of a child developing acute otitis media.

_____

_____

_____

**5.** Discuss the characteristics that increase the risk of a child having difficulty with the development of speech or language, or having learning difficulties.

_____

_____

_____

# SECTION II: APPLYING YOUR KNOWLEDGE

## Activity E  CASE STUDY

Brandon, age 6 months, has been brought to the pediatrician's office for a well-baby checkup. Brandon's mother tells the nurse that she is concerned about Brandon's left eye. She tells the nurse that Brandon's eyes do not seem to be looking in the same place. Upon assessment the nurse finds asymmetry of the corneal light reflex. Brandon is referred for further assessment to an ophthalmologist.

1. Brandon is diagnosed with amblyopia. What information would the nurse know to include in a teaching plan for Brandon's family at this first visit?

   _____

   _____

   _____

2. Why is it important to treat amblyopia as soon as it is found and what treatments might be used in the treatment of Brandon's condition?

   _____

   _____

   _____

# SECTION III: PRACTICING FOR NCLEX

## Activity F  NCLEX-STYLE QUESTIONS

*Answer the following questions.*

1. The nurse is caring for a 2-year-old girl with persistent otitis media with effusion. Which of the following interventions is most important to the developmental health of the child?

   **a.** Informing the parents to avoid nonprescription drugs

   **b.** Telling parents not to smoke in the house

   **c.** Educating the parents about proper antibiotic use

   **d.** Reassessing for language acquisition

2. The nurse is explaining information to the parents of a 3-year-old boy who may have strabismus. Which of the following examinations would the nurse expect to assist with first in order to find out if he has strabismus?

   **a.** Refractive examination

   **b.** Visual acuity test

   **c.** Corneal light reflex test

   **d.** Ophthalmologic examination

3. The nurse is caring for a 10-year-old girl with acute periorbital cellulitis. Which of the following will be the primary nursing intervention (therapy) for this disorder?

   **a.** Application of heated aqua pad to site

   **b.** Administering Rocephin IV as ordered

   **c.** Administering Morphine Sulfate as ordered

   **d.** Monitoring for increased intracranial pressure

4. The nurse is caring for a 24-month-old boy with regressed retinopathy of prematurity. Which of the following interventions would be priority for this child?

   **a.** Assessing the child for asymmetric corneal light reflex

   **b.** Observing for rubbing or shutting the eyes or squinting

   **c.** Referring the child to the local district of Early Intervention

   **d.** Teaching the parents to check how the child's glasses fit

5. The nurse is caring for an 8-year-old boy with otitis media with effusion. Which of the following situations may have caused this disorder?

   **a.** He frequently goes swimming

   **b.** He has good attendance at school

   **c.** He is experiencing recurrent nasal congestion

   **d.** He had recent bacterial conjunctivitis

6. The nurse is caring for a 7-year-old girl in an outpatient clinic diagnosed with amblyopia that is unrelated to any other disorder. Which of the following interventions would be most helpful at this time?

   a. Discouraging the child from roughhousing

   b. Explaining postsurgical treatment of the eye

   c. Ensuring follow-up visits with the ophthalmologist

   d. Educating parents on how to use prescribed atropine drops

7. The nurse is teaching the parents of a 4-year-old boy with strabismus. Teaching for the parents would include:

   a. The need for ultraviolet-protective glasses postoperatively

   b. The importance of completing the full course of oral antibiotics

   c. The possibility that multiple operations may be necessary

   d. That it is critical to comply with patching as prescribed

8. The nurse is educating the parents of a 5-year-old girl with infectious conjunctivitis about the disorder. Which of the following is most important to prevent the spread of the disorder?

   a. Properly applying the prescribed antibiotic

   b. Staying home from school

   c. Washing hands frequently

   d. Keeping hands away from eyes

9. A 10-year-old boy has just been treated for otitis externa and now the nurse is teaching the boy and his parents about prevention. Which of the following recommendations would be included as part of the education?

   a. Using alcohol and vinegar for soreness

   b. Using cotton swabs to keep the inner ear dry

   c. Using a hair dryer on cool to dry the ears

   d. Washing his hair only when necessary

10. The nurse is teaching parents of a 9-year-old girl about the importance of her wearing her prescribed glasses. Which of the following subjects is least important to promoting compliance?

   a. Getting scheduled eye examinations on time

   b. Checking condition and fit of glasses monthly

   c. Watching for signs that prescription needs changing

   d. Encouraging the use of eye protection for sports

11. The pediatric office nurse notes that several of the young children that are waiting to see the physician may have conjunctivitis. Which of the following findings are consistent with bacterial conjunctivitis?

   a. Only the right eye is involved.

   b. The drainage is yellow and thick.

   c. The drainage is white.

   d. There is clear, watery drainage from both eyes.

   e. The child suffers from seasonal allergies.

12. A child has been diagnosed with bacterial conjunctivitis. Which of the following statements by the child's parent indicate the need for further education?

   a. "I'll continue to use Visine to help with the redness."

   b. "All of us at home need to wash our hands really well."

   c. "We should not use a towel that he has used."

   d. "He can go back to school in 4 hours after that thick yellow drainage is gone."

   e. "This is really contagious."

   24 to 48h

13. The young child has been diagnosed with a corneal abrasion. Which of the following findings are most consistent with this diagnosis?

    a. The child's pupils are equal, round, reactive to light and accommodation.

    b. The child denies any eye pain.

    c. The child complains that it hurts to look towards bright light.

    d. The child has a large purple bruise over the eye and edema on the eyelid.

    e. The child's eye is draining clear fluid and the child says it feels like it is full of tears.

14. The nurse works in a pediatrician office. Which of the following children who have been diagnosed with acute otitis media does the nurse expect the physician to treat with antibiotics?

    a. The 12-year-old child is complaining that he has some mild ear pain with a temperature of 101.4 F.

    b. The 8-year-old child who is crying due to ear pain and has a temperature of 103 F.

    c. The 2-month-old child who is having difficulty sleeping and has a fever of 102.6 F.

    d. The 5-month-old child who is fussy and pulling at her ears.

    e. The 22-month-old who is irritable with the presence of purulent drainage from her right ear.

# Nursing Care of the Child with a Respiratory Disorder

## Learning Objectives

- Distinguish between the anatomy and physiology of the respiratory system in children versus adults.
- Identify various factors associated with respiratory illness in infants and children.
- Discuss common laboratory and other diagnostic tests useful in the diagnosis of respiratory conditions.
- Describe nursing care related to common medications and other treatments used for management and palliation of respiratory conditions.
- Recognize risk factors associated with various respiratory disorders.
- Distinguish different respiratory disorders based on their signs and symptoms.
- Discuss nursing interventions commonly used for respiratory illnesses.
- Devise an individualized nursing care plan for the child with a respiratory disorder.
- Develop child/family teaching plans for the child with a respiratory disorder.
- Describe the psychosocial impact of chronic respiratory disorders on children.

## SECTION I: ASSESSING YOUR UNDERSTANDING

### Activity A FILL IN THE BLANKS

1. A _____ is a surgical construction of a respiratory opening in the trachea.

2. Allergic rhinitis is associated with _____ dermatitis and asthma.

3. Cough and _____ are symptoms of influenza for both children and adults.

4. Pulse oximetry is an _____ measurement of oxygen saturation in arterial blood.

5. Auscultation of the lungs might reveal _____ or rales in the younger child with pneumonia.

6. Tuberculin skin testing is also known as a _____ test.

7. Pseudoephedrine is an example of a _____ used for the treatment of runny or stuffy nose associated with the common cold.

## Activity B  LABELING

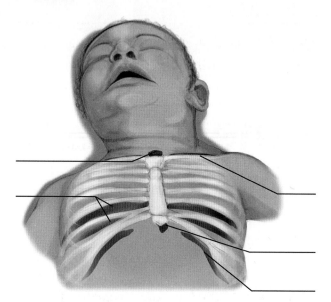

Label the image using the following terms:

Intercostal
Substernal
Supraclavicular
Subcostal
Suprasternal

## Activity C  MATCHING

*Match the term in Column A with the proper definition in Column B.*

**Column A**

_____ 1. Nasal cannula

_____ 2. Non-rebreather mask

_____ 3. Partial rebreather mask

_____ 4. Simple face mask

_____ 5. Venturi mask

**Column B**

a. Minimum flow rate of 6 L/min

b. Oxygen reservoir bag

c. Mixes room air and oxygen

d. Must have patent nasal passages

e. One-way valve

## Activity D  SEQUENCING

*Place the following steps for using a bulb syringe in the proper order:*

1. Clean the bulb syringe

2. Compress the bulb

3. Empty the bulb

4. Instill saline nose drops

5. Place the bulb in the nose

6. Release pressure on bulb

7. Remove the bulb from nose

8. Tilt the infant's head back

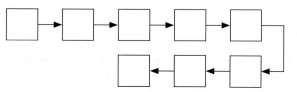

## Activity E  SHORT ANSWERS

*Briefly answer the following.*

1. Discuss common signs and symptoms that are seen with sinusitis.

_____

_____

_____

2. Discuss common laboratory and diagnostic tests that the nurse anticipates to be ordered for a child suspected of having cystic fibrosis and identify findings that indicate cystic fibrosis.

_____

_____

_____

3. Compare the similarities and differences of croup and epiglottitis.

_____

_____

_____

4. Discuss the therapeutic management of the common cold.

_____

_____

_____

5. What is the most common cause of bronchiolitis and discuss the peak incidence of the disorder.

_____

_____

_____

# SECTION II: APPLYING YOUR KNOWLEDGE

## Activity F   CASE STUDY

James Jackson, an 8-year-old boy, is admitted to the pediatric hospital because of dyspnea, coughing, and wheezing. James states "my chest feels really tight." Physical findings include pallor, tachypnea, tachycardia, and bilateral wheezing on auscultation. This is the first time James has experienced these symptoms.

1. What health history information is important for the nurse to collect?

   _____

   _____

   _____

2. List four nursing diagnoses that would pertain to James. Prioritize and provide rationale.

   James has been diagnosed with asthma and is prescribed a bronchodilator and a metered dose inhaler while in the health care facility and for home. His breathing becomes easier and he states the tightness has gone away.

   _____

   _____

   _____

3. Since this is James' first episode of asthma, what will be important discharge teaching for him and his family?

   _____

   _____

   _____

# SECTION III: PRACTICING FOR NCLEX

## Activity G   NCLEX-STYLE QUESTIONS

*Answer the following questions.*

1. The nurse is assessing several children. Which child is most at risk for dysphagia?
   a. A 7-month-old with erythematous rash
   b. An 8-year-old with fever and fatigue
   c. A 4-year-old with pharyngitis
   d. A 2-month-old with toxic appearance

2. The nurse is caring for a 14-month-old boy with cystic fibrosis. Which of these signs of ineffective family coping requires the most urgent intervention?
   a. Compliance with therapy is diminished
   b. The family becomes over vigilant
   c. The child feels fearful and isolated
   d. Siblings are jealous and worried

3. The nurse is taking a health history for a 3-year-old girl suspected of having pneumonia who presents with a fever, chest pain, and cough. Which of the following is a risk factor for pneumonia?
   a. The child is a triplet
   b. The child was a postmaturity date infant
   c. The child has diabetes
   d. The child attends day care

4. The nurse is auscultating the lungs of a lethargic, irritable 6-year-old boy and hears wheezing. The nurse will most likely be including which teaching point if the child is suspected of having asthma.

   a. "I'm going to have the respiratory therapist get some of the mucus from your lungs."

   b. "I'm going to have this hospital worker take a picture of your lungs."

   c. "We're going to go take a look at your lungs to see if there are any sores on them."

   d. "I'm going to hold your hand while the phlebotomist gets blood from your arm."

5. The nurse is caring for a 3-year-old girl who is cyanotic and breathing rapidly. Which of the following would best relieve these symptoms?

   a. Suctioning

   b. Oxygen

   c. Saline lavage

   d. Saline gargles

6. The nurse knows that respiratory disorders in children are sometimes attributed to differences in anatomy and physiology. Which of the following is an accurate statement?

   a. Adults have twice as many alveoli as newborns

   b. The tongue is proportionately smaller in infants than in adults

   c. Infants consume twice as much oxygen as adults

   d. Hypoxemia occurs later in children than adults

7. The nurse is caring for a 5-year-old girl who shows signs and symptoms of epiglottis. The nurse recognizes a common complication of the disorder is for the child to:

   a. Complain of ear pain

   b. Experience nuchal rigidity

   c. Have unilateral breath sounds upon auscultation

   d. Be at risk for respiratory distress

8. The nurse is developing a teaching plan for the parents of a 10-year-old boy with cystic fibrosis. The plan should include teaching of:

   a. Use of a flutter valve device

   b. Use of a metered dose inhaler

   c. Proper use of a nebulizer

   d. How to work a peak flow meter

9. The nurse is caring for a neonate being treated for respiratory distress syndrome who is on a ventilator. Early assessment of the complication of mucus plugging can be determined by:

   a. Promoting adequate gas exchange

   b. Monitoring for adequate lung expansion

   c. Maintaining adequate fluid volume

   d. Preventing infection

10. The nurse is caring for a 10-year-old girl with allergic rhinitis. Which intervention helps prevent secondary bacterial infection?

    a. Using normal saline nasal washes

    b. Teaching parents how to avoid allergens

    c. Discussing anti-inflammatory nasal sprays

    d. Teaching parents about oral antihistamines

11. The young child is wearing a nasal cannula. The oxygen is set at 3 L/minute. Calculate how much oxygen the child is receiving?

12. The child has been diagnosed with asthma and the child's physician is using a stepwise approach. Rank the following in order of occurrence as the child's condition worsens.

    a. The nurse administers a medium-dose inhaled corticosteroid and salmeterol

    b. The nurse administers albuterol as needed

    c. The nurse administers a medium-dose inhaled corticosteroid

    d. The nurse administers a low-dose inhaled corticosteroid

13. The student nurse is discussing the differences between children's respiratory systems and adults'. Which of the following statements by the student nurse are accurate? Select all that apply.

    a. "Children are less likely to develop problems associated with swelling of the airways."

    b. "When compared to adults, children's tongues are proportionally smaller."

    c. "The only time that newborns can breathe through their mouths is when they cry."

    d. "A newborn's respiratory tract is drier because the newborn doesn't make very much mucus."

    e. "Children under the age of 6 years are more prone to developing sinus infections."

14. The young child has been diagnosed with group A streptococcal pharyngitis. The physician orders amoxicillin 45 mg/kg in three equally divided doses. The child weighs 23 pounds. Calculate how many milligrams the child will receive with each dose of amoxicillin (round to the nearest whole milligram).

15. The child has been admitted to the hospital with a possible diagnosis of pneumonia. Which of the following findings are consistent with this diagnosis?

    a. The child's temperature is 98.4 F

    b. The child's chest X-ray indicates the presence of perihilar infiltrates

    c. The child's white blood cell count is elevated

    d. The child's respiratory rate is rapid

    e. The child is producing yellow purulent sputum

# Nursing Care of the Child with a Cardiovascular Disorder

## Learning Objectives

- Compare anatomic and physiologic differences of the cardiovascular system in infants and children versus adults.
- Describe nursing care related to common laboratory and diagnostic tests used in the medical diagnosis of pediatric cardiovascular conditions.
- Distinguish cardiovascular disorders common in infants, children, and adolescents.
- Identify appropriate nursing assessments and interventions related to medications and treatments for pediatric cardiovascular disorders.
- Develop an individualized nursing care plan for the child with a cardiovascular disorder.
- Describe the psychosocial impact of chronic cardiovascular disorders on children.
- Devise a nutrition plan for the child with cardiovascular disease.
- Develop patient/family teaching plans for the child with a cardiovascular disorder.

## SECTION I: ASSESSING YOUR UNDERSTANDING

### Activity A   FILL IN THE BLANKS

1. Cardiac _angiography_ is the radiographic study of the heart and coronary vessels after injection of contrast medium.

2. Cardiac catheterization may be categorized as diagnostic, interventional, or _electrophysiology_.

3. Coarctation of the aorta is defined as _narrowing_ of the aorta.

4. Examples of defects with increased _pulmonary_ blood flow are patent ductus arteriosus (PDA), atrial septal defect (ASD), and ventricular septal defect (VSD).

5. Eighty percent of all cases of heart failure in children with congenital heart defects occur by the age of _6 months_.

6. Cardiac disorders that are not congenital are considered _acquired_ disorders.

7. _Rheumatic fever_ is a delayed disorder resulting from group A streptococcal pharyngeal infection.

## Activity B MATCHING

*Match the term in Column A with the proper definition in Column B.*

**Column A**

b 1. Alprostadil

a 2. Furosemide

d 3. Heparin

c 4. Ace inhibitors

e 5. Niacin

**Column B**

a. Management of edema associated with heart failure

b. Temporary maintenance of ductus arterious patency in infants with ductal-dependent congenital heart defects

c. Management of hypertension

d. Prophylaxis and treatment of thromboembolic disorders especially after cardiac surgery

e. Medication to lower blood cholesterol levels

## Activity C SEQUENCING

*Place the following changes that occur in the cardiopulmonary system immediately following birth in proper order:*

1. Drop in pulmonary artery pressure

2. Reduction of pulmonary vascular resistance to blood flow

3. Decreased pressure in the right atrium

4. Lungs inflate

5. Closure of the ductus arteriosis

6. Closure of the foramen ovale

4 → 2 → 1 → 3 → 6 → 5

→ Lungs inflate
→ Reduction of pulmonary vascular resistance to blood flow
→ Drop in pulmonary vascular resistance to blood flow
→ Decrease pressure in ® atrium
→ Closure Foramen ovale / Closure ductus arteriosis.

## Activity D SHORT ANSWERS

*Briefly answer the following.*

1. Describe the action and indications for digoxin (Lanoxin). What are the key considerations when administering digoxin?

_____

_____

_____

2. Heart murmurs must be evaluated on the basis of what characteristics?

_____

_____

_____

3. What are the three types of atrial septal defects?

_____

_____

_____

4. Discuss the incidence of ventricular septal defect (VSD) and common assessment findings.

_____

_____

_____

5. What are the risk factors for the development of infective endocarditis?

_____

_____

_____

# SECTION II: APPLYING YOUR KNOWLEDGE

## Activity E CASE STUDY

The nurse is caring for a 2-year-old girl who was admitted to the hospital to undergo a cardiac catheterization for a suspected cardiac defect.

1. Discuss preprocedure nursing care for the child and family.

_____

_____

_____

2. Discuss postprocedure nursing care following a cardiac catheterization.

_____

_____

_____

# SECTION III: PRACTICING FOR NCLEX

## Activity F NCLEX-STYLE QUESTIONS

*Answer the following questions.*

1. The nurse is caring for an 8-month-old infant with a suspected congenital heart defect. The nurse examines the child and documents the following expected finding:
   a. Steady weight gain since birth
   b. Softening of the nail beds
   c. Appropriate mastery of developmental milestones
   d. Intact rooting reflex

2. The nurse is assessing the heart rate of a healthy 6-month-old. The nurse would expect which heart rate range?
   a. 60 to 68 bpm
   b. 70 to 80 bpm
   c. 80 to 105 bpm
   d. 120 to 130 bpm

3. The nurse is conducting a physical examination of a 7-year-old girl prior to a cardiac catheterization. The nurse knows to pay particular attention to assessing the child's pedal pulses. How can the nurse best facilitate their assessment after the procedure?
   a. Mark the location of the child's peripheral pulses with an indelible marker
   b. Mark the child's pedal pulses with an indelible marker, then document
   c. Document the location and quality of the child's pedal pulses
   d. Assess the location and quality of the child's peripheral pulses

4. The nurse is assessing the past medical history of an infant with a suspected cardiovascular disorder. Which of the following responses by the mother warrants further investigation?
   a. "His Apgar score was an eight"
   b. "I was really nauseous throughout my whole pregnancy"
   c. "I am on a low dose of lithium"
   d. "I had the flu during my last trimester"

5. A nurse is assessing the skin of a 12-year-old with suspected right ventricular heart failure. Which of the following findings would the nurse expect to note?
   a. Edema of the lower extremities
   b. Edema of the face
   c. Edema in the presacral region
   d. Edema of the hands

6. A nurse is palpating the pulse of a child with suspected aortic regurgitation. Which of the following assessment findings would the nurse expect to note?
   a. Appropriate mastery of developmental milestones
   b. Bounding pulse
   c. Preference to resting on the right side
   d. Pitting periorbital edema

7. The nurse is conducting a physical examination of a baby with a suspected cardiovascular disorder. Which of the following assessment findings is suggestive of sudden ventricular distention?

   a. Decreased blood pressure

   b. A heart murmur

   c. Cool, clammy, pale extremities

   d. Accentuated third heart sound

8. The nurse performs a cardiac assessment and notes a loud heart murmur with a precordial thrill. This murmur would be classified as a:

   a. Grade I

   b. Grade II

   c. Grade III

   d. Grade IV

9. The nurse is assessing the blood pressure of an adolescent. Which blood pressure measurement would be expected for a healthy 13-year-old boy?

   a. 80/40 mm Hg

   b. 80 to 100/64 mm Hg

   c. 94 to 112/56 to 60 mm Hg

   d. 100 to 120/50 to 70 mm Hg

10. The nurse is auscultating heart sounds of a child with a mitral valve prolapse. The nurse would expect which assessment finding?

    a. A mild to late ejection click at the apex

    b. Abnormal splitting of S2 sounds

    c. Clicks on the upper left sternal border

    d. Intensifying of S2 sounds

11. The infant has been hospitalized and develops hypercyanosis. The physician has ordered the nurse to administer 0.1 mg of morphine sulfate per every kilogram of the infant's body weight. The infant weighs 15.2 pounds. Calculate the infant's morphine sulfate dose. Round your answer to the nearest tenth.

    0.7

12. The young child had a chest tube placed during cardiac surgery. Which of the following findings may indicate the development of cardiac tamponade? Select all that apply.

    a. The chest tube drainage had been averaging 15 to 25 mL out per hour and now there is no drainage from the chest tube

    b. The child's heart rate has increased from 88 beats per minute to 126 beats per minute

    c. The child's right atrial filling pressure has decreased

    d. The child is resting quietly

    e. The child's apical heart rate is strong and easily auscultated

13. The pediatric nurse has digoxin ordered for each of the five children. The nurse will withhold digoxin for which of the following children? Select all that apply.

    a. The 4-month-old child's apical heart rate is 102 beats per minute

    b. The 12-year-old's digoxin level was 0.9 ng/mL from a blood draw this morning

    c. The 16-year-old child has a heart rate of 54 beats per minute

    d. The 2-year-old child has a digoxin level of 2.4 ng/mL from a blood draw this morning

    e. The 5-year-old child has developed vomiting, diarrhea and is difficult to arouse

14. Identify which of the following findings are major criteria used to help the physician diagnose acute rheumatic fever? Select all that apply.

    a. The young child has an elevated erythrocyte sedimentation rate

    b. The young child has a temperature of 101.2 F

    c. The child has painless nodules located on his wrists

    d. The child has developed pericarditis with the presence of a new heart murmur

    e. The child has developed heart block with a prolonged PR interval

**15.** The child has returned to the nurse's unit following a cardiac catheterization. The insertion site is located at the right groin. Peripheral pulses were easily palpated in bilateral lower extremities prior to the procedure. Which of the following findings should be reported to the child's physician?

a. The right groin is soft without edema

b. The child's right foot is cool with a pulse assessed only with the use of a Doppler

c. The child has a temperature of 102.4 °F

d. The child is complaining of nausea

e. The child has a runny nose

# Nursing Care of the Child with a Gastrointestinal Disorder

## Learning Objectives

- Compare the differences in the anatomy and physiology of the gastrointestinal system between children and adults.
- Discuss common medical treatments for infants and children with gastrointestinal disorders.
- Discuss common laboratory and diagnostic tests used to identify disorders of the gastrointestinal tract.
- Discuss medication therapy used in infants and children with gastrointestinal disorders.
- Recognize risk factors associated with various gastrointestinal illnesses.
- Differentiate between acute and chronic gastrointestinal disorders.
- Distinguish common gastrointestinal illnesses of childhood.
- Discuss nursing interventions commonly used for gastrointestinal illnesses.
- Devise an individualized nursing care plan for infants/children with a gastrointestinal disorder.
- Develop teaching plans for family/patient education for children with gastrointestinal illnesses.
- Describe the psychosocial impact that chronic gastrointestinal illnesses have on children.

## SECTION I: ASSESSING YOUR UNDERSTANDING

### Activity A FILL IN THE BLANKS

1. Vomiting is a reflex with three different phases. The first phase is the prodromal period, the second phase is _Retching_, and the third phase is vomiting.

2. Biliary _atresia_ is an absence of some or all of the major biliary ducts, resulting in obstruction of bile flow.

3. Chronic diarrhea is diarrhea that lasts for more than ___2___ weeks.

4. Oral candidiasis is a _fungal_ infection of the oral mucosa.

5. Cholelithiasis is the presence of _stones_ in the gallbladder.

6. _Probiotic_ supplementation while a child is taking antibiotics for other disorders may reduce the incidence of antibiotic-related diarrhea.

7. The proximal segment of the bowel telescoping into a more distal segment of the bowel is known as _intussusception_

**Activity B** LABELING

*Identify which is the colostomy and which is the ileostomy.*

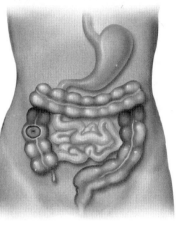 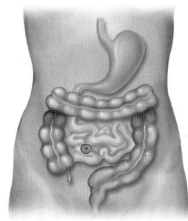

*colostomy*                    *Ileostomy*

**Activity C** MATCHING

*Match the term in Column A with the proper definition in Column B.*

**Column A**

*b* 1. Bowel prep
*C* 2. Cleansing enema
*d* 3. Icteric
*a* 4. Total parenteral nutrition (TPN)
*e* 5. Ostomy

**Column B**

a. Long-term NPO status, swallowing or absorption difficulties

b. Colonoscopy or bowel surgery

c. Severe constipation or impaction

d. Jaundiced or yellow in color

e. Imperforate anus, gastroschisis, Hirschsprung's disease

**Activity D** SEQUENCING

*Place the steps of abdominal assessment in the proper sequence.*

1. Palpation
2. Inspection
3. Percussion
4. Auscultation

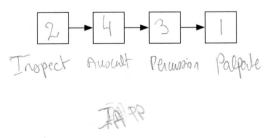

```
2 → 4 → 3 → 1
```

*Inspect  Auscult  Percussion  Palpate*

*IA PP*

**Activity E** SHORT ANSWERS

*Briefly answer the following.*

1. What does the acronym S.T.O.M.A. stand for?

   *Set up equipment*
   *Take off the pouch (obscure the stoma*
   *and mark the new pouch backing Apply new po*

2. Infants and children repeatedly put objects to their mouth for exploration. Why is this considered a risk factor for gastrointestinal illnesses?

   *mouth highly vascular Infection*

3. How is acute hepatitis typically treated?

   *Rest / hydration / nutrition*

4. What complications are of most concern during infancy for the child with a cleft palate?

   *Feeding issues*
   *gagging / choking, nasal regurgitation,*

5. Discuss the signs and symptoms that would indicate that an infant had pyloric stenosis.

   *Forceful, nonbillious vomiting*
   *non related to feeding position*
   *wt loss / Lethargy / most common*
   *after 2 to 4w*

*Dhard movable "olive like" area palpated RUQ*

# SECTION II: APPLYING YOUR KNOWLEDGE

## Activity F CASE STUDY

Nico Taylor, a 1-month-old boy who was born at 33 weeks gestation is seen in your clinic. His birth weight was 4 pounds 12 ounces and length was 18 inches. At his 2 week check-up he weighed 5 pounds 4 ounces and was 18.5 inches in length. His mother reports that he has always spit up quite a bit, but eats well. A few days ago she noted increased irritability with a hoarse cry and arching of his back with feedings. On physical exam he weighs 4 pounds 14 ounces with a length of 19 inches. His head is round with a sunken anterior fontanel, and his mucous membranes are sticky. Heart rate is 152 without a murmur, and breath sounds are clear with a respiratory rate of 42. His abdomen is soft and nondistended with positive bowel sounds in all four quadrants. Nico's skin turgor is poor.

1. Which part of your physical assessment findings is concerning to you?

   _____

   _____

   _____

2. What interventions are anticipated for Nico?

   _____

   _____

   _____

3. How would you evaluate Nico's progress?

   _____

   _____

   _____

4. Nico is diagnosed with gastroesophageal reflux. What education will you provide for the family regarding Nico's care?

   _____

   _____

   _____

# SECTION III: PRACTICING FOR NCLEX

## Activity G NCLEX-STYLE QUESTIONS

*Answer the following questions.*

1. A 4-month-old has had a fever, vomiting, and loose watery stools every few hours for 2 days. The mother calls the physician's office and asks the nurse what she should do. What is the most appropriate response from the nurse?

   a. "Do not give the child anything to drink for 4r hours. If the fever goes down and the loose stools stop, you can resume breastfeeding."

   b. "Continue breastfeeding as you have been doing. The fluid from the breast milk is important to maintain fluid balance."

   c. "Give a clear pediatric electrolyte replacement for the next few hours, then call back to report on how your daughter is doing."

   d. "Bring her to the office today so we can evaluate her fluid balance and determine how we can treat her."

2. The nurse is caring for a 13-year-old girl with suspected autoimmune hepatitis. The girl inquires about the testing required to evaluate the condition. How should the nurse respond?

   a. "You will most likely have a blood test to check for certain antibodies."

   b. "You will most likely have an ultrasound evaluation."

   c. "You will most likely have viral studies."

   d. "You will most likely be tested for ammonia levels."

3. The nurse is obtaining the history of an infant with a suspected intestinal obstruction. Which of the following responses regarding newborn stool patterns would indicate a need for further evaluation for Hirschsprung's disease?

   a. The infant passed a meconium stool in the first 24 to 48 hours of life

   b. The infant has had diarrhea for 3 days

   c. The infant has been constipated and passing gas for 2 days

   d. The infant passed a meconium plug

4. A nurse is caring for a 6-year-old girl recently diagnosed with celiac disease and is discussing dietary restrictions with the girl's mother. Which of the following responses indicates a need for further teaching?

   a. "My daughter is eating more vegetables."

   b. "There is gluten hidden in unexpected foods."

   c. "There are many types of flour besides wheat."

   d. "My daughter can eat any kind of fruit."

5. The nurse is providing instructions to the parents of a 10-year-old boy who has undergone a barium swallow/upper and lower GI for suspected inflammatory bowel disease. Which of the following instructions is most important?

   a. "Please be aware of any signs of infection."

   b. "It is very important to drink lots of water and fluids after the test is finished."

   c. "Your child could have diarrhea for several days afterward."

   d. "Your child might have lighter stools for the next few days."

6. A nurse is caring for a 13-year-old boy recently diagnosed with Crohn's disease. He says he feels isolated and that there is no one who understands the challenges of his disease. How should the nurse respond?

   a. "You need to remember that Crohn's disease goes into periods of remission."

   b. "This is something that you will eventually accept with time."

   c. "There are a lot of kids experiencing similar feelings at the Crohn's support group."

   d. "You have to go to a support group; it will be very helpful."

7. The nurse is assessing a 10-day-old infant for dehydration. Which of the following findings indicates severe dehydration?

   a. Pale and slightly dry mucosa

   b. Blood pressure of 80/42

   c. Tenting of skin

   d. Soft and flat fontanels

8. A nurse is caring for a 6-year-old boy with a history of encopresis. What is the best way to approach the parents to assess for proper laxative use?

   a. "Tell me about his daily stool patterns."

   b. "Are you giving him the laxatives properly?"

   c. "Are the laxatives working?"

   d. "Describe his bowel movements for the past week."

9. Which of the following exhibits features most suggestive of ulcerative colitis rather than Crohn's disease?

   a. A 16-year-old female with continuous distribution of disease in the colon, distal to proximal

   b. A 14-year-old female with full-thickness chronic inflammation of the intestinal mucosa

   c. An 18-year-old male with abdominal pain

   d. A 12-year-old with oral temperature of 101.6 F

10. The nurse is conducting a physical examination of an infant with suspected pyloric stenosis. Which of the following findings indicates pyloric stenosis?

    a. Olive-shaped mass in upper right abdomen

    b. Perianal fissures and skin tags

    c. Abdominal pain and irritability

    d. Hard, moveable "olive-like mass" in the upper right quadrant

11. The infant is listless with sunken fontanels and has been diagnosed with dehydration. The infant is still producing at least 1 mL/kg each hour of urine. The infant weighs 13.2 pounds. At the minimum, how many milliliters of urine will the infant produce during the next 8-hour shift?

48

12. The young child has been diagnosed with hepatitis B. Which of the following statements by the child's mother indicates that further education is required?

    a. "We went swimming in a local lake 2 months ago and I just knew she drank some of the lake water."

    b. "Could I have this virus in my body, too?"

    c. "The virus is the reason her skin looks a little yellowish."

    d. "The only way you can get this virus is from intravenous drug use."

    e. "Her fever and rash are probably related to this virus."

13. The adolescent child has been diagnosed with gastroesophageal reflux disease. Which of the following statements by the child indicates that adequate learning has occurred?

    a. "This famotidine may make me tired."

    b. "The omeprazole could give me a headache."

    c. "It sounds like the physician is reluctant to give me a prokinetic because of the side effects."

    d. "I will probably need a laxative because of the omeprazole."

    e. "I should try to lie down right after I eat."

14. The child has been diagnosed with severe dehydration. The physician has ordered the nurse to administer a bolus of 20 mL/kg of normal saline over a 2-hour period. The child weighs 63.5 pounds. How should the nurse set the child's intravenous administration pump? (mL/hour) Round to the nearest whole number.    289 mL/hr

15. The newborn was diagnosed with esophageal atresia. Which of the following findings is most consistent with this condition?

    a. The newborn's mouth was very dry.

    b. The newborn coughed excessively during attempts to feed.

    c. The newborn's skin was very jaundiced.

    d. Coarse crackles were auscultated throughout all lung fields.

    e. With X-ray, the nasogastric tube that the nurse attempted to insert previously was found coiled in the upper esophagus.

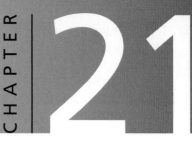

# CHAPTER 21

# Nursing Care of the Child with a Genitourinary Disorder

## Learning Objectives

- Compare anatomic and physiologic differences of the genitourinary system in infants and children versus adults.
- Describe nursing care related to common laboratory and diagnostic testing used in the medical diagnosis of pediatric genitourinary conditions.
- Distinguish genitourinary disorders common in infants, children, and adolescents.
- Identify appropriate nursing assessments and interventions related to medications and treatments for pediatric genitourinary disorders.
- Develop an individualized nursing care plan for the child with a genitourinary disorder.
- Describe the psychosocial impact of chronic genitourinary disorders on children.
- Devise a nutrition plan for the child with renal insufficiency.
- Develop child/family teaching plans for the child with a genitourinary disorder.

## SECTION I: ASSESSING YOUR UNDERSTANDING

### Activity A  FILL IN THE BLANKS

1. Cytotoxic drugs cause bone marrow _Suppression_.

2. Human chorionic gonadotropin is used to precipitate _testicular_ descent.

3. A creatinine (serum) clearance test is used to diagnose impaired _renal_ function.

4. Urodynamic studies measures the urine _flow_ during micturition.

5. Desmopressin is a medication commonly used to treat nocturnal _enuresis_.

6. Bladder capacity of the newborn is _30mL_.

### Activity B  LABELING

*Indicate which image represents:*

1. Hypospadias
2. Epispadias

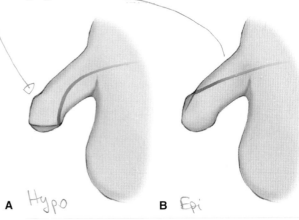

A  _Hypo_          B  _Epi_

## Activity C  MATCHING

*Match the term in Column A with the proper definition in Column B.*

**Column A**

_e_ **1.** Anuria

_d_ **2.** Anascara

_a_ **3.** Menorrhagia

_b_ **4.** Oliguria

_c_ **5.** Hyperlipidemia

**Column B**

**a.** Profuse menstrual bleeding

**b.** Significant decrease in urinary output

**c.** Elevated lipid levels in the blood stream

**d.** Severe generalized edema

**e.** Absence of urine formation

*Match the treatment in Column A with the appropriate indication in Column B.*

**Column A**

_c_ **1.** Peritoneal dialysis

_d_ **2.** Foley catheter

_b_ **3.** Nephrostomy tube

_a_ **4.** Bladder augmentation

**Column B**

**a.** Decreased bladder capacity

**b.** Used to drain an obstructed kidney

**c.** Acute or chronic renal failure

**d.** Unable to void postoperatively

## Activity D  SEQUENCING

*Review the steps of care needed for the child scheduled to undergo a voiding cystourethrogram (VCUG)*

**1.** Bladder filled with contrast material

**2.** Insertion of urinary catheter

**3.** Bladder emptied

**4.** Child scanned with fluoroscope

**5.** Fluoroscope completed

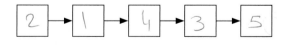

2 → 1 → 4 → 3 → 5

## Activity E  SHORT ANSWERS

*Briefly answer the following.*

**1.** How will the urine appear after a bladder augmentation is done?

contain mucous

**2.** What are the key nursing implications following cystoscopy?

Encourage fluids / burning sensation @ voiding and urine may appear rinse

**3.** What medications/ supplements are commonly used to treat the complications of end-stage renal disease?

Vit D/ $Ca^{2+}$ to correct hypocalcemia and hyper Phosphat
Ferrous for anemia / Bicitra or $NaCO_3$ to correct acidosis
Multi V / Erythropoietin to stimulate RBC

**4.** Discuss testicular torsion.

Can result in ischemia if/left untreated / most commonly boy age 12 to 18 y

**5.** The nurse has completed the newborn assessment for a baby boy. The assessment reveals the right testicle is undescended. How will this condition be managed?

@ 6 month testicle need to descent
Otherwise surgery needed

# SECTION II: APPLYING YOUR KNOWLEDGE

## Activity F  CASE STUDY

Corey Bond is a 5-year-old introduced female. She was brought to the clinic by her mother. She presented with fever and lethargy for the past 24 hours. A urinalysis and culture confirmed that Corey has a urinary tract infection. This is Corey's first urinary tract infection and her mother is concerned and states "I do not understand how a 5-year-old can get a urinary tract infection?"

1.  How will you address the mother's concerns?

    _____

    _____

    _____

2.  Corey is started on oral antibiotics at home. What education can you provide the family regarding treatment and providing comfort?

    _____

    _____

    _____

3.  What can Corey and her family do to try to prevent the recurrence of a urinary tract infection?

    _____

    _____

    _____

# SECTION III: PRACTICING FOR NCLEX

## Activity G  NCLEX-STYLE QUESTIONS

*Answer the following questions.*

1.  The nurse is caring for a 10-year-old girl presenting with fever, dysuria, flank pain, urgency, and hematuria. The nurse would expect to help obtain which of the following tests first to reveal preliminary information about the urinary tract?
    a.  Total protein, globulin, and albumin
    b.  Creatinine clearance
    c.  Urinalysis
    d.  Urine culture and sensitivity

2.  The nurse is caring for a 12-year-old boy diagnosed with acute glomerulonephritis. When reviewing the boy's health history which of the following will likely be noted?
    a.  The boy has a history of recurrent urinary tract infections
    b.  The boy has a family history of renal disorders
    c.  The boy has a recent history of an upper respiratory infection.
    d.  The boy has a history of hypotension.

3.  The nurse is caring for a child who is undergoing peritoneal dialysis. Immediately after draining the dialysate, what is the immediate action the nurse should take?
    a.  Empty the old dialysate
    b.  Weigh the old dialysate
    c.  Weigh the new dialysate
    d.  Start the process over again with a fresh bag

4.  A nurse is caring for a 12-year-old girl recently diagnosed with end-stage renal disease. The nurse is discussing dietary restrictions with the girl's mother. Which of the following responses indicates a need for further teaching?
    a.  "My daughter can eat what she wants when she is hooked to the machine."
    b.  "My daughter must avoid a high sodium diet."
    c.  "She needs to restrict her potassium intake."
    d.  "She can eat whatever she wants on dialysis days."

5.  The nurse is administering cyclophosphamide as ordered for a 12-year-old boy with nephrotic syndrome. Which of the following instructions is most accurate regarding administration of this cytotoxic drug?
    a.  Administer in the evening on an empty stomach
    b.  Provide adequate hydration and encourage voiding
    c.  Administer in the morning, encourage fluids and voiding during and after administration
    d.  Encourage fluids, adequate food intake, and voiding before and after administration

6. A nurse is caring for a 10-year-old boy with nocturnal enuresis with no physiologic cause. He says he is embarrassed and wishes he could stop the bedwetting immediately. How should the nurse respond?

   a. "You will grow out of this eventually; you just need to be patient."

   b. "There are several things we can do to help you achieve this goal."

   c. "There are almost 5 million people that have enuresis."

   d. "The pull-ups look just like underwear; no one has to know."

7. The nurse is assessing an infant with suspected hemolytic uremic syndrome. Which of the following characteristics of this condition would the nurse expect to assess, including information from the chart review?

   a. Hemolytic anemia, acute renal failure, and hypotension

   b. Dirty green colored urine, elevated erythrocyte sedimentation, and depressed serum complement level

   c. Hemolytic anemia, thrombocytopenia, and acute renal failure

   d. Thrombocytopenia, hemolytic anemia, and nocturia several times each night

8. A nurse is caring for a 13-year-old boy with end-stage renal disease who is preparing to have his hemodialysis treatment in the dialysis unit. Which of the following is the appropriate nursing action?

   a. Administer his routine medications as scheduled

   b. Take his blood pressure measurement in extremity with AV fistula

   c. Withhold his routine medication until after dialysis is completed

   d. Assess the Tenckhoff catheter site

9. The nurse is conducting a follow-up visit for a 13-year-old girl who has been treated for pelvic inflammatory disease. Which of the following remarks indicates a need for further teaching?

   a. "I should be tested for other sexually transmitted diseases."

   b. "Douching is not necessary and can cause bacteria to flourish."

   c. "I cannot have sex again until my partner is treated."

   d. "My partner needs to be treated with antibiotics."

10. The nurse is caring for a child who receives dialysis via an AV fistula. Which of the following findings indicates an immediate need to notify the physician?

    a. Presence of a bruit

    b. Presence of a thrill

    c. Dialysate without fibrin or cloudiness

    d. Absence of a thrill

11. The nurse is caring for a child diagnosed with hydronephrosis. Which of the following manifestations is consistent with complications of the disorder?

    a. Hypertension

    b. Hypotension

    c. Hypothermia

    d. Tachycardia

12. The nurse is caring for a child who has been admitted to the acute care facility with manifestations consistent with hydronephrosis. Which of the following diagnostic tests can the nurse anticipate will be performed to confirm diagnosis? Select all that apply.

    a. Intravenous pyelogram (IVP)

    b. Urinalysis

    c. Voiding cystourethrogram (VCUG)

    d. Complete blood cell count

    e. Renal ultrasound

13. The nurse is caring for the parents of a newborn who has an undescended testicle. Which of the following comments by the parents indicates understanding of the condition?

    a. "Our son may need surgery on his testes before we are discharged to go home."

    b. "Our son may have to go through life without two testes."

    c. "Our son's condition may resolve on its own."

    d. "Our son will likely have a high risk of cancer in his teen years as a result of this condition."

14. The nurse is caring for a child with epididymitis. When planning care which of the following interventions may be included?
    a. Scrotal elevation
    b. Warm compresses
    c. Corticosteroid therapy
    d. Catheterization

15. The nurse is planning the discharge instructions for the parents of a 1-month-old child who has had a circumcision completed.

Which of the following should be included in the education provided?
    a. Use Vaseline on the head of the penis for the first 2 weeks after the procedure.
    b. Report any bleeding to the physician.
    c. Reduce the child's fluid intake to reduce voiding during the first 24 hours.
    d. Report redness or swelling on the penile shaft.

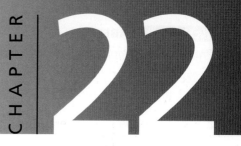

# Nursing Care of the Child with a Neuromuscular Disorder

## Learning Objectives

- Compare differences between the anatomy and physiology of the neuromuscular system in children versus adults.
- Identify nursing interventions related to common laboratory and diagnostic tests used in the diagnosis and management of neuromuscular conditions.
- Identify appropriate nursing assessments and interventions related to medications and treatments used for childhood neuromuscular conditions.
- Distinguish various neuromuscular illnesses occurring in childhood.
- Devise an individualized nursing care plan for the child with a neuromuscular disorder.
- Develop patient/family teaching plans for the child with a neuromuscular disorder.
- Describe the psychosocial impact of chronic neuromuscular disorders on the growth and development of children.

## SECTION I: ASSESSING YOUR UNDERSTANDING

### Activity A  FILL IN THE BLANKS

1. Dermatomyositis is a(n) _autoimmune_ disease that results in inflammation of the muscles or associated tissues.

2. Due to hypertonicity, sustained _clonus_ may be present after forced dorsiflexion.

3. Atrophy is a _decrease_ or wasting in size of a muscle.

4. Spasticity is _involuntary_ muscle contractions that are not coordinated with other muscles.

5. Decreased muscle tone is called _hypotonia_.

6. The structural disorders of spina bifida occulta, meningocele, and myelomeningocele are all considered _neural tube defect_

7. _Guillaume barré_ syndrome is also called acute inflammatory demyelinating polyradiculoneuropathy.

## Activity B  LABELING

*Provide the appropriate labels for the following images.*

1. Normal spine
2. Spine showing spina bifida occulta
3. Spine showing meningocele
4. Spine showing myelomeningocele

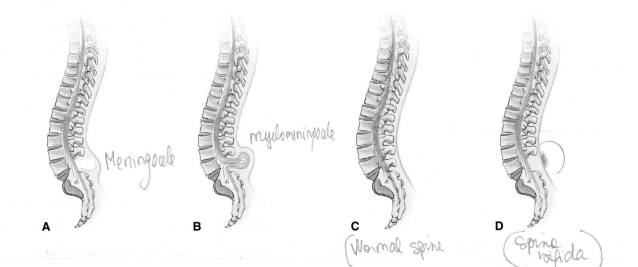

Meningocele

myelomeningocele

A          B          C          D

(Normal spine)       (Spine bifida)

## Activity C  MATCHING

*Match the medication in Column A with the appropriate action in Column B.*

**Column A**

<u>a</u>  1. Baclofen

<u>c</u>  2. Corticosteroids

<u>d</u>  3. Botulin toxin

<u>b</u>  4. Benzodiazepines

<u>e</u>  5. Oxybutynin

**Column B**

a. Central acting skel-
   etal muscle relaxant

b. Anticonvulsant

c. Anti-inflammatory

d. Neurotoxin

e. Antispasmodic

## Activity D  SHORT ANSWERS

*Briefly answer the following.*

1. What are the four classifications of cerebral
   palsy? Which is the most common form?
   Which is the rarest form?

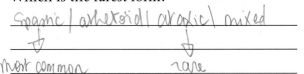

   Spastic / athetoid / ataxic / mixed

   most common          rare

2. According to the text, what is the appropriate
   nursing management focus for a child with
   myelomeningocele?

   focus on preventing infection / bowel/bladder
   nutrition / latex allergic R

3. What are the common symptoms of Guillain–
   Barré syndrome in children?

   Pain in lower extremities

4. What factors increase the risk of a fetus developing a neural tube defect?

   lack prenatal care / lack of folic acid
   anticonvulsant use

5. Discuss the commonalities of the various forms of muscular dystrophy. What is the most common childhood type of muscular dystrophy?

_Duchenne / inherited progressive muscle waste_

# SECTION II: APPLYING YOUR KNOWLEDGE

## Activity E  CASE STUDY

Elijah Jefferson, a 2-year-old boy, was recently diagnosed with cerebral palsy (CP). He was born at 28 weeks gestation after a complicated and prolonged delivery. Elijah's parents have many questions and concerns about their son's diagnosis. They ask "Can Elijah outgrow this disorder with proper physical and occupational therapy?"

1. How can you help Elijah's parents to have an accurate perception of CP?

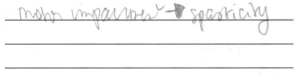

_(abnormal) motor pattern) Motor associated c brain anoxia_
_non progressive abnormal brain function_

2. What are some assessment findings on exam that are characteristic of CP?

_____

_____

_____

3. Discuss the focus of nursing management when caring for a child with CP.

_motor impairment → spasticity_

_____

_____

# SECTION III: PRACTICING FOR NCLEX

## Activity F  NCLEX-STYLE QUESTIONS

*Answer the following questions.*

1. The nurse is taking the history of a 4-year-old boy. His mother mentions that he seems weaker and unable to keep up with his 6-year-old sister on the playground. Which of the following questions will elicit the most helpful information?

    a. "Has he achieved his developmental milestones on time?"

    b. "Would you please describe the weakness you are seeing in your son?"

    c. "Do you think he is simply fatigued?"

    d. "Has his pace of achieving milestones diminished?"

2. The nurse is conducting a physical examination of a 9-month-old baby with a suspected neuromuscular disorder. Which of the following findings would warrant further evaluation?

    a. Presence of symmetrical spontaneous movement

    b. Absence of Moro reflex

    c. Absence of tonic neck reflex

    d. Presence of Moro reflex

3. The nurse is conducting a wellness examination of a 6-month-old child. The mother points out some dimpling and skin discoloration in the child's lumbosacral area. How should the nurse respond?

    a. "This could be an indicator of spina bifida; we need to evaluate this further."

    b. "This can be considered a normal variant with no indication of a problem; however, the doctor will want to take a closer look."

    c. "Dimpling, skin discoloration, and abnormal patches of hair are often indicators of spina bifida occulta."

    d. "This is often an indicator of spina bifida occulta as opposed to spina bifida cystica."

4. A nurse is caring for an infant with a meningocele. Which of the following would alert the nurse that the lesion is increasing in size?

   a. Leaking cerebrospinal fluid

   b. Increasing ICP

   c. Constipation and bladder dysfunction

   d. Increasing head circumference

5. A nurse is teaching the parents of a boy with a neurogenic bladder about clean intermittent catheterization. Which of the following responses indicates a need for further teaching?

   a. "We must be careful to use latex-free catheters."

   b. "The very first step is to apply water-based lubricant to the catheter."

   c. "My son may someday learn how to do this for himself."

   d. "We need to soak the catheter in a vinegar and water solution daily."

6. A nurse is caring for a 13-year-old boy with Duchenne muscular dystrophy. He says he feels isolated and that there is no one who understands the challenges of his disease. How should the nurse respond?

   a. "You need to remain as active as possible and have a positive attitude."

   b. "There are many things that you can do like crafts, computers or art."

   c. "There are a lot of kids with the same type of muscular dystrophy you have at the MDA support group."

   d. "You have to go to a support group; it will be very helpful."

7. The nurse is conducting a physical examination of a 10-year-old boy with a suspected neuromuscular disorder. Which of the following is a sign of Duchenne muscular dystrophy?

   a. Walking on the toes or balls of the feet with a rolling or waddling gait

   b. Appearance of smaller than normal calf muscles

   c. Signs of hydrocephalus

   d. Lordosis

8. A nurse is caring for a 2-year-old girl with cerebral palsy. The child is having difficulty with proper nutrition and is not gaining adequate weight. How can the nurse elicit additional information to establish a diagnosis?

   a. "Let's see if she is dehydrated and we'll assess her respiratory system."

   b. "Does she have difficulty swallowing or chewing?"

   c. "Does she like to feed herself or do you feed her?"

   d. "Lets offer her a snack now and you can tell me about her diet on a typical day."

9. The nurse is caring for a 5-year-old child with Guillain–Barré syndrome. Which of the following would be the best way to assess the level of paralysis?

   a. Gentle tickling

   b. Observe for symmetrical flaccid weakness

   c. Monitor for ataxia

   d. Inquire about sensory disturbances

10. The nurse is providing presurgical care for a newborn with myelomeningocele. Which of the following is the central nursing priority?

    a. Maintain infant's body temperature

    b. Prevent rupture or leaking of cerebrospinal fluid

    c. Maintain infant in prone position

    d. Keep lesion free from fecal matter or urine

11. The child has a meningocele and a neurogenic bladder. Which of the following topics should the nurse include in the teaching plan when educating the child and the child's caregivers? Select all that apply.

    a. How and when to administer oxybutynin chloride

    b. The importance of antibiotic use to prevent urinary tract infections from occurring

    c. How and when to perform clean intermittent urinary catheterization

    d. Signs and symptoms of a urinary tract infection

    e. Different types of surgeries used to treat this condition

12. The nurse is assessing a young boy who has been brought to the physician for mobility and balance issues by his parents. Which of the following findings is positively associated with the presence of Duchenne muscular dystrophy? Select all that apply.
    a. Serum creatine kinase levels are elevated
    b. An electromyogram demonstrates the problem is within the nerves, not the muscles
    c. A muscle biopsy shows an absence of dystrophin
    d. The child is unable to rise easily into a standing position when placed on the floor
    e. Genetic testing indicates the presence of a gene associated with spinal muscular atrophy

13. The nurse learns that the child has been admitted with clinical manifestations associated with cholinergic crisis. Which of the following findings is associated with this condition? Select all that apply.
    a. The child exhibits diaphoresis
    b. The child's apical heart rate is 52 beats per minute
    c. The child's blood pressure is 172/94
    d. The child is complaining that his muscles are very weak
    e. The child is drooling excessively

14. The young girl has been prescribed corticosteroids for dermatomyositis. Which of the following statements by her mother indicates the need for further education? Select all that apply.
    a. "I give it to her first thing in the morning before breakfast."
    b. "We are taking her to Disney in the summer."
    c. "The physician said when it's time for her to stop taking this medication; he will gradually start reducing her dose."
    d. "She's got to take this medication to help with the calcium deposits that can form."
    e. "She might recover completely from this condition."

15. The young child has been diagnosed with Guillain–Barré syndrome and it is progressing in a classic manner. Rank the following sequence of events in the order that they typically occur.
    a. The child states that it is difficult to move his arms
    b. The child states that it is difficult to move his legs
    c. The child is having difficulty producing facial expressions
    d. The child complains of numbness and tingling in his toes

# Nursing Care of the Child with a Musculoskeletal Disorder

## Learning Objectives

- Compare the anatomy and physiology of the musculoskeletal system in children and adults.
- Identify nursing interventions related to common laboratory and diagnostic tests used in the diagnosis and management of musculoskeletal disorders.
- Identify appropriate nursing assessments and interventions related to medications and treatments for common childhood musculoskeletal disorders.
- Distinguish various musculoskeletal disorders occurring in childhood.
- Devise an individualized nursing care plan for the child with a musculoskeletal disorder.
- Develop child/family teaching plans for the child with a musculoskeletal disorder.
- Describe the impact of chronic musculoskeletal disorders on the growth and development of children.

## SECTION I: ASSESSING YOUR UNDERSTANDING

### Activity A FILL IN THE BLANKS

1. Kyphosis refers to excessive _Convex_ curvature of the spine resulting in a humpback appearance.

2. The _Epiphysis_ is where ossification of new bone occurs.

3. An external _Fixation_ is a device that holds bones together externally.

4. Transient _synovitis_ of the hip is the most common cause of hip pain in children.

5. Osteomyelitis is a _B_ infection of the bone and soft tissue surrounding the bone.

6. _Ossification_, the conversion of cartilage to bone, continues throughout childhood and is complete at adolescence.

7. The newborn's feet may display in-toeing, also known as metatarsus _Adductus_ as a result of in utero positioning.

## Activity B LABELING

*Label the types of traction.*

a. Dunlop side-arm 00-90
b. Cervical skin traction
c. Russell's traction
d. 90-90 traction
e. Halo traction

f. Side-arm 90-90
g. Balanced suspension traction
h. Bryant's traction
i. Buck's traction
j. Cervical skeletal tongs

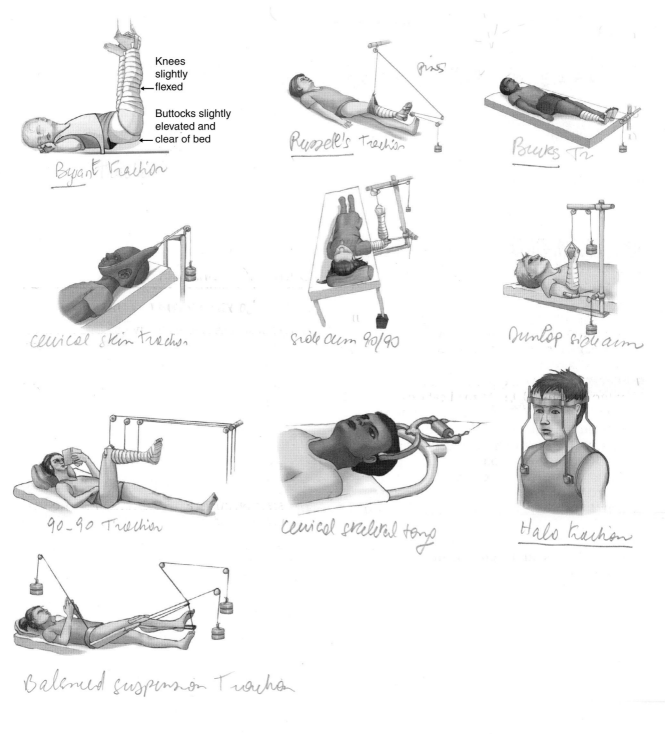

## Activity C MATCHING

*Match the medication in Column A with the appropriate indication in Column B.*

**Column A**

*d* **1.** Bisphosphonate-IV

*c* **2.** Narcotic analgesics

*e* **3.** Nonsteroidal anti-inflammatory drugs

*b* **4.** Benzodiazepines

*a* **5.** Acetaminophen

**Column B**

**a.** Relief of mild pain if used alone

**b.** Treatment of muscle spasms

**c.** Relief of moderate to severe pain

**d.** Decrease incidence of fractures

**e.** Relief of mild to moderate pain

## Activity D SEQUENCING

*Place the following parts of a physical examination of a child with a suspected clavicle injury in the proper sequence*

**1.** Gently palpate clavicles

**2.** Observe for any noticeable deformity

**3.** Palpate neurovascular status of fingers

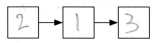

## Activity E SHORT ANSWERS

*Briefly answer the following.*

**1.** Explain the difference between dislocation, subluxation, and frank dislocation in relation to developmental dysplasia of the hip (DDH).

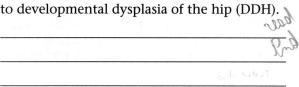

_____

_____

_____

**2.** List and explain the four types of fractures seen in children.

_____

_____

_____

**3.** What should be included in the teaching guidelines for a parent with a child with osteogenesis imperfecta?

_____

_____

_____

**4.** You are the nurse providing instructions to a 10-year-old boy, and his parents, who has just had an arm cast removed following a fracture. What are important instructions for his care?

_____

_____

_____

**5.** What is torticollis and what type of exercises are necessary to treat the disorder?

_____

_____

_____

# SECTION II: APPLYING YOUR KNOWLEDGE

### Activity F  CASE STUDY

You are caring for a 2-year-old boy who was brought to the clinic by his mother. He presented with right arm bruising, swelling, and wrist point tenderness. An X-ray confirmed he had a right wrist fracture. The doctor decided he needed a cast.

1. What assessments and interventions should you perform before application of the cast?

   _____

   _____

   _____

2. What assessments and interventions should you perform after application of the cast?

   _____

   _____

   _____

3. What education will the family need for home care of their son?

   _____

   _____

   _____

# SECTION III: PRACTICING FOR NCLEX

### Activity G  NCLEX-STYLE QUESTIONS

*Answer the following questions.*

1. A nurse is assisting the parents of a child who requires a Pavlik harness. The parents are apprehensive about how to care for their baby. The nurse should stress which of the following teaching points?

   a. "The baby needs the harness only for 2 to 3 weeks."

   b. "It is important that the harness be worn continuously."

   c. "The harness does not hurt the baby."

   d. "Let me teach you how to make appropriate adjustments to the harness."

2. The nurse is conducting a routine physical examination of a newborn to screen for developmental DDH. The nurse correctly assesses the infant by placing the infant:

   a. In a prone position, noting asymmetry of the thigh or gluteal folds.

   b. With both legs extended and observes the hip and knee joint relationship.

   c. With both legs extended and observes the feet.

   d. In a supine position with both legs extended and observes the tibia/fibula.

3. A 5-year-old child is in traction and at risk for impaired skin integrity due to pressure. Which of the following is the most effective intervention?

   a. Inspect the child's skin for rashes, redness, irritation, or pressure sores.

   b. Apply lotion to dry skin.

   c. Gently massage the child's back to stimulate circulation.

   d. Keep the child's skin clean and dry.

4. A nurse is conducting a physical examination of an infant with suspected metatarsus adductus. Which of the following findings would indicate Type II metatarsus adductus? The forefoot is:

   a. Inverted and turned slightly upward

   b. Flexible past neutral actively and passively

   c. Flexible passively past neutral, but only to midline actively

   d. Rigid, does not correct to midline even with passive stretching

5. A nurse is providing instructions for home cast care. Which of the following responses by the parent indicates a need for further teaching?

   a. "We must avoid causing depressions in the cast."

   b. "Pale, cool, or blue skin coloration is to be expected."

   c. "The casted arm must be kept still."

   d. "We need be aware of odor or drainage from the cast."

6. A nurse is caring for a 6-year-old boy with a fractured ulna. He is fearful about the casting process and is resisting treatment. How should the nurse respond?
   a. "The application of the cast will not hurt."
   b. "Would you like to pick out your favorite color?"
   c. "Look over there at the neon fish in our aquarium."
   d. "Will you please take this medicine for pain?"

7. The nurse is providing postoperative care for a boy who has undergone surgical correction for pectus excavatum. The nurse should emphasize which of the following to the child and his parents?
   a. "Please watch for signs of infection."
   b. "Be sure to monitor his vital capacity."
   c. "Do not allow him to lie on either side."
   d. "Do not allow him to lie on his stomach."

8. A nurse is caring for an 11-year-old with an Ilizarov fixator and is providing teaching regarding pin care. The nurse should provide which of the following instructions?
   a. "Cleansing by showering should be sufficient."
   b. "You must clean the pin sites with saline."
   c. "The pin site should be cleaned with anti-bacterial solution."
   d. "Please make sure that the pin site is cleansed with betadine swabs after showering."

9. The nurse is caring for an infant girl in an outpatient setting. The infant has just been diagnosed with DDH. The mother is very upset about the diagnosis and blames herself for her daughter's condition. Which of the following would best address the mother's concerns?
   a. "There are simple noninvasive treatment options."
   b. "Your daughter will likely wear a Pavlik harness."
   c. "Don't worry; this is a relatively common diagnosis."
   d. "This is not your fault and we will help you with her care and treatment."

10. The nurse is conducting a physical examination of a newborn with suspected osteogenesis imperfecta. Which of the following is a common finding?
    a. Foot is drawn up and inward
    b. Sole of foot faces backwards
    c. Dimpled skin, hair in lumbar region
    d. Blue sclera

11. The young child is experiencing muscle spasms and has been given lorazepam. Which of the following statements by the child indicate that the child may be experiencing some common side effects? Select all that apply.
    a. "I feel sort of dizzy."
    b. "I need to take a nap."
    c. "My muscle cramps are getting worse."
    d. "I think I'm going to throw up."
    e. "My belly hurts."

12. The young boy has fractured his left leg and has had a cast applied. The nurse educates the boy and his parents prior to discharge from the hospital. The parents should call the physician when which of the following occurs? Select all that apply.
    a. The boy experiences mild pain when wiggling his toes.
    b. The boy has had a fever of greater than 102 F for the last 36 hours.
    c. New drainage is seeping out from under the cast.
    d. The outside of the boy's cast got wet and had to be dried using a hair dryer.
    e. The boy's toes are light blue and very swollen.

13. The child has been diagnosed with rickets. The child's mother is educated about the importance of providing the child with 10 μg micrograms (400 International Units) of an oral vitamin D supplement each day. The child's mother purchases over-the-counter vitamin D drops. The supplement is noted to contain 5 μg of vitamin D in each 0.5 mL. How much of the supplement should the mother administer to the child each day?

1 mL

14. The child has been diagnosed with slipped capital femoral epiphysis. Which of the following characteristics about the patient is risk factor associated with the development of this condition? Select all that apply.

    a. The child is noted to be underweight by the nurse.
    b. The child is 13 years old.
    c. The child is African American.
    d. The child's parents state that the child has recently experienced a "growth spurt."
    e. The child is male.

15. Identify which of the following images is a greenstick fracture.

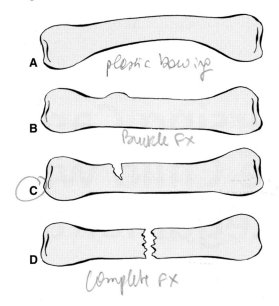

A  plastic bowing

B  Buckle Fx

C  

D  complete Fx

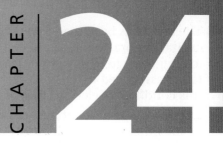

# CHAPTER 24

# Nursing Care of the Child with an Integumentary Disorder

## Learning Objectives

- Compare anatomic and physiologic differences of the integumentary system in infants and children versus adults.
- Describe nursing care related to common laboratory and diagnostic tests used in the medical diagnosis of integumentary disorders in infants, children, and adolescents.
- Distinguish integumentary disorders common in infants, children, and adolescents.
- Identify appropriate nursing assessments and interventions related to pediatric integumentary disorders.
- Develop an individualized nursing care plan for the child with an integumentary disorder.
- Describe the psychosocial impact of a chronic integumentary disorder on children or adolescents.
- Develop patient/family teaching plans for the child with an integumentary disorder.

## SECTION I: ASSESSING YOUR UNDERSTANDING

### Activity A FILL IN THE BLANKS

1. Diaper wearing _decrease_ the skin's pH, activating fecal enzymes that further contribute to skin maceration.

2. Serum _IgE_ may be elevated in the child with atopic dermatitis.

3. Urticaria is a type I _Hypersensitivity_ reaction.

4. Seborrhea in infants is commonly referred to as _cradle cap_

5. Acne neonatorum occurs as a response to the presence of maternal _Androgens_.

### Activity B MATCHING

*Match the term in Column A with the correct definition in Column B.*

**Column A**

_b_ 1. Annular

_c_ 2. Papule

_d_ 3. Vesicle

_a_ 4. Macule

_e_ 5. Scaling

**Column B**

a. A flat discolored area on the skin

b. In a circle or ring shape

c. Small raised bump on the skin

d. A fluid-filled bump on the skin

e. Flaking of the skin

**Column A**

____d____ **1.** Silver
sulfadiazine 1%

____c____ **2.** Isotretinoin

____a____ **3.** Coal tar
preparations

____b____ **4.** Benzoyl
peroxide

**Column B**

**a.** Psoriasis, atopic
dermatitis

**b.** Mild acne vulgaris

**c.** Cystic acne

**d.** Burns

### Activity C SEQUENCING

*List in order the stages in the progression of an impetigo lesion.*

**1.** Formation of a crust on an ulcer-like base

**2.** Papules

**3.** Painless pustules with an erythematous border

**4.** Honey-colored exudate

**5.** Vesicles

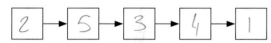

2 → 5 → 3 → 4 → 1

### Activity D SHORT ANSWERS

*Briefly answer the following.*

**1.** Review the different cutaneous reactions commonly found in dark-skinned children compared to children with lighter skin.

**2.** According to the text, what are the four criteria used to describe lesions?

Linear refers to lesions in a line

Shape: the lesions are round, oval, annular

morbilliform refers to rosy maculopapular rash. Target lesions
look just like a bull-eye

**3.** What are the differences between bullous impetigo and non-bullous impetigo?

Impetigo is readily recognizable skin rash

Non bullous

Trauma / atopic dermatitis
skin trauma

Bullous

Sporadic occurence pattern
Dvp in intact skin result
from toxin production
of staphylococcus aureus

**4.** List the risk factors that are associated with the development of pressure ulcers. What sites are more prone for pressure ulcer development?

occipital upon / toe /

wheelchair sacral / hip area

**5.** Explain the relationship between puberty and acne vulgaris.

50% to 85% between 12 and 16 y

Androgenous hr stimulate sebaceous glands

## SECTION II: APPLYING YOUR KNOWLEDGE

### Activity E CASE STUDY

Eva Lopez is a 1-year-old child. She has presented at the ambulatory care clinic with reports of itching and scratching that is worse at night. The assessment reveals dry patches of skin. She has evidence of bleeding at the wrists from scratching. A diagnosis of atopic dermatitis (eczema) is made.

**1.** The mother states, "I do not understand why the rash comes and goes and only seems to appear after Eva has been scratching?" Address the mother's concerns.

**2.** What education will the family need to help manage atopic dermatitis?

Promote skin hydration

# SECTION III: PRACTICING FOR NCLEX

### Activity F NCLEX-STYLE QUESTIONS

*Answer the following questions.*

1. The nurse is conducting a primary survey of a child with burns. Which of the following assessment findings points to airway injury from burn or smoke inhalation?
   a. Burns on hands
   b. Cervical spine injury
   c. Stridor
   d. Internal injuries

2. The nurse is conducting a physical examination of a child with severe burns. Which of the following internal physiologic manifestations would the nurse expect to occur first?
   a. Insulin resistance
   b. Hypermetabolic response with increased cardiac output
   c. Decrease in cardiac output
   d. Increased protein catabolism

3. The nurse is caring for a 10-month-old with a rash. The child's mother reports that the onset was abrupt. The nurse assesses diffuse erythema and skin tenderness with, ruptured bullae in the axillary area with red weeping surface. The nurse suspects which of the following bacterial infections?
   a. Folliculitis   *red raised hair follicles*
   b. Impetigo   *red macules/bullous eruptions on erythematous base*
   c. Non-bullous impetigo   *(papule progressing to vesicles then painless pustules*
   d. Scalded skin syndrome

4. A nurse providing teaching on ways to promote skin hydration for the parents of an infant with atopic dermatitis. Which of the following responses indicates a need for further teaching?
   a. "We need to avoid any skin product containing perfumes, dyes, or fragrances."
   b. "We should use a mild soap for sensitive skin."
   c. "We should bathe our child in hot water, twice a day."
   d. "We should use soap to clean only dirty areas."

5. A nurse is caring for a child with tinea pedis. Which of the following assessment findings would the nurse expect to note?
   a. Red scaling rash on soles and between the toes
   b. Patches of scaling in the scalp with central hair loss   *T capitis*
   c. Inflamed boggy mass filled with pustules   *T capitis*
   d. Erythema, scaling, maceration in the inguinal creases and inner thighs   *T cruris*

6. A nurse assessing a 6-month-old girl with an integumentary disorder. The nurse notes three virtually identically sized, round red circles with scaling that are symmetrically spaced on both of the girl's inner thighs. What should the nurse ask the mother?   *nickel dermatitis*
   a. "Has she been exposed to poison ivy?"
   b. "Does she wear sleepers with metal snaps?"
   c. "Do you change her diapers regularly?"
   d. "Tell me about your family history of allergies."

7. The nurse is conducting a physical examination of a boy with erythema multiforme. Which of the following assessment findings would the nurse expect to note?
   a. Lesions over the hands and feet, and extensor surfaces of the extremities with spread to the trunk
   b. Thick or flaky/greasy yellow scales   *Seborrhea*
   c. Silvery or yellow-white scale plaques and sharply demarcated borders   *psoriasis*
   d. Superficial tan or hypopigmented oval shaped scaly lesions especially on upper back and chest and proximal arms   *tinea versi*

8. A nurse is caring for a child with a wasp sting. What is the priority nursing intervention?
   a. Remove jewelry or restrictive clothing
   b. Apply ice intermittently
   c. Administer the diphenhydramine per protocol
   d. Cleanse wound with mild soap and water

9. The nurse is examining a child for indications of frostbite and notes blistering with erythema and edema. The nurse notes which of the following degrees of frostbite?

   a. First degree frostbite  *white plaque*

   **b.** Second degree frostbite  *erythema / Edema*

   c. Third degree frostbite  *hemorrhagic blister*

   d. Fourth degree frostbite  *Nail necrosis / flaughring*

10. The nurse is providing teaching on ways to maintaining skin integrity and preventing infection for the parents of a boy with atopic dermatitis. Which of the following responses indicates a need for further teaching?

    **a.** "We should avoid using petroleum jelly."

    b. "We should keep his fingernails short and clean."

    c. "We should avoid tight clothing and heat."

    d. "We need to develop ways to prevent him from scratching."

11. The nurse is providing education to the parents of a teenaged boy diagnosed with impetigo. Which of the following statements by the boy indicates the need for further education?

    **a.** "I will need to cover my son's skin lesions with bandages until it has healed."

    b. "It is important to remove the crusts before applying any topical medications."

    c. "This condition is contagious."  *Bacterial infection*

    d. "My son can continue to attend school while he is taking the prescribed antibiotics."

12. A 16-year-old male who has diagnosed with tinea pedis questions the nurse about how he may have contracted the condition. What information may be provided to the boy by the nurse?  *(fungal infection)*

    a. "It is unlikely you will be able to determine the cause of the infection."

    b. "This condition is common in individuals with lowered immunity."

    **c.** "You may have gotten the condition from a community shower or gym area."

    d. "You likely had an infection in another area of your body and it has spread."

13. The nurse is discussing the use of over-the-counter ointments to manage a mild case of diaper rash. What ingredients should the nurse instruct the parents to look for in a compound? Select all that apply.

    **a.** Vitamin A

    **b.** Zinc

    **c.** Vitamin D

    d. Vitamin $B_6$

    e. Vitamin $B_{12}$

14. The nurse is discussing dietary intake with the parents of a 4-year-old child who has been diagnosed with atopic dermatitis. Later nurse notes the menu selection made by the parents for the child. Which selection indicates the need for further instruction?

    **a.** Peanut butter and jelly sandwich

    b. Chicken nuggets

    c. Tomato soup

    d. Carrot and celery sticks

15. The nurse is developing the plan of care for a 3-year-old child diagnosed with atopic dermatitis. When reviewing the desired patient outcomes which of the following are common focuses for a child with this diagnosis? Select all that apply.

    a. Pain management

    **b.** Promotion of skin hydration

    **c.** Maintenance of skin integrity

    d. Reduction in anxiety

    **e.** Prevention of infection

# CHAPTER 25

# Nursing Care of the Child with a Hematologic Disorder

## Learning Objectives

- Identify major hematologic disorders that affect children.
- Determine priority assessment information for children with hematologic disorders.
- Analyze laboratory data in relation to normal findings and report abnormal findings.
- Provide nursing diagnoses appropriate for the child and family with hematologic disorders.
- Identify priority interventions for children with hematologic disorders.
- Develop a teaching plan for the family of children with hematologic disorders.
- Identify resources for children and families with hematologic disorders or nutrition deficits.

## SECTION I: ASSESSING YOUR UNDERSTANDING

### Activity A  FILL IN THE BLANKS

1. The complete blood count is also called the CBC or _hemogram_.

2. Anemia is the reduction of red blood cells or hemoglobin in the total blood _volume_.

3. Erythropoietin is a hormone produced by the _kidneys_ that stimulates the production of red blood cells.

4. Mean corpuscular volume (MCV) is a measure of the average _size_ of the RBC.

5. Heme is iron surrounded by _Protoporphyrin_

6. _Mean Platelet volume_ is the measurement of the size of the platelets.

7. If the levels of RBCs and Hgb are lower than normal _Anemia_ is present.

**Activity B  LABELING**

*Place the following labels in the appropriate location on the diagram.*

1. Multipotent stem cell
2. Neutrophil
3. Lymphocyte
4. Monocyte
5. Megakaryocyte/erythroid progenitor

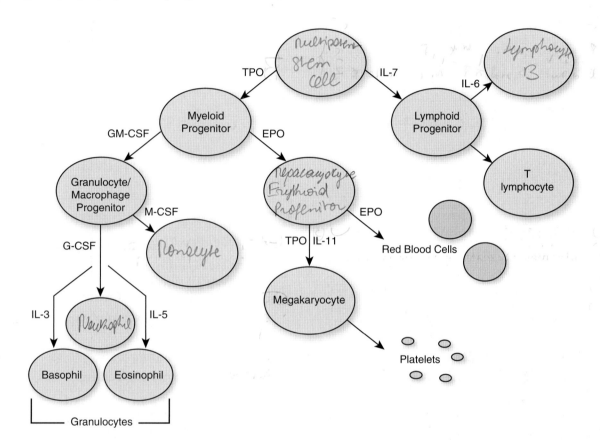

**Activity C  MATCHING**

*Match the medication in Column A with the appropriate indication in Column B.*

**Column A**

___e___ 1. Factor VII

___c___ 2. Deferoxamine

___d___ 3. Intravenous immune globulin (IVIG)

___b___ 4. Penicillin

___a___ 5. Chelating agents

**Column B**

a. Blood lead levels greater than 45 µg/dL

b. Prophylaxis of infection in asplenia

c. Iron toxicity

d. Idiopathic thrombocytopenic purpura

e. Hemophilia

**Activity D  SHORT ANSWERS**

*Briefly answer the following.*

1. Explain the difference between folic acid deficiency and pernicious anemia. What is the appropriate management for each?

| Folic acid | Pernicious anemia |
|---|---|
| ↑ diet intake iron (malabsorption from medication such as Dilantin/ parasitic infection | Deficiency Vit B12 |

2. According to the American Academy of Pediatrics, what is the recommended action for a blood lead level of 20 to 44 µg/dL?

*repeat lab within week*

*educate on lead exposure*

3. Signs of changes in the hematologic system are often subtle and overlooked. What are some of the first signs of a problem developing?

*pallor/ (bruising) (flushing)*

4. Discuss the incidence of sickle cell anemia.

*African American/ Mediterranean/ Indian Descent*

5. Discuss how iron deficiency anemia occurs and which age groups it is most prevalent in.

*Children between 6 to 20 M*

# SECTION II: APPLYING YOUR KNOWLEDGE

## Activity E CASE STUDY

Jayda Johnson, 15-months-old, is brought to the clinic for a routine exam. Her parents state she has been irritable lately. Assessment findings reveal pallor of the mucous membranes and conjunctivae, heart rate of 120 and a heart murmur heard upon auscultation.

1. What other assessment information about the home environment is important for the nurse to gather.

2. Lab results revealed hemoglobin of 10 g/dL and hematocrit of 29%. The physician decides to start Jayda on a daily dose of ferrous sulfate. What instructions should be given to the child's parents?

3. What sociocultural influences may be related to the child's condition?

# SECTION III: PRACTICING FOR NCLEX

## Activity F NCLEX-STYLE QUESTIONS

*Answer the following questions.*

1. The nurse is caring for a child with DIC. The nurse notices signs of neurological deficit. The appropriate nursing action is to:
   a. Continue to monitor neurological signs
   b. Notify the physician
   c. Evaluate respiratory status
   d. Inspect for signs of bleeding

2. The nurse is examining the hands of a child with suspected iron deficiency anemia. Which of the following would the nurse expect to find?
   a. Capillary refill in less than 2 seconds
   b. Pink palms and nail beds
   c. Absence of bruising
   d. Spooning of nails
      *(convex shape)*

3. The nurse is evaluating the complete blood count of a 7-year-old child with a suspected hematological disorder. Which of the following findings would be associated with an elevated mean corpuscular volume (MCV)?

    a. Macrocytic RBCs

    b. Decreased WBCs

    c. Platelet count of 250,000

    d. Hgb of 11.2 g/dL

4. A nurse is caring for a newborn whose screening test result indicates the possibility of SCA or sickle cell trait. The nurse would expect the test result to be confirmed by which of the following lab tests:

    a. Reticulocyte count

    b. Peripheral blood smear

    c. Erythrocyte sedimentation rate

    d. Hemoglobin electrophoresis    *Hgb*

5. A nurse is providing dietary interventions for a 5-year-old with an iron deficiency. Which of the following responses indicates a need for further teaching?

    a. "Red meat is a good option; he loves the hamburgers from the drive-thru."

    b. "He will enjoy tuna casserole and eggs"

    c. "There are many iron fortified cereals that he likes"

    d. "I must encourage a variety of iron-rich foods that he likes"

6. A nurse is caring for a 7-year-old boy with hemophilia who requires an infusion of factor VIII. He is fearful about the process and is resisting treatment. How should the nurse respond?

    a. "Would you like to administer the infusion?"

    b. "Would you help me dilute this and mix it up?"

    c. "Will you help me apply this band-aid?"

    d. "Please be brave; we need to stop the bleeding"

7. The nurse is providing teaching about iron supplement administration to the parents of a 10-month-old child. It is critical that the nurse emphasize which of the following teaching points to the parents?

    a. "You must precisely measure the amount of iron"

    b. "Your child may become constipated from the iron"

    c. "Please give him plenty of fluids and encourage fiber"

    d. "Place the liquid behind the teeth; the pigment can cause staining"

8. A nurse in the emergency department is examining a 6-month-old with symmetrical swelling of the hands and feet. The nurse immediately suspects:

    a. Cooley's anemia

    b. ITP

    c. Sickle cell disease    *(Vaso Occlusive event)*

    d. Hemophilia

9. The nurse is caring for a child with aplastic anemia. The nurse is reviewing the child's blood work and notes the granulocyte count about 500, platelets over 20,000, and the reticulocyte count is over 1%. The parents ask if these values have any significance. The nurse is correct in responding:

    a. "The doctor will discuss these findings with you when he comes to the hospital."

    b. "These values will help us monitor the disease."

    c. "These labs are just common labs for children with this disease."

    d. "I'm really not allowed to discuss these findings with you."

10. The nurse is caring for an 18-month-old with suspected iron deficiency anemia. Which of the following lab results confirms the diagnosis?
    a. Increased hemoglobin and hematocrit, increased reticulocyte count, microcytosis, and hypochromia
    b. Increased serum iron and ferritin levels: decreased FEP level, microcytosis and hypochromia
    c. Decreased hemoglobin and hematocrit, decreased reticulocyte count, microcytosis, and hypochromia, decreased serum iron and ferritin levels and increase FEP level
    d. Increased hemoglobin and hematocrit, increased reticulocyte, microcytosis and hypochromia, increased serum iron and ferritin levels and decreased FEP level

11. The blood cell becomes an erythrocyte. Rank the following steps in the proper order of occurrence.

    *d, c, a, b*

    a. The myeloid cell becomes a megakaryocyte ③
    b. Erythropoietin helps the cell turn into a red blood cell ④
    c. Thrombopoietin acts on the cell ②
    d. The bone marrow releases a stem cell ①

12. The young girl has been diagnosed with a hematologic disorder. Her erythrocyte count is below normal. The mean corpuscular volume is below normal. The girl's mean corpuscular hemoglobin concentration is below normal. Which of the following statements by the girl's nurse is true regarding this girl? Select all that apply.
    a. "She's anemic."
    b. "Her red blood cells are macrocytic."
    c. "Her red blood cells are hypochromic."
    d. "The amount of hemoglobin in her red blood cells is very dilute."
    e. "Her red blood cells are smaller than normal."

13. The young boy has had his spleen surgically removed. Which of the following statements by the boy's parents prior to discharge indicates that an adequate amount of learning has occurred?
    a. "If he gets a fever, I'm going to call our physician right away."
    b. "If he does get sick, then we'll need to put on his medic alert bracelet."
    c. "Before he goes to the dentist, we'll make sure he gets antibiotics."
    d. "He's going to need several vaccines."
    e. "He's going to get really good at washing his hands."

14. The child has anemia and iron supplements will be administered by his parents at home. Which of the following statements by the child's parents indicates that further education is required?
    a. "It's better if I give the iron with orange juice."
    b. "I can give the iron mixed with chocolate milk." *absorption reduced c̄ milk*
    c. "If the iron is mixed in a drink, then he should drink it with a straw."
    d. "He may develop diarrhea." *Iron constipate*
    e. "His urine may look dark."

15. The child has been diagnosed with severe iron deficiency anemia. The child requires 5 mg/kg of elemental iron per day in three equally divided doses. The child weighs 47.3 pounds. How many milligrams of elemental iron should the child receive with each dose? Round to the nearest whole number.

# CHAPTER 26

# Nursing Care of the Child with an Immunologic Disorder

## Learning Objectives

- Explain anatomic and physiologic differences of the immune system in infants and children versus adults.
- Describe nursing care related to common laboratory and diagnostic testing used in the medical diagnosis of pediatric immune and autoimmune disorders.
- Distinguish immune, autoimmune, and allergic disorders common in infants, children, and adolescents.
- Identify appropriate nursing assessments and interventions related to medications and treatments for pediatric immune, autoimmune, and allergic disorders.
- Develop an individualized nursing care plan for the child with an immune or autoimmune disorder.
- Describe the psychosocial impact of chronic immune disorders on children.
- Devise a nutrition plan for the child with immunodeficiency.
- Develop patient/family teaching plans for the child with an immune or autoimmune disorder.

## SECTION I: ASSESSING YOUR UNDERSTANDING

### Activity A FILL IN THE BLANKS

1. In systemic lupus erythematosus (SLE), auto-antibodies react with the child's _self antigens_ to form immune complexes.

2. _Chemotaxis_ is the movement of white blood cells to an inflamed or infected area of the body in response to chemicals released by neutrophils, monocytes, and the suffering tissue.

3. Primary immune deficiencies such as SCID and Wiskott–Aldrich syndrome are cured only by _bone marrow_ or stem cell transplantation.

4. The malar rash of SLE resembles the shape of a _Butterfly_.

5. For most children only allergies to fish, shellfish, tree nuts, and _peanuts_ persist into adulthood.

6. A _Maculopopular_ rash is often an early sign of a graft-versus-host disease that is developing in response to a bone marrow or stem cell transplant.

7. HIV infects the CD4 cells, also known as the _T helper_ cells.

## Activity B MATCHING

*Match the medication in Column A with the appropriate indication in Column B.*

**Column A**

_e_ 1. Cyclophosphamide

_d_ 2. Protease inhibitors

_b_ 3. Cyclosporine A

_a_ 4. Methotrexate

_c_ 5. NSAIDs

**Column B**

a. Severe polyarticular juvenile idiopathic arthritis (JIA)

b. Prevention of rejection of renal transplants

c. JIA

d. Treatment of HIV as part of 3-drug regimen

e. Severe SLE

## Activity C SEQUENCING

*Place the following anaphylaxis treatment priorities in the proper sequence.*

1. Administration of corticosteroids

2. Injection of intramuscular epinephrine

3. Administration of intravenous diphenhydramine

4. Assessment of airway and support of the airway, breathing, and circulation

4 → 2 → 3 → 1

## Activity D SHORT ANSWERS

*Briefly answer the following.*

1. What is the complement in relation to the immune system?

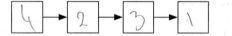
*[handwritten]* Work antibodies / proper destruction B production inflammation regulation of immune RE

2. Which laboratory test for HIV requires serial testing? Why?

*[handwritten]* Elisa

3. Why are skin test responses (such as PPD for tuberculosis detection) diminished until about 1 year of age?

*[handwritten]* Kids decrease ability to produce an inflammatory response

4. Discuss what is meant by the statement, "Children acquire HIV infection either vertically or horizontally."

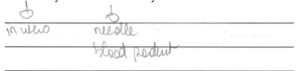
*[handwritten]* in utero    needle    blood product

5. What is avascular necrosis and what group of patients are at an increased risk of developing this complication?

*[handwritten]* Avascular necrosis ← ↑ dose corticosteroid causing bone damage

# SECTION II: APPLYING YOUR KNOWLEDGE

## Activity E CASE STUDY

A 15-year-old female presents with complaints of pain and swelling in her joints, weight gain, and fatigue. After further assessment the physician suspects SLE.

1. What laboratory and diagnostic tests may you expect the physician to order?

*[handwritten]* CBC ↓Hgb ↓Hct ↓Platelet ↓WBC C3 C4 ↓

2. The mother asks, "Will these tests confirm whether or not my daughter has lupus?" How would you respond?

3. If the diagnosis is confirmed, what education will be necessary for the girl and her mother?

_____

_____

_____

# SECTION III: PRACTICING FOR NCLEX

**Activity F** **NCLEX-STYLE QUESTIONS**

*Answer the following questions.*

1. The nurse is caring for a 6-month-old boy with Wiskott–Aldrich syndrome. The nurse teaches the parents which of the following:
   a. "Don't use a tub bath for daily cleansing"
   b. "Don't encourage a pacifier due to possible oral malformation"
   c. "Do not insert anything in the rectum"
   d. "Do not use a sponge bath for light cleaning"

2. The nurse is preparing to administer intravenous immunoglobulin (IVIG) for a child who has not had an IVIG infusion in over 10 weeks. The nurse knows to first:
   a. Begin infusion slowly increasing to prescribed rate
   b. Assess for adverse reaction
   c. Obtain baseline physical assessment
   d. Premedicate with acetaminophen or diphenhydramine

3. The nurse is providing instructions to the parents of a child with a severe peanut allergy. Which of the following statements by the parents indicates a need for further teaching about the use of the EpiPen Jr.®?
   a. "We must massage the area for 10 seconds after administration"
   b. "We must make sure that the black tip is pointed downward"
   c. "The EpiPen Jr.® should be jabbed into the upper arm"
   d. "The EpiPen Jr.® must be held firmly for 10 seconds"

4. A nurse is caring for an infant whose mother is HIV positive. The nurse knows that which of the following diagnostic test results will be positive even if the child is not infected with the virus:
   a. Erythrocyte sedimentation rate
   b. Immunoglobulin electrophoresis
   c. Polymerase chain reaction test
   d. Enzyme-linked immunosorbant assay

5. A nurse is providing dietary interventions for a 12-year-old with a shellfish allergy. Which of the following responses indicates a need for further teaching?
   a. "He will likely outgrow this"
   b. "He must avoid lobster and shrimp"
   c. "We must order carefully when dining out"
   d. "Wheezing is a sign of a severe reaction"

6. A nurse is conducting a physical examination of a 12-year-old girl with suspected SLE. How would the nurse best interview the girl?
   a. "Do you notice any wheezing when you breathe or a runny nose?"
   b. "Do you have any shoulder pain or abdominal tenderness?"
   c. "Tell me if you have noticed any new bruising or different color patterns on your skin"
   d. "Have you noticed any hair loss or redness on your face?"

7. The nurse is providing teaching about food substitutions when cooking for the child with an allergy to eggs. Which of the following responses indicates a need for further teaching?
   a. "I must not feed my child eggs in any form"
   b. "I can use the egg white when baking, but not the yolk"
   c. "1 tsp yeast and ¼ cups warm water is a substitute in baked goods"
   d. "1 teaspoon baking powder equals one egg in a recipe"

8. A nurse in the emergency department is examining an 18-month-old with lip edema, urticaria, stridor, and tachycardia. The nurse immediately suspects:
   a. Severe polyarticular JIA
   b. Anaphylaxis
   c. SLE
   d. SCID

9. The nurse is providing teaching for the parents of a child with a latex allergy. The nurse tells the client to avoid which of the following foods?

   a. Blueberries

   b. Pumpkin

   c. Banana

   d. Pomegranate

10. The nurse is caring for a child with JIA. There is involvement of five or more small joints and it is affecting the body symmetrically. This tells the nurse which of the following?

    a. The child has polyarticular JIA

    b. The child has systemic JIA

    c. The child has pauciarticular JIA

    d. The child is at risk for anaphylaxis

11. The child has a peanut allergy and accidentally ate food that contained peanuts. Which of the following findings are clinical manifestations of anaphylaxis? Select all that apply.

    a. The child's pulse is 52 beats per minute

    b. The child states that his tongue feels "too big" for his mouth

    c. The child has developed hives on his face and trunk

    d. The child states he feels might "throw up"

    e. The child states that he feels like he might faint

12. The nurse is preparing to administer the child's dose of IVIG. Which of the following activities by the nurse indicates the need for further education? Select all that apply.

    a. The nurse is preparing to administer the medication ventrogluteal site as an intramuscular injection

    b. The nurse takes baseline vital signs and will monitor the vital signs during the infusion

    c. The nurse is prepared to give acetaminophen to the child

    d. The nurse is prepared to give diphenhydramine to the child

    e. The nurse has mixed the medication with the child's intravenous antibiotic

13. The nurse is assessing children in a physician's office. Which of the following children may have a primary immunodeficiency?

    a. The child has been diagnosed with six episodes of acute otitis media during the previous year

    b. The child is 3 years old and has oral thrush that is unresolved with treatment

    c. The child has been admitted to the hospital three times within the last year with pneumonia

    d. The child has been diagnosed with a severe case of acute sinusitis during the last year

    e. The child has taken antibiotics for the last 3 months without evidence of clearing of the infection

14. The young child is diagnosed with acute otitis media. The child's mother states that the child had a severe reaction to penicillin in the past. Which of the following statements by the nurse indicates that further education is required? Select all that apply.

    a. "You may want to look into desensitization techniques."

    b. "It is important for you to share this information with any future physician."

    c. "Here is your prescription for cephalexin from the physician."

    d. "Here is your prescription from the physician for penicillin V."

    e. "Desensitization procedures are performed in an acute care setting."

15. The young girl has been diagnosed with JIA and has been prescribed methotrexate. Which of the following statements by the child's parent indicates that adequate learning has occurred?

    a. "We'll need to bring her back in for some lab tests after she starts methotrexate."

    b. "She can take methotrexate with yogurt or chocolate milk."

    c. "She may start feeling better by next week."

    d. "Swimming sounds like a good exercise for her."

    e. "A warm bath before bed might help her sleep better."

# CHAPTER 27

# Nursing Care of the Child with an Endocrine Disorder

## Learning Objectives

- Describe the major components and functions of a child's endocrine system.
- Differentiate between the anatomic and physiologic differences of the endocrine system in children and adults.
- Identify the essential assessment elements, common diagnostic procedures, and laboratory tests associated with the diagnosis of endocrine disorders in children.
- Identify the common medications and treatment modalities used for palliation of endocrine disorders in children.
- Distinguish specific disorders of the endocrine system affecting children.
- Link the clinical manifestations of specific disorders in the endocrine system of a child with the appropriate nursing diagnoses.
- Establish the nursing outcomes, evaluative criteria, and interventions for a child with specific disorders in the endocrine system.
- Develop child/family teaching plans for the child with an endocrine disorder.

## SECTION I: ASSESSING YOUR UNDERSTANDING

### Activity A FILL IN THE BLANKS

1. Insulin is developed and secreted by beta cells, located in the islets of _Langerhans_ in the pancreas.

2. Ophthalmic changes, due to hyperthyroidism, include _enophthalmus_, which is less pronounced in children.

3. The most common initial symptoms of diabetes mellitus reported are _polyuria_ and polydipsia.

4. Twitching of the extremities, referred to as _tetany_, is related to hypocalcemia in children with hypoparathyroidism.

5. Slow, deep _Kussmaul_ respirations are characteristic of air hunger during metabolic acidosis.

6. Dwarfism is due to a growth hormone _deficiency_.

7. The presence of a goiter is typically associated with _hyperthyroidism_.

## Activity B LABELING

*Circle the areas on the body corresponding with insulin injection sites.*

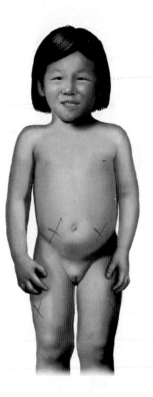
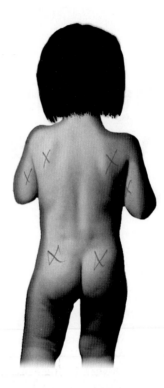

## Activity C MATCHING

*Match the gland in Column A with the proper word or phrase in Column B.*

**Column A**

_e_ **1.** Adrenal gland

_c_ **2.** Pancreas

_b_ **3.** Parathyroid

_a_ **4.** Thymus

_d_ **5.** Thyroid

**Column B**

**a.** Humoral factors

**b.** Calcium and phosphorus concentration

**c.** Glucagon and somatostatin

**d.** Calcium and phosphorus homeostasis

**e.** Mineralocorticoids

## Activity D SEQUENCING

*Place the following insulin types in the proper order of their onset times:*

**1.** Lispro

**2.** NPH

**3.** Regular

**4.** Ultralente

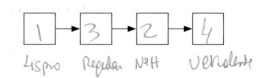

## Activity E SHORT ANSWERS

*Briefly answer the following.*

1. What are the teaching topics needed to educate parents of children with diabetes mellitus?

_____

_____

_____

2. List signs and symptoms of hypothyroidism and hyperthyroidism.

_____

_____

_____

3. What are the nursing implications when teaching, discussing, and caring for children with diabetes mellitus in the following age groups: (a) infants and toddlers, (b) preschoolers, (c) school age, (d) and adolescent?

_____

_____

_____

4. Discuss how *Healthy People 2020* suggests addressing the goal of reducing the annual number of new cases of diagnosed diabetes in the population.

_____

_____

_____

5. What teaching points should the nurse discuss with the parents of a child receiving growth hormone in regards to possible adverse reactions?

_____

_____

_____

# SECTION II: APPLYING YOUR KNOWLEDGE

## Activity F CASE STUDY

A 12-year-old boy is admitted to the pediatric unit with weakness, fatigue, blurred vision, headaches, and mood and behavior changes. After further assessment he was diagnosed with diabetes mellitus type 2 (DM type 2). His mother states, "I know a little about diabetes and I thought type 2 diabetes was seen only in adults?"

1. How would you address the mother's question?

_____

_____

_____

2. What will be the focus of your nursing management for Carlos and his family?

_____

_____

_____

3. What challenges may you anticipate with educating Carlos?

_____

_____

_____

# SECTION III: PRACTICING FOR NCLEX

**Activity G** **NCLEX-STYLE QUESTIONS**

*Answer the following questions.*

1. The nurse is providing acute care for an 11-year-old boy with hypoparathyroidism. Which of the following is the priority intervention?

   a. Providing administration of calcium and vitamin D

   b. Ensuring patency of the IV site to prevent tissue damage

   c. Monitoring fluid intake and urinary calcium output

   d. Administering intravenous calcium gluconate as ordered

2. The nurse is assessing a 4-year-old girl with ambiguous genitalia. Which of the following findings would be consistent with congenital adrenal hyperplasia?

   a. Auscultation reveals irregular heartbeat

   b. Observing pubic hair and hirsutism

   c. Palpation elicits pain from constipation

   d. Observing hyperpigmentation of the skin

3. The nurse is assessing a 7-year-old girl who complains of headache, is irritable, and vomiting. Her health history reveals she has had meningitis. Which of the following is the priority intervention?

   a. Notifying the physician of the neurologic findings

   b. Setting up safety precautions to prevent injury

   c. Monitoring urine volume and specific gravity

   d. Restoring fluid balance with IV sodium chloride

4. The nurse is caring for a 4-year-old boy during a growth hormone stimulation test. Which of the following is a priority task for the care of this child?

   a. Providing a wet washcloth to suck on

   b. Educating family about side effects

   c. Monitoring blood glucose levels

   d. Monitoring intake and output

5. The nurse is assessing a 1-month-old girl who, according to the mother, doesn't eat well. Which of the following assessments would suggest the child has congenital hypothyroidism?

   a. Mother reports frequent diarrhea

   b. Observation of an enlarged tongue

   c. Auscultation reveals tachycardia

   d. Palpation reveals warm, moist skin

6. The nurse is caring for an obese 15-year-old girl who missed two periods and is afraid she is pregnant. Which of the following findings would indicate polycystic ovary syndrome?

   a. Observation of acanthosis nigricans

   b. Complains of blurred vision and headaches

   c. Auscultation reveals increased respiratory rate

   d. Palpation reveals hypertrophy and weakness

7. The nurse is assessing a 16-year-old boy who has had long-term corticosteroid therapy. Which of the following findings, along with the use of the corticosteroids, would indicate Cushing's disease?

   a. History of rapid weight gain

   b. Observing a round, child-like face

   c. Observing high weight to height ratio

   d. Observing delayed dentition

8. The nurse is caring for a 10-year-old girl with hyperparathyroidism. Which of the following would be a primary nursing diagnosis for this child?

   a. Disturbed body image related to hormone dysfunction

   b. Imbalanced nutrition: more than body requirements

   c. Deficient fluid volume related to electrolyte imbalance

   d. Deficient knowledge related to treatment of the disease

9. The nurse is teaching an 11-year-old boy and his family how to manage his diabetes. Which of the following does not focus on glucose management?

   a. Teaching that 50% of daily calories should be carbohydrates

   b. Instructing the child to rotate injection sites to decrease scar formation

   c. Encouraging the child to maintain the proper injection schedule

   d. Promoting higher levels of exercise than previously maintained

10. The nurse is caring for a 12-year-old girl with hypothyroidism. Which of the following will be part of the nurse's teaching plan for the child and family?

    a. Educating how to recognize vitamin D toxicity

    b. Teaching how to maintain fluid intake regimens

    c. Teaching to administer methimazole with meals

    d. Instructing to report irritability or anxiety

11. The child has developed hypothyroidism and has been prescribed sodium L-thyroxine. The starting dose is 12 mg/kg of body weight each day. The child weighs 72 pounds. Calculate the child's dose in micrograms and round to the nearest whole number.

12. Rank the different types of insulin based on their duration of action beginning with the shortest to the longest duration.

    a. Humulin N

    b. Lispro

    c. Lantus

    d. Humulin R

    b d A c

13. The young child has been diagnosed with a secondary growth hormone deficiency. The child weighs 58 pounds. The physician orders the child to receive 0.2 mg of growth hormone for each kilogram of body weight per week, divided into daily doses. How many milligrams of growth hormone would the child receive with each dose? Round to the thousandths place.

14. Which of the following male/female may have delayed puberty? Select all that apply.

    a. The 14-year old female has not developed breasts

    b. The 13-year old female has no pubic hair

    c. The 15-year old male has had no changes to the size of testicles

    d. The 14-year old male has no pubic hair

    e. The 13-year old male has no changes in the appearance of his scrotum

15. The child may have developed thyroid storm. Which of the following are clinical manifestations of thyroid storm? Select all that apply.

    a. The child's temperature is 103.2F

    b. The child's linen is wet and the child complains of feeling "sweaty"

    c. The child's apical heart rate is 172 beats per minute

    d. The child states he feels very tired and wants to take a nap

    e. The child has been mild-mannered and compliant

# CHAPTER 28

# Nursing Care of the Child with a Neoplastic Disorder

## Learning Objectives

- Compare childhood and adult cancers.
- Describe nursing care related to common laboratory and diagnostic testing used in the medical diagnosis of pediatric cancer.
- Identify types of cancer common in infants, children, and adolescents.
- Identify appropriate nursing assessments and interventions related to medications and treatments for pediatric cancer.
- Develop an individualized nursing care plan for the child with cancer.
- Describe the psychosocial impact of cancer on children and their families.
- Devise a nutrition plan for the child with cancer.
- Develop child/family teaching plans for the child with cancer.

## SECTION I: ASSESSING YOUR UNDERSTANDING

### Activity A  FILL IN THE BLANKS

1. Presence of a tumor in the _mediastinal_ region can cause a child with cancer to complain of chest pain or shortness of breath.

2. Retinoblastoma may be identified by the presence of _leukocoria_ in one or both eyes

3. Untreated, neutropenia can lead to _sepsis_ and should be treated with IV antibiotics immediately.

4. Nursing care for a child receiving treatment for cancer focuses on _prevention_ and palliation of side effects.

5. Bone cancer may be treated with a combination of _limb salvage_ procedure, radiation, and chemotherapy.

6. _Leukemia_ is the most frequently occurring type of childhood cancer.

7. A _clinical trial_ is a carefully designed research study that assesses the effectiveness of a treatment as well as its acute and long-term effects on the patient.

## Activity B   LABELING

*Place an X on the most common locations where rhabdomyosarcoma occurs.*

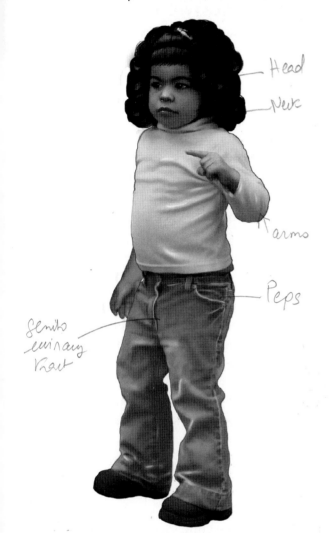

Head

Neck

arms

Peps

Genito
urinary
tract

## Activity C   MATCHING

*Match the medical treatment in Column A with the proper word or phrase in Column B.*

**Column A**

__c__ **1.** Biopsy

__b__ **2.** Central venous catheter

__d__ **3.** Implanted port

__e__ **4.** Leukapheresis

__a__ **5.** Radiation therapy

**Column B**

**a.** High-energy X-ray

**b.** Long-term IV medication

**c.** May be done with needle

**d.** Vena cava or subclavian vein

**e.** White blood cell extraction

## Activity D   SEQUENCING

*Place the following phases of the cell cycle in the proper order:*

**1.** G0

**2.** G1

**3.** G2

**4.** M

**5.** S

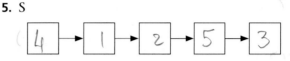

| 4 | 1 | 2 | 5 | 3 |

## Activity E   SHORT ANSWERS

*Briefly answer the following.*

**1.** Describe the signs and symptoms of rhabdomyosarcoma based on the location of the tumor.

_____

_____

_____

**2.** Name the eight drugs discussed in this chapter that help prevent or palliate the effects of chemotherapy and other tests and therapies.

_____

_____

_____

**3.** Name the five kinds of imaging used to diagnose cancer. Briefly describe how they work, what information they provide, and what the nursing implications are.

_____

_____

_____

**4.** Discuss three ways how childhood cancer differs from adult cancer.

_____

_____

_____

**5.** Discuss how chemotherapy agents work in relation to the cell cycle.

_____

_____

_____

# SECTION II: APPLYING YOUR KNOWLEDGE

## Activity F   CASE STUDY

A 4-year-old boy is brought to the clinic by his parents due to fever. After further assessment the diagnosis of acute lymphoblastic leukemia (ALL) was confirmed. The child was admitted to your unit and started on treatment immediately. Upon assessment and review of his lab work today you find his temperature to be 101.2°F, HR 100, RR 24. His absolute neutrophil count (ANC) is <500.

1. What will be your priority nursing interventions?

   _____

   _____

   _____

2. One week later, John is ready to be discharged home and will receive his treatment in the outpatient setting. What education will you review with the family regarding preventing infection?

   _____

   _____

   _____

3. The mother asks, "How can we help John's development not fall behind other children his age?"

   _____

   _____

   _____

# SECTION III: PRACTICING FOR NCLEX

## Activity G   NCLEX-STYLE QUESTIONS

*Answer the following questions.*

1. The nurse is teaching the parents of a 15-year-old boy who is being treated for acute myelogenous leukemia about the side effects of chemotherapy. For which of the following symptoms should the parents seek medical care immediately?

   **a.** Earache, stiff neck, or sore throat

   **b.** Blisters, ulcers, or a rash appear

   **c.** A temperature of 101°F or greater

   **d.** Difficulty or pain when swallowing

2. The nurse is assessing a 2-year-old girl whose parents noticed that one of her pupils appeared to be white. Which of the following findings is typical of retinoblastoma? (Select all that apply)

   **a.** Observation of eyes reveals yellow discharge

   **b.** Parents report that the child has headaches

   **c.** Observation confirms cat's eye reflex in pupil

   **d.** Assessment discloses hyphema in one eye

   **e.** Usually diagnosed when the child is over the age of 7 years

3. The nurse is providing preoperative care for a 7-year-old boy with a brain tumor and his parents. Which of the following is the priority intervention?

   **a.** Assessing the child's level of consciousness

   **b.** Providing a tour of the intensive care unit

   **c.** Educating the child and parents about shunts

   **d.** Having him talk to a child who has had this surgery

4. The nurse is assessing a 14-year-old girl with a tumor. Which of the following findings would indicate Ewing's sarcoma?

   a. Child complains of dull bone pain just below her knee

   b. Palpation reveals swelling and redness on the right ribs

   c. Child complains of persistent pain from minor ankle injury

   d. Palpation discloses asymptomatic mass on the upper back

5. The nurse is teaching a group of 13-year-old boys and girls about screening and prevention of reproductive cancers. Which of the following subjects would not be included in the nurse's teaching plan? (Select all that apply)

   a. Self examination is an effective screening method for testicular cancer

   b. Testicular cancer is one of the most difficult cancers to cure

   c. A papanicolaou smear does not require parent consent in most states

   d. Sexually transmitted disease is a risk factor for cervical cancer

   e. Provide information regarding the benefits of receiving the HPV vaccine

6. The nurse is caring for a 4-year-old boy following surgical removal of a stage I neuroblastoma. Which of the following interventions will be most appropriate for this child?

   a. Applying aloe vera lotion to irradiated areas of skin

   b. Administering antiemetics as prescribed for nausea

   c. Giving medications as ordered via least invasive route

   d. Maintaining isolation as prescribed to avoid infection

7. The nurse is caring for a 6-year-old girl with leukemia who is having an oncological emergency. Which of the following signs and symptoms would indicate hyperleukocytosis?

   a. Bradycardia and distinct S1 and S2 sounds

   b. Wheezing and diminished breath sounds

   c. Respiratory distress and poor perfusion

   d. Tachycardia and respiratory distress

8. The nurse is assessing a 3-year-old boy whose mother complains that he is listless and has been having trouble swallowing. Which of the following findings would suggest the child has a brain tumor?

   a. Observation reveals nystagmus and head tilt

   b. Vital signs show blood pressure measures 120/80

   c. Examination shows temperature of 38.5°C and headache

   d. Observation reveals a cough and labored breathing

9. The nurse is assessing a 4-year-old girl whose mother complains that she is not eating well, is losing weight, and has started vomiting after eating. Which of the following risk factors from the health history would suggest the child may have a Wilm's tumor?

   a. The child has Down syndrome

   b. The child has Beckwith–Wiedemann syndrome

   c. The child has Schwachman syndrome

   d. There is a family history of neurofibromatosis

10. The nurse is educating the parents of a 16-year-old boy who has just been diagnosed with Hodgkin's disease. Which of the following subjects would be most appropriate at this time?

    a. Describing the two ways of staging the disease

    b. Telling about the drugs and side effects of chemotherapy

    c. Informing the parents about postoperative care

    d. Explaining how to care for skin after radiation therapy

11. The child has been diagnosed with cancer and is being treated with chemotherapy. Which of the following findings are most likely common side effects of this type of treatment? Select all that apply.

    a. The child's mother states, "It seems like he catches every bug that comes along."

    b. The child's teeth are enlarged

    c. The child has no hair on his head

    d. The child's mother states that she often has to repeat herself because he can't hear very well

    e. The child is complaining of feeling nauseated

12. The child has been prescribed chemotherapy. In order to properly calculate the child's dose, the nurse must first figure the child's body surface area (BSA). The child is 130 cm tall and weighs 27 kg. Calculate the child's BSA and round to the hundredths place.

13. The child has been diagnosed with leukemia. Rank the following medications used to treat leukemia in order based on the stage of treatment.

    a. The child is receiving chemotherapy through an intrathecal catheter

    b. The child is receiving high doses of mercaptopurine and methotrexate

    c. The child is receiving low doses of mercaptopurine and methotrexate

    d. The child is receiving vincristine through an intravenous line and oral steroids

14. The physician requests the nurse to calculate the child's ANC. The complete blood count indicates that the child's "segs" are 14%, bands are 9%, and white blood cells (WBC) are 15,000. Calculate the child's absolute neutrophil count.

15. The child has been admitted to the hospital. Her absolute neutrophil count is 450 and the child has been placed in neutropenic precautions. Which of the following nursing interventions indicates that the nurse requires further education? Select all that apply.

    a. The child has been placed in a semiprivate room

    b. The child is being transported to radiology for an X-ray and the nurse places gloves on the child's hands

    c. The nurse monitors the child's vital signs every 2 to 4 hours

    d. The nurse assesses the child for clinical manifestations of an infection every 4 to 8 hours

    e. The nurse carefully washes his hands before and after providing care for the child

# CHAPTER 29

# Nursing Care of the Child with a Genetic Disorder

## Learning Objectives

- Discuss various inheritance patterns, including nontraditional patterns of inheritance.
- Discuss ethical and legal issues associated with genetic testing.
- Discuss genetic counseling and the role of the nurse.
- Discuss the nurse's role and responsibilities when caring for a child diagnosed with a genetic disorder and his/her family.
- Identify nursing interventions related to common laboratory and diagnostic tests used in the diagnosis and management of genetic conditions.
- Distinguish various genetic disorders occurring in childhood.
- Devise an individualized nursing care plan for the child with a genetic disorder.
- Develop child/family teaching plans for the child with a genetic disorder.

## SECTION I: ASSESSING YOUR UNDERSTANDING

### Activity A  FILL IN THE BLANKS

1. Many time genes for the same trait have two or more _____ or versions that may be expressed.

2. Close blood relationship, referred to as _____, is a risk factor for genetic disorders.

3. The physical appearance, or _____, is the expression of a dominant gene or two recessive genes.

4. When a child receives different genes from the mother and father for the same trait, the child's genes are _____, and usually the dominant gene will be expressed.

5. Trisomy 21 is a disorder caused by _____ or an error in cell division during meiosis.

6. The _____ of an organism is its entire hereditary information encoded in the DNA.

7. A _____ is a long, continuous strand of DNA that carries genetic information.

## Activity B MATCHING

*Match the disorder in Column A with the phrase in Column B*

**Column A**

_____ **1.** Achondroplasia

_____ **2.** Apert syndrome

_____ **3.** CHARGE syndrome

_____ **4.** Marfan syndrome

_____ **5.** VATER association

**Column B**

**a.** No single feature present in all individuals

**b.** Not a diagnosis

**c.** Disorder of connective tissue

**d.** Disordered growth

**e.** Older paternal age

## Activity C SHORT ANSWERS

*Briefly answer the following.*

**1.** Describe at least five major complications a child with Down syndrome can experience.

_____

_____

_____

**2.** Summarize the guiding principles for nurses providing support and education to families of children with genetic abnormalities.

_____

_____

_____

**3.** Briefly describe how the four errors of metabolism disorders are associated with specific odors of a child's excretions.

_____

_____

_____

**4.** Discuss the incidence of Trisomy 21.

_____

_____

_____

**5.** What are the common clinical manifestations that would alert the nurse to the likelihood that an infant has Trisomy 13?

_____

_____

_____

# SECTION II: APPLYING YOUR KNOWLEDGE

## Activity D CASE STUDY

A 1-week-old baby girl named Chloe is seen in your clinic secondary to abnormal newborn screening results. Her mother states, "Chloe has been doing great. She eats well, every 2 to 3 hours. I do not understand why we are here today. The nurse called and mentioned something about an inborn error of metabolism. I do not understand what that is and how Chloe could have that? She is not even sick."

**1.** How would you address the mother's concerns?

_____

_____

_____

**2.** The newborn screen came back positive for a fatty acid oxidation disorder, medium-chain acyl-CoA dehydrogenase deficiency. After further testing the diagnosis was confirmed. What education and nursing management will you provide?

_____

_____

_____

# SECTION III: PRACTICING FOR NCLEX

## Activity E NCLEX-STYLE QUESTIONS

*Answer the following questions.*

1. The nurse is assessing a newborn boy. Which of the following findings would indicate the possibility of the disorder neurofibromatosis? (Select all that apply)
   a. History shows a grandparent had neurofibromatosis
   b. Measurement shows a slightly larger head size
   c. Inspection discloses several café au lait spots on the trunk
   d. Observation reveals freckles on the lower extremities
   e. Abnormal curvature of the spine

2. The nurse is caring for a 9-year-old girl with Marfan syndrome. Which of the following interventions would be part of the nursing plan of care for this child? (Select all that apply)
   a. Arranging for respiratory therapy at home
   b. Promoting annual ophthalmology examinations
   c. Monitoring for bone and joint problems
   d. Encourage use of antibiotics before dentistry
   e. Including in home physical therapy

3. The nurse is examining an 8-year-old boy with chromosomal abnormalities. Which of the following signs and symptoms suggest the boy has Angelman syndrome?
   a. Palpation discloses reduced muscular tonicity
   b. Observation reveals moonlike round face
   c. History shows surgery for cleft palate repair
   d. Observation shows jerky ataxic movement

4. The nurse is counseling a couple who are concerned that the woman has achondroplasia in her family. The woman is not affected. Which of the following statements by the couple indicates the need for more teaching?
   a. "If the mother has the gene, then there is a 50% chance of passing it on."
   b. "If the father doesn't have the gene, then his son won't have achondroplasia."
   c. "If the father has the gene, then there is a 50% chance of passing it on."
   d. "Since neither one of us has the disorder, we won't pass it on."

5. The nurse is caring for an 8-year-old girl who has just been diagnosed with fragile X syndrome. Which of the following interventions would be the priority?
   a. Explain care required due to the disorder
   b. Assess family's ability to learn about the disorder
   c. Educate the family about available resources
   d. Screen to determine current level of functioning

6. The nurse is assessing a 2-week-old boy who was born at home and has not had metabolic screening. Which of the following signs or symptoms would indicate phenylketonuria?
   a. Palpation reveals increased reflex action
   b. Observation shows signs of jaundice
   c. Detection of a musty odor to the urine
   d. The parents report the child has seizures

7. The nurse is examining a 2-year-old girl with Vater association. Which of the following signs or symptoms would be noted?
   a. Observation that the child has a hearing aid
   b. Inspection reveals underdeveloped labia
   c. Assessment of the eye reveals a cleft in the iris
   d. History of corrective surgery for anal atresia

8. The nurse is assessing infants in the newborn nursery. Which of the following assessments would be indicative of a major anomaly?

   a. A 12-hour Caucasian male with café au lait macules on his trunk

   b. A 16-hour African American male with polydactyly

   c. A set of Indian identical twin females with syndactyly

   d. A 4-hour Asian female with protruding ears

9. The nurse is caring for a newborn girl with galactosemia. Which of the following interventions will be necessary for her health?

   a. Adhering to a low phenylalanine diet

   b. Eliminating dairy products from her diet

   c. Eating frequent meals and never fasting

   d. Lifetime supplementation with thiamine

10. The nurse is assessing a 3-year-old boy with Sturge–Weber syndrome. Which of the following findings is most indicative of the disorder?

    a. Record shows the boy has seizures

    b. Observation shows behavior problems

    c. Inspection reveals a port wine stain

    d. Observation indicates mild retardation

11. The nurse is interviewing parents after their newborn was diagnosed with a genetic disorder. Which of the following statements by the mother is associated with risk factors of genetic disorders? (Select all that apply)

    a. "Our obstetrician told us that I wasn't making enough amniotic fluid during this pregnancy."

    b. "My husband is 55 years old."

    c. "Our alpha-fetoprotein came back negative when I was 18 weeks pregnant."

    d. "My sister's baby was born with trisomy 18."

    e. "He is our first child."

12. The 14-year-old boy may have Klinefelter syndrome. Which of the following findings is associated with this genetic disorder? (Select all that apply)

    a. He has a long trunk and short legs

    b. He is shorter than average for his age

    c. He has been diagnosed with dyslexia

    d. His scrotum is smaller than normal

    e. He has developed a significant amount of breast tissue

13. The experienced pediatric nurse is quizzing a student nurse regarding the appearance of a newborn with trisomy 18. Which of the following statements by the student nurse indicates the need for further education? (Select all that apply)

    a. "This newborn may have a very small head."

    b. "This newborn may have extra fingers or toes."

    c. "This newborn may have a major heart problem."

    d. "This newborn may have webbed fingers and toes."

    e. "This newborn may have ears that look like they are placed low."

14. The nursing student is studying patterns of inheritance regarding genetic disorders. The student demonstrates understanding when recognizing that monogetic disorders include which of the following? (Select all that apply)

    a. Autosomal dominant

    b. Autosomal recessive

    c. X-linked dominant

    d. Mitochondrial inheritance

    e. Genomic imprinting

15. The experienced nurse works for an obstetrician. Which of the following couples may benefit from genetic counseling? (Select all that apply)

    a. The mother-to-be is 29 years old

    b. The father-to-be is 58 years old

    c. The parents-to-be are cousins

    d. The parents-to-be are African American

    e. The parents-to-be have a child who was born blind and deaf

# CHAPTER 30

# Nursing Care of the Child with a Cognitive or Mental Health Disorder

## Learning Objectives

- Discuss the impact of alterations in mental health upon the growth and development of infants, children, and adolescents.
- Describe the techniques used to evaluate the status of mental health in children.
- Identify appropriate nursing assessments and interventions related to therapy and medications for the treatment of childhood and adolescent mental health disorders.
- Distinguish mental health disorders common in infants, children, and adolescents.
- Develop an individualized nursing care plan for the child with a mental health disorder.
- Develop child/family teaching plans for the child with a mental health disorder.

# SECTION I: ASSESSING YOUR UNDERSTANDING

### Activity A  FILL IN THE BLANKS

1. Purging is self-induced vomiting or evacuation of the _____.

2. For a diagnosis of attention-deficit/hyperactivity disorder (ADHD), the symptoms of impulsivity and hyperactivity begin before 7 years of age and must persist longer than _____ months.

3. Children with _____ experience difficulty with reading, writing, and spelling.

4. Burns that appear in a _____ or glove pattern are highly suspicious of inflicted burns.

5. _____ is defined as failure to provide a child with appropriate food, clothing, shelter, medical care, and schooling.

6. A disorder in which an adult meets her own psychological needs by having an ill child is known as _____.

7. Pervasive developmental disorder is another name for _____.

## Activity B  LABELING

*Mark an X on all of the areas that indicate injury sites that are suspicious for abuse.*

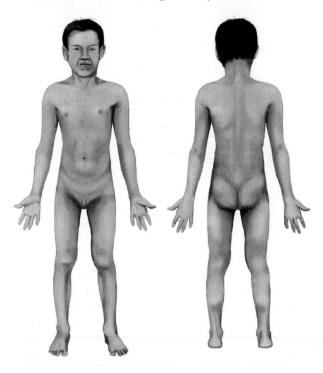

## Activity C  MATCHING

*Match the term in Column A with the proper definition in Column B*

**Column A**

_____ **1.** Affect

_____ **2.** Anxiety

_____ **3.** Binging

_____ **4.** Dysgraphia

_____ **5.** Dyscalculia

**Column B**

**a.** Feelings of dread, worry, discomfort

**b.** Emotional reaction associated with an experience

**c.** Problems with math and computation

**d.** Rapid excessive consumption of food or drink

**e.** Difficulty producing the written word

## Activity D  SHORT ANSWERS

*Briefly answer the following.*

1. What are some common behavior management techniques that can be utilized in the hospital, clinic, classroom, or home setting?

   _____

   _____

   _____

2. According to the text, what common laboratory and diagnostic studies are ordered for the assessment of abuse?

   _____

   _____

   _____

3. What is generalized anxiety disorder?

   _____

   _____

   _____

4. Discuss the data that should be collected if the nurse suspects an adolescent patient is suffering from depression.

   _____

   _____

   _____

5. What are the common classifications of medications used to treat ADHD and what is the intended goal of medication treatment?

   _____

   _____

   _____

# SECTION II: APPLYING YOUR KNOWLEDGE

## Activity E CASE STUDY

Elisa, a 6-month-old female is seen in your clinic for her wellness check-up. Her mother states "I have seen so much about autism in the news lately. What is autism and how would I know if Elisa has this disorder?"

**1.** How would you explain autism to Elisa's mother?

_____

_____

_____

**2.** What signs and symptoms would be exhibited by an infant or toddler who has autism?

_____

_____

_____

# SECTION III: PRACTICING FOR NCLEX

## Activity F NCLEX-STYLE QUESTIONS

*Answer the following questions.*

**1.** The nurse is conducting a well child assessment of a 3-year-old. Which of the following statements by the parents would warrant further investigation?

a. "He spends a lot of time playing with his little cars"

b. "He spends hours repeatedly lining up his cars"

c. "He is very active and keeps very busy"

d. "He would rather run around than sit on my lap and read a book"

**2.** The mother of a 10-year-old boy with attention deficit/hyperactivity disorder contacts the school nurse. She is upset because her son has been made to feel different by his peers because he has to visit the nurse's office for a lunch time dose of medication. The boy is threatening to stop taking his medication. How should the nurse respond?

a. "He should ignore the children, he needs this medication"

b. "I can have the teacher speak with the other children"

c. "You may want to talk to your physician about an extended release medication"

d. "Remind him that his schoolwork may deteriorate"

**3.** The nurse is conducting an examination of a boy with Tourette's syndrome. Which of the following would the nurse expect to observe?

a. Toe walking

b. Sudden, rapid stereotypical sounds

c. Spinning and hand flapping

d. Lack of eye contact

**4.** A nurse is providing a routine wellness examination and follow-up for a 3-year-old recently diagnosed with autism spectrum disorder. Which of the following responses indicates a need for additional referral or follow-up?

a. "We have recently completed his individualized education plan"

b. "We really like the treatment plan that has been created by his school"

c. "We try to be flexible and change his routine from day to day"

d. "We have a couple of baby sitters who know how to handle his needs"

**5.** A nurse is caring for a child with intellectual disability. The medical chart indicates an IQ of 37. The nurse understands that the degree of disability is classified as which of the following?

a. Mild

b. Moderate

c. Severe

d. Profound

6. A nurse is caring for a 10-year-old intellectually disabled girl hospitalized for a scheduled cholecystectomy. The girl expresses fear related to her hospitalization and unfamiliar surroundings. How should the nurse respond?

   a. "Don't worry, you will be going home soon"

   b. "Tell me about a typical day at home"

   c. "Have you talked to your parents about this?"

   d. "Do you want some art supplies?"

7. The nurse is caring for a girl with anorexia who has been hospitalized with unstable vital signs and food refusal. The girl requires enteral nutrition. The nurse is alert for which of the complications that signal re-feeding syndrome?

   a. Cardiac arrhythmias, confusion, seizures

   b. Orthostatic hypotension

   c. Hypothermia and irregular pulse

   d. Bradycardia with ectopy

8. A nurse is conducting a physical examination of an adolescent girl with suspected bulimia. Which of the following assessment findings would the nurse expect to note?

   a. Eroded dental enamel

   b. Dry sallow skin

   c. Soft sparse body hair

   d. Thinning scalp hair

9. The nurse is examining a child with fetal alcohol syndrome. Which of the following assessment findings would the nurse expect to note?

   a. Macrocephaly

   b. Low nasal bridge with short upturned nose

   c. Clubbing of fingers

   d. Short filtrum with thick upper lip

10. The nurse is providing teaching about medication management of attention deficit hyperactivity disorder. Which of the following responses indicates a need for further teaching?

    a. "We should give it to him after he eats breakfast"

    b. "This may cause him to have difficulty sleeping"

    c. "If he takes this medicine he will no longer have ADHD"

    d. "We should see an improvement in his schoolwork"

11. The school-aged child has been diagnosed with dysgraphia and dyslexia. Which of the following findings may be present? Select all that apply.

    a. The child experiences difficulty when asked to hop on one foot

    b. The child experiences difficulty when asked to add and subtract numbers

    c. The child experiences difficulty when asked to jump rope

    d. The child experiences difficulty when asked to write words

    e. The child experiences difficulty when asked to spell his name

12. The 18-month-old toddler has been brought into the pediatrician's office by his parents. Which of the following findings are warning signs that the toddler may be autistic based on what he should be able to do according to his age? Select all that apply.

    a. The parents stated that the toddler has never "babbled"

    b. The toddler does not exhibit attempts to communicate by pointing to objects

    c. The child does not use any words

    d. The child does not speak in short sentences

    e. The child cannot jump rope

13. The child has been diagnosed with attention deficit hyperactivity disorder and has been prescribed Ritalin (methylphenidate). Which of the following findings are most likely adverse effects related to this type of medication? Select all that apply.

    a. The child has gained weight since beginning Ritalin

    b. The child complains that his head hurts at times

    c. The child's parents state that he sleeps much longer than he used to

    d. The child has been more irritable since beginning Ritalin

    e. The child complains that he has developed abdominal pain

**14.** The child has been diagnosed with a mental health disorder and the child's parents are beginning to incorporate behavior management techniques. Which of the following statements by the child's parent indicates the need for further education? Select all that apply.

   **a.** "I use a higher pitched voice when I communicate with her."

   **b.** "I am quick to point out the things that she does that make me crazy."

   **c.** "We have set some boundaries that are nonnegotiable."

   **d.** "We tell her when she is doing something well."

   **e.** "We're trying to make her accountable and responsible for her own behavior."

**15.** The parents of an adolescent are concerned about his mental health and have brought the adolescent into the physician's office for an evaluation. Which of the following statements by the child's parents indicates that the child may have a mental health disorder? Select all that apply.

   **a.** "He has started sleeping for only 3 hours each night."

   **b.** "He has lost 10 pounds over the last 4 months."

   **c.** "He hangs out with the same kids he always has."

   **d.** "He used to be a straight-A student and now he's bringing home Cs and Ds."

   **e.** "He still enjoys playing a lot of baseball."

# CHAPTER 31

# Nursing Care during a Pediatric Emergency

## Learning Objectives

- Identify various factors contributing to emergency situations among infants and children.
- Discuss common treatments and medications used during pediatric emergencies.
- Conduct a health history of a child in an emergency situation, specific to the emergency.
- Perform a rapid cardiopulmonary assessment.
- Discuss common laboratory and other diagnostic tests used during pediatric emergencies.
- Integrate the principles of the American Heart Association (AHA) and Pediatric Advanced Life Support (PALS) in the comprehensive management of pediatric emergencies, such as respiratory arrest, shock, cardiac arrest, near drowning, poisoning, and trauma.

# SECTION I: ASSESSING YOUR UNDERSTANDING

### Activity A  FILL IN THE BLANKS

1. Children as old as 18 years of age should be managed using the _pediatric_ advanced life support guidelines.

2. Use the mnemonic _LEAN_ to remember which drugs may be given via the tracheal route

3. The assessment and management of the _Airway_ of a prearresting or arresting child is always the first intervention in a pediatric emergency situation.

4. A nonreactive _pupil_ indicates the need for immediate relief of increased intracranial pressure.

5. Circumoral pallor or _cyanosis_ is a late and often ominous sign of respiratory distress.

6. To open the airway of a victim suspected of having a neck injury the rescuer should utilize the _jaw thrust_ technique.

7. The best place to check the pulse in a child is either at the _femoral_ or carotid site.

## Activity B LABELING

*Identify the arrhythmia by placing the proper arrhythmia type under the appropriate illustration*

1. Supraventricular tachycardia
2. Ventricular tachycardia
3. Sinus tachycardia
4. Coarse ventricular fibrillation

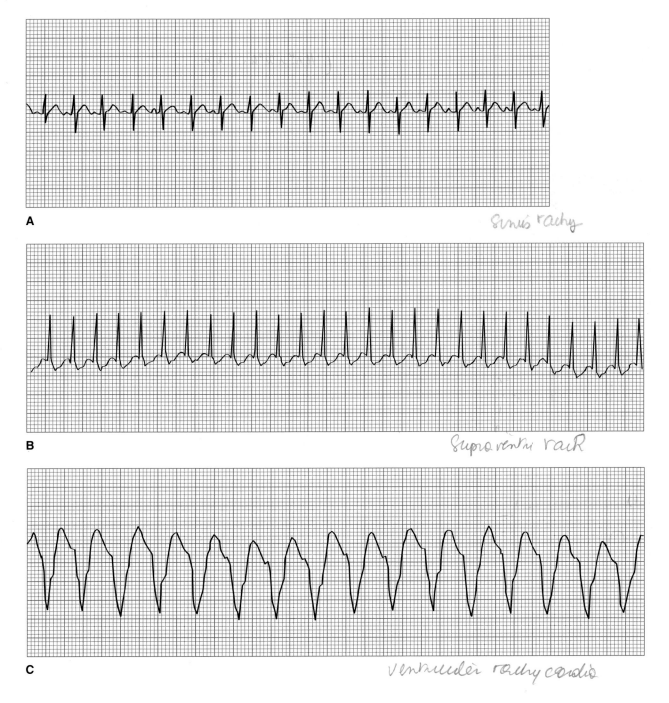

A

*Sinus tachy*

B

*Supraventri tach*

C

*Ventricular tachycardia*

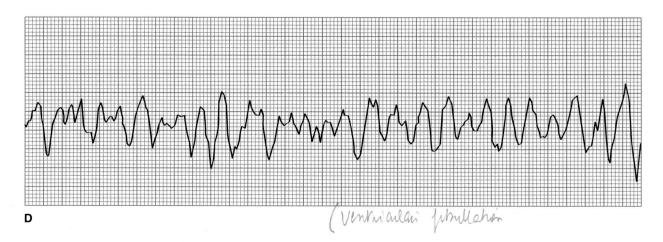

**D**    *(Ventricular fibrillation)*

1. Supraventricular tachycardia (SVT): note rate above 220, abnormal P waves, no beat-to-beat variability.
2. Ventricular tachycardia: rapid and regular rhythm, wide QRS without P waves.
3. Sinus tachycardia: normal QRS and P waves, mild beat-to-beat variability.
4. Coarse ventricular fibrillation: chaotic electrical activity.

**Activity C** MATCHING

*Match the test in Column A with the correct statement in Column B*

| Column A | Column B |
|---|---|
| *c* 1. Arterial blood gas | a. Usually available in emergency department |
| *a* 2. Chest X-ray | b. Accompany the child to observe and manage |
| *b* 3. Computerized tomography | c. Never delay resuscitation efforts pending results |
| *e* 4. Toxicology panel | d. Notify lab of drugs the child is taking |
| *d* 5. Urinalysis | e. Standards vary with agency used |

**Activity D** SEQUENCING

*Place the following CPR steps in the proper order:*

1. Administer 100% oxygen   3
2. Evaluate heart rate and pulses   *end*
3. Look, listen, feel for respirations   4
4. Position to open airway   1
5. Suction   2

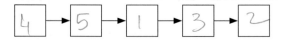

$$4 \rightarrow 5 \rightarrow 1 \rightarrow 3 \rightarrow 2$$

**Activity E** SHORT ANSWERS

*Briefly answer the following.*

1. Describe rates of compression to breaths and the hand positions used with CPR for infants and children for both one-person and two-person CPR.

_____

_____

_____

2. Describe how to distinguish SVT from sinus tachycardia.

_____

_____

_____

3. Describe the proper procedure for one person to ventilate a child with a bag valve mask.

_____ 10 L/min

Size bag according to Broselow tape

_____

**4.** What is the purpose of using cricoid pressure during resuscitation?

_____

_____

_____

**5.** Discuss the mnemonic "DOPE" in regards to a child who is intubated.

D isplacement

O bstruction

P neumothorax

E quipment failure

# SECTION II: APPLYING YOUR KNOWLEDGE

### Activity F CASE STUDY

A nurse is providing training for pediatric emergencies to a day care staff, including CPR, use of a defibrillator, poisonings, and near-drowning interventions. One of the day care providers states that she didn't think automatic external defibrillators (AEDs) were used for children. Another day care provider questions how the chain of survival is different for children compared to adults since she was certified in adult CPR several months ago.

**1.** How would you respond to the question regarding the use of AEDs with children?

_____

_____

_____

**2.** How does the chain of survival for children differ from the chain of survival for adults?

_____

_____

_____

# SECTION III: PRACTICING FOR NCLEX

### Activity G NCLEX-STYLE QUESTIONS

*Answer the following questions.*

**1.** A 6-year-old girl who is being treated for shock is pulseless with an irregular heart rate of 32 BPM. Choose the priority intervention:
- **a.** Give three doses of epinephrine
- **b.** Administer doses defibrillator shocks in a row
- **c.** Initiate cardiac compressions
- **d.** Defibrillate once followed by three cycles of CPR

**2.** The parents of a 7-month-old boy with a broken arm agree on how the accident happened. Which account would lead the nurse to suspect child abuse?
- **a.** "He was climbing out of his crib and fell."
- **b.** "He fell out of a shopping cart in the store."
- **c.** "Mom turned and he fell from changing table."
- **d.** "The gate was open and he fell down three steps."

**3.** A 3-year-old girl had a near-drowning incident when she fell into a wading pool. Which intervention would be of the highest priority?
- **a.** Suctioning the upper airway to ensure airway patency
- **b.** Inserting a nasogastric tube to decompress stomach
- **c.** Covering the child with warming blankets
- **d.** Assuring the child stays still during an X-ray

**4.** A 2-year-old boy is in respiratory distress. Which nursing assessment finding would suggest the child aspirated a foreign body?
- **a.** Hearing dullness when percussing the lungs
- **b.** Noting absent breath sounds in one lung
- **c.** Auscultating a low-pitched, grating breath sound
- **d.** Hearing a hyperresonant sound on percussion

5. The nurse is ventilating a 9-year-old girl with a bag valve mask. Which action would most likely reduce the effectiveness of ventilation?

 a. Checking the tail for free flow of oxygen

 b. Setting the oxygen flow rate at 15 L/minute

 c. Pressing down on the mask below the mouth

 d. Referring to Broselow tape for bag size

6. The nurse is examining a 10-year-old boy with tachypnea and increased work of breathing. Which finding is a late sign that the child is in shock?

 a. Blood pressure slightly less than normal

 b. Equally strong central and distal pulses

 c. Significantly decreased skin elasticity

 d. Delayed capillary refill with cool extremities

7. The nurse is examining a 10-month-old girl who has fallen from the back porch. Which assessment will directly follow evaluation of the "ABCs?"

 a. Observing skin color and perfusion

 b. Palpating the abdomen for soreness

 c. Auscultating for bowel sounds

 d. Palpating the anterior fontanel

8. The nurse is caring for a 10-month-old infant with signs of respiratory distress. Which is the best way to maintain this child's airway?

 a. Placing the hand under the neck

 b. Inserting a small towel under shoulders

 c. Using the head tilt chin lift technique

 d. Employing the jaw-thrust maneuver

9. The nurse is caring for a 4-year-old boy who is receiving mechanical ventilation. Which is the priority intervention when moving this child?

 a. Auscultating the lungs for equal air entry

 b. Checking the $CO_2$ monitor for a yellow display

 c. Watching for disconnections in the breathing circuit

 d. Monitoring the pulse oximeter for oxygen saturation

10. CPR is in progress on an 8-year-old boy who is in shock. Which is the priority nursing intervention?

 a. Using a large bore catheter for peripheral venous access

 b. Inserting an indwelling urinary catheter to measure urine output

 c. Attaining central venous access via the femoral route

 d. Drawing a blood sample for arterial blood gas analysis

11. The child needs a tracheal tube placed. The child is 8 years old. Calculate the size of the tracheal tube that should be used for this child.

12. The nurse must calculate the adolescent's cardiac output. The child's heart rate is 76 beats per minute and the stroke volume is 75 mL. Calculate the child's cardiac output.

13. The child's physician requests that the nurse should notify her if the child's urine output is less than 1 mL/kg of body weight each hour. The child weighs 56 pounds. Calculate the minimum amount of urine output the child should produce each hour. Round to the nearest whole number.

14. The child's ability to perfuse well is poor due to inadequate circulation. The physician writes an order for the child to receive 20 mL of normal saline for each kilogram of body weight. The child will receive the normal saline as a bolus through a central intravenous line. The child weighs 78 pounds. Calculate the amount of normal saline the nurse should administer as a bolus. Round to the nearest whole number.

15. The nurse has been monitoring the child's vital signs. The child is 7 years old. Calculate the child's minimum acceptable systolic blood pressure.

# Answers

## CHAPTER 1

### SECTION I: ASSESSING YOUR UNDERSTANDING

#### Activity A FILL IN THE BLANKS

1. Unintentional
2. Specialty
3. Anticipatory
4. Mortality
5. Guardians

#### Activity B MATCHING

1. d    2. e     3. c     4. b     5. a

#### Activity C SEQUENCING

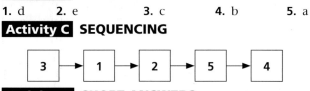

$$3 \rightarrow 1 \rightarrow 2 \rightarrow 5 \rightarrow 4$$

#### Activity D SHORT ANSWERS

1. The primary level of service focuses on health promotion and illness prevention and typically occurs in the community. Provided in clinics, offices, schools, homes, and child care facilities.

   The secondary level of service is generally provided in acute treatment centers that focus on diagnosis and treatment of illness.

   The tertiary level of service involves restorative, rehabilitative, or quality-of-life care issues provided in rehabilitation, hospice, and home care settings.
2. The components of case management are as follows:
   - Collaborative process involving assessment, planning, implementation, coordination, monitoring, and evaluation
   - Advocacy, communication, and resource management
   - Patient-focused comprehensive care across a continuum
   - Coordinated care with an interdisciplinary approach
3. The standards are assessment, diagnosis, outcomes identification, planning, implementation, and evaluation. The purpose of the standards is to specify

what is adequate and effective for general pediatric nursing and to promote consistency in practice.
4. Healthy People originated in 1979. The principle behind the report was to set national objectives and provide a means to monitor progress. The report incorporates input from public health and prevention experts; federal, state, and local governments; and more than 2,000 organizations.
5. Child mortality is defined as the number of deaths per 100,000 population in children between 1 and 14 years of age. The mortality rate for children between ages 1 and 4 years was 29.4 per 100,000 with the leading cause of death being unintentional injuries followed by congenital malformations. The mortality rate for children ages 5 to 14 years was 16.3 per 100,000 with the leading cause, again unintentional injuries followed by cancer. Other causes of childhood mortality include suicide, homicide, diseases of the heart, influenza, and pneumonia.

### SECTION II: APPLYING YOUR KNOWLEDGE

#### Activity E CASE STUDY

1. Barriers may include financial barriers such as lack of insurance, not enough insurance, or inability to pay for services. Sociocultural and ethnic factors can contribute to barriers to health care. Overall, white, non-Hispanic children were more likely than African American and Hispanic children to be in very good or excellent health (America's Children, 2002). Lack of transportation, the need for both parents to work, and genetic factors also pose barriers to health care. Knowledge barriers, including lack of understanding of child health prevention services, also exist. Rising health care costs resulting in cost containment creates barriers. Eighty-five percent of employed families are under some type of managed health care plan or health maintenance organization (known as HMOs). This prospective payment system based on diagnosis-related groups (known as DRGs) limits the amounts of health care. This includes the reimbursement from Medicaid so the trend is to discharge as soon as possible and deliver care in the home or through

community-based services. The overall plans may improve access to preventive services but limit the access to specialty care, which greatly impacts children with chronic or long-term illnesses.

2. The primary role will be that of caregiver (providing direct nursing care to Isabelle and her family during this hospital stay), advocate (safeguard and advance the interests of Isabelle and her family by knowing their needs and resources, informing them of their rights and options, and assisting them to make informed choices/decisions regarding Isabelle's care), educator (instruct and counsel Isabelle and her family on the health care setting, procedures, condition and other areas to maintain optimal health), and manager (manage the delivery of health care services to Isabelle to encourage quality, cost-effectiveness, and continuity of care for the best outcome for her and her family). Other important roles will include researcher (utilize and integrate research to establish evidence-based practice for children and their families), coordinator (provide basic organizing functions to coordinate care for Isabelle and her family), collaborator (integrate the care for Isabelle with interdisciplinary health care team members), communicator (ensure communication with Isabelle and her family is appropriate and based on age and developmental level), and consultant (work as a consultant to ensure Isabelle and her family's needs are met such as facilitating support groups or discussing with school nurse the plan of care for Isabelle if appropriate)

# SECTION III: PRACTICING FOR NCLEX

## Activity F NCLEX-STYLE QUESTIONS

1. **Answer: c**
   RATIONALE: Recommending that the child wears a protective helmet best supports the goals of Healthy People 2010 because unintentional injury is a leading cause of mortality and morbidity for children. Good diet, frequent hand washing, and proper head lice treatment are important but do not affect child health status as much as injury prevention does.

2. **Answer: c**
   RATIONALE: Assessing the child's daily oxygen supplement needs addresses the child's physical health but not the contemporary issue of quality of life. Helping the child modify trendy clothing to his needs, consulting with the school nurse, and adapting technologies for use outside of the home will improve the child's quality of life by building independence and self-esteem.

3. **Answer: a**
   RATIONALE: Reminding the mother that the child will imitate her parents may prevent the child from imitating dangerous behavior, but this is less likely to be a danger. Explaining how to

toddler proof the house helps prevent injury to the child. Explaining how to teach self hand washing helps to prevent infection. Describing self-care for brushing teeth helps prevent dental caries. These interventions help avoid common health problems.

4. **Answer: d**
   RATIONALE: Helping the family save money on therapy equipment is a consumer assistance activity, but it does not empower these health care consumers. The pediatric nurse is uniquely positioned to empower this family by performing the role of educator regarding therapy, by being an advocate regarding their wishes to get a lung transplant, and by keeping them informed as equal partners in family-centered care.

5. **Answer: b**
   RATIONALE: It is important to log-off whenever leaving the computer. The person that shares the nurse's log-on session may get called away from the computer leaving the nurse responsible for any breech in security. Keeping IDs and passwords confidential is basic computer security. E-mail is not a safe way to transmit confidential information for transmittal. Printing is safer. Closing patient files before stepping away from the computer helps ensure privacy.

6. **Answer: b**
   RATIONALE: One of the factors associated with childhood injuries is parental drug or alcohol abuse. This is the leading cause for child mortality. Low-birth-weight babies are at higher risk for infant mortality. Foreign-born adoption is a factor for childhood morbidity. The child's hostility toward other children may be an environmental or psychosocial factor for childhood morbidity.

7. **Answer: d**
   RATIONALE: Making phone calls to the parents of the children who were determined to need counseling is least important to the nursing plan of care. It is, no doubt, mandatory for the nurse to inform and support the parents. However, this intervention is the least important based on the nursing diagnosis of the children's need for counseling, the intervention to arrange for a counselor, and the adaptation of the intervention by providing counseling for the friends of the injured child.

8. **Answer: a**
   RATIONALE: The fact that the child has asthma is a factor for morbidity. The other findings, single parenthood, young maternal age at birth, and child abuse, are factors for child mortality.

9. **Answer: b**
   RATIONALE: The nurse would not prescribe services. If the nurse's evaluation and monitoring disclosed a needed service that would improve the child's outcome, the nurse would advocate for the child.

Other activities involved in care management include facilitating the doctor's diagnosis and treatment plan, Helping the family access the services they need and evaluating the child's progress toward recovery.

10. **Answer: d**
RATIONALE: The leading cause for hospitalization, by far, for this child's age group is pregnancy and childbirth. Mental illness is second and is a growing concern. Respiratory diseases and obesity are major concerns, but lesser than responsible sexual behavior.

11. **Answer: b**
RATIONALE: The leading cause of death in adolescents is accidents. Educational programs focusing on prevention of accidents and reduction of risk factors would be most beneficial in this age group.

12. **Answer: d**
RATIONALE: An increasing number of children are being diagnosed with mental health disorders. The best way to determine the reliability of the teacher's concerns would be to determine the behaviors being noticed.

13. **Answer: b**
RATIONALE: Family-centered care involves a mutually beneficial partnership between the child, the family, and health care professionals (O'Malley, Brown, & Krug, 2008). It applies to the planning, delivery, and evaluation of health care for children of all ages in any setting.

14. **Answer: d**
RATIONALE: The consent of a parent or guardian is required for completion of a surgical procedure such as a circumcision. The parent in the case is under age. She may, however, consent for health care treatment of her child.

15. **Answer: d**
RATIONALE: Requests of the parents and child must be documented. The surgeon does not have the automatic authority to override the parents' wishes. The child is under age and does not have decision-making authority.

# CHAPTER 2

## SECTION I: ASSESSING YOUR UNDERSTANDING

### Activity A FILL IN THE BLANKS

1. Discipline
2. Easy
3. Competence
4. Resilience
5. Suicide

### Activity B MATCHING

**1.** b  **2.** e  **3.** c  **4.** a  **5.** d

### Activity C SEQUENCING

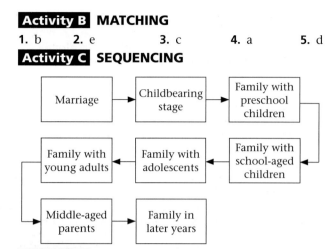

### Activity D SHORT ANSWERS

1. For positive reinforcement to be effective, feedback must be immediate, consistent, and frequent.
2. Answers may include strong commitment to school and academic performance; involvement in social activities, feelings of connectedness to family or other adults outside the family; ability to discuss problems with parents or a supportive adult; and consistent presence of a parent at least once during the day.
3. Last rites or special burial customs are associated with, Hindu, Judaism (Orthodox and Conservative), Islam, and Roman Catholic.

## SECTION II: APPLYING YOUR KNOWLEDGE

### Activity E CASE STUDY

1. The nurse should include a variety of points in the interaction. There are different parenting styles and they vary based on the amount of control exerted over the child during parenting. The husband appears to fit into the authoritarian parenting style in which the parent expects obedience from the children without questioning the rules for the family. The parent also expects the children to accept the family beliefs and values. Whatever the style of parenting, it is important that caregiving is sensitive and responsive in order to promote appropriate physical, neurophysiologic, and psychological development.

   With the recent change in family structure it can be difficult for Joel, especially if there are differing views and practices related to discipline. It may be helpful to discuss this with Joel's stepfather. Parenting is more effective if parents adjust their style to meet the needs of their children at different developmental levels and temperaments. The American Academy of Pediatrics (1998) suggests three components: (1) maintain a positive, supportive, nurturing caregiver–child relationship; (2) provide positive reinforcement techniques to increase the desirable behaviors; and (3) remove the positive reinforcement techniques or use punishment to reduce or eliminate undesirable behaviors. Corporal punishment, such as spanking, may stop the negative behavior but it also increases the chance for physical injury, may lead to altered caregiver–child relationships, and may lead to the child becoming accustomed to the form resulting in the need to increase the intensity to achieve the same affects. Some positive strategies for effective discipline include setting clear, consistent, and developmentally appropriate expected behaviors. It is important to provide age appropriate explanations of the consequences if the child has unacceptable behavior. Always administer the consequence soon after the unacceptable behavior. Make sure the consequence is appropriate to the age of the child and situation. Stay calm but firm without showing anger when administering consequences. Catch the child displaying appropriate behavior and praise the child. Ensure the environment is set to assist the child in accomplishing the appropriate behavior.

2. The recent changes in family structure, especially if there are different views and practices related to child care and health practices, may result in conflict. Initial response to these changes varies with each child but more than one-third of children are troubled and distressed 5 years after the divorce of their parents with depression being the most common symptom (Behrman & Kliegman, 2004). It is important as a parent to understand this and place the children's interest in the forefront. This can help minimize the negative impacts that occur for children.

# SECTION III: PRACTICING FOR NCLEX

**Activity F** NCLEX-STYLE QUESTIONS

1. **Answer: c**
   Children living with their grandparents may experience emotional stress if the biological parents are in and out of the child's life. Teaching basic child care skills is appropriate for the adolescent family. Determining the decision maker is important with an extended family, and financial aid is important for single parents.

2. **Answer: a**
   It would be most appropriate to assess the parent's coping abilities because they are in the wrong stage of the family life cycle to be having another child. Providing anticipatory guidance, describing the nutritional value of breastfeeding, and promoting the importance of vaccinations are interventions for younger parents.

3. **Answer: d**
   The nurse would focus on the father for decisions about the course of treatment. Assuring medications are received on time is the family health manager's role. Staying with the child in the hospital will be handled by the family nurturer. All clinical input will be provided to the family gatekeeper for dissemination.

4. **Answer: b**
   It is important to make the consequence known before the bad behavior. This way the child has the opportunity to avoid misbehaving. Effective discipline is performed in close proximity to the misbehavior. It is important to set a good example and avoid hypocritical behavior.

5. **Answer: c**
   In the Arab American culture, women are subordinate to men and children are subordinate to the parents. The nurse would deal directly and exclusively with the father. This family would not place much emphasis on preventative care either. Inquiring about folk remedies used may be needed with African American families. Coordinating care through the mother is appropriate with a Hispanic family.

6. **Answer: c**
   Suggesting that the parents provide a place where the child can roughhouse would be best for the child and them. Disciplining him for running in the house, encouraging him to do quiet activities, and spanking him if he has a tantrum are counter to his temperament.

7. **Answer: d**
   Both parents together should discuss with the children how things will work after the divorce. The children should not be expected to act like adults because they are not. Tell them about the divorce ahead of time, and tell them the reasons in nonjudgmental terms that they can understand.

8. **Answer: a**
   The physiological health of the children is of the greatest importance. Assessment of the family's psychological and emotional status should not be overlooked. If mother needs support, a referral to Parents without Partners may be helpful.

9. **Answer: b**
   If the mother's partner is being verbally abusive of the child, there is risk of physical violence. There could be a number of reasons other than violence to dread going home. Strictness is not necessarily a sign of abuse. The boyfriend's absence may only be a sign or irresponsibility and not of a violent nature.

10. **Answer: b**
    Going home early from shopping if the child misbehaves is an example of extinction

discipline. Positive reinforcement is eliminated for inappropriate behavior. Going out for ice cream, praising her for polite behavior, and letting her go to a friend's house are all types of positive reinforcement.

**11. Answer: c**
Secondhand smoke and other pollutants is a health hazard for children. A recent study found that residual tobacco smoke and carcinogens remain after a cigarette is extinguished (referred to as thirdhand smoke). These toxins cling to the smoker's hair and clothes and can be present on any surface in the house, such as carpet and cushions. Children are particularly susceptible to third-hand smoke since they breathe near, crawl, touch and mouth contaminated surfaces (Winickoff et al., 2009).

**12. Answer: d**
Medicaid is a joint federal and state program that provides health insurance to low-income parents and their children. It is state administered and each state has its own set of guidelines.

**13. Answer: b**
African American traditional beliefs include the use of prayer and laying on of hands to promote a return to health and reduction of discomfort.

**14. Answer: a**
The Arab American traditions typically have the male as being superior. Information in most cases will be passed to the man for consent first.

**15. Answer: c**
The Native American beliefs often hold hot and cold as being potential cause for illnesses.

# CHAPTER 3

## SECTION I: ASSESSING YOUR UNDERSTANDING

### Activity A FILL IN THE BLANKS

1. Colic
2. Anticipatory
3. Prolactin
4. Colostrums
5. Separate
6. Development
7. 12 to 18

### Activity B LABELING

UPPER
Central incisor 8-12 months
Lateral incisor 9-13 months
Cuspid 16-22 months
First molar 13-19 months
Second molar 25-33 months

LOWER
Second molar 25-33 months
First molar 13-19 months
Cuspid 16-22 months
Lateral incisor 9-13 months
Central incisor 8-12 months

### Activity C MATCHING

**Question 1**

**1.** f  **2.** a  **3.** b  **4.** e  **5.** d  **6.** c

**Question 2**

**1.** b  **2.** a  **3.** d  **4.** c  **5.** e

### Activity D SEQUENCING

5 → 4 → 1 → 3 → 2

### Activity E SHORT ANSWERS

1. Encourage breastfeeding in all mothers beginning with the prenatal visit if applicable. Provide accurate education related to breastfeeding.

   Be available for questions or problems related to initiation and continuation of breastfeeding. Consult lactation consultant as needed or available.

   Encourage pumping of breast milk when mother returns to work in order to continue breastfeeding.

   Refer to local breastfeeding support groups such as La Leche League.

2. Breastfeeding or feeding of expressed human milk is recommended for all infants, including sick or premature newborns (with rare exceptions). The exceptions include infants with galactosemia, maternal use of illicit drugs and a few prescription medications, maternal untreated active tuberculosis, and maternal human immunodeficiency virus (HIV) infection in developed countries.

3. Early cues of hunger in a baby include making sucking motions, sucking on hands, or putting the fist to the chin.

4. When assessing the growth and development of a premature infant, use the infant's adjusted age to determine expected outcomes. To determine adjusted age, subtract the number of weeks that the infant was premature from the infant's chronological age.

5. Primitive reflexes are subcortical and involve a whole-body response. Selected primitive reflexes present at birth include moro, root, suck, asymmetric tonic neck, plantar and palmar grasp, step, and Babinski. Except for the Babinski, which disappears around 1 year of age, these primitive reflexes diminish over the first few months of life, giving way to protective reflexes.

6. The heart doubles in size over the first year of life. As the cardiovascular system matures, the average pulse rate decreases from 120 to 140 in the newborn to about 100 in the 1-year-old. Blood pressure steadily increases over the first 12 months of life, from an average of 60/40 in the newborn to 100/50 in the 12-month-old. The peripheral capillaries are closer to the surface of the skin, thus making the newborn and young infant more susceptible to heat loss. Over the first year of life, thermoregulation (the body's ability to stabilize body temperature) becomes more effective: the peripheral capillaries constrict in response to a cold environment and dilate in response to heat.

## SECTION II: APPLYING YOUR KNOWLEDGE
### Activity F CASE STUDY

1. The discussion should include the following points:
Play is the work of children and is the natural way they learn. It is critical to their development. It allows them to explore their environment, practice new skills, and problem solve. They practice gross, fine motor and language skills through play. Young infants love to watch people's faces and will often appear to mimic the expressions they see. Parents can talk to and sing to their child while participating in the daily activities that infants need such as feeding, bathing, and changing. As infants become older, toys may be geared toward the motor skills or language skills that are developing currently. Appropriate toys for this age group include: fabric or board books, different types of music, easy to hold toys that do things or make noise (fancy rattles), floating, squirting bath toys, and soft dolls or animals. Books are also very important toys for infants. Reading aloud and sharing books during early infancy are critical to the development of neural networks that are important in the later tasks of reading and word recognition. Reading books increases listening comprehension. Infants demonstrate their excitement about picture books by kicking and waving their arms and babbling when looking at them. Reading to all ages of infants is appropriate and the older infant develops fine motor skills as he learns to turn book pages. Reading picture books and simple stories to infants starts a good habit that should be continued throughout childhood.

2. The discussion should include the following points:
Erikson's stage of psychosocial development is trust versus mistrust. Development of a sense of trust is crucial in the first year, as it serves as the foundation for later psychosocial tasks. The parent or primary caregiver is in a position to significantly impact the infant's development of a sense of trust. When the infant's needs are consistently met, the infant develops this sense of trust. Caregivers respond to these basic needs by feeding, changing diapers, and cleaning, touching, holding, and talking to infants. If the parent or caregiver is inconsistent in meeting the infant's needs in a timely manner, then over time the infant develops a sense of mistrust. As the infant gets older, the nervous system matures. The infant begins to realize a separation between self and caregivers. The infant learns to tolerate small amounts of frustration, and learns to trust the caregivers even if gratification is delayed, because the infant understands that needs will eventually be provided.

The first stage of Jean Piaget's theory of cognitive development is referred to as the sensorimotor stage (birth to 2 years). Infants learn about themselves and the world around them through developing sensory and motor capacities. Infants between 4 and 8 months repeat actions to achieve wanted results, such as shaking a rattle to hear the noise it makes. At this age their actions are purposeful, though do not always have an end goal in mind.

3. The discussion should include the following points:
Inability to sit with assistance, does not turn to locate sound, crosses eyes most of the time, does not laugh or squeal, does not smile or seem to enjoy people.

## SECTION III: PRACTICING FOR NCLEX
### Activity G NCLEX-STYLE QUESTIONS

1. **Answer: c**
The child's head size is large for his adjusted age of 4 months which would be cause for concern. Normal growth would be 3.6 inches. At 10 pounds, 2 ounces, the child is the right weight for a 4-month-old adjusted age. Palmar grasp reflex disappears between 4 and 6 months adjusted age, so this would not be a concern yet. The child is of average weight for a 4-month-old adjusted age.

2. **Answer: a**
Urging the parents to get time away from the child would be most helpful in the short term, particularly if the parents are stressed. Educating the parents about when colic stops would help them see an end to the stress. Observing how the parents

respond to the child helps to determine if the parent/child relationship was altered. Assessing the parents' care and feeding skills may identify other causes for the crying.

3. **Answer: d**
   The normal newborn may lose up to 10% of their birth weight. The baby in question has lost just below this amount. This will likely not require hospitalization. Expressing to the mother that her baby will likely be hospitalized is rash and will most likely not occur.

4. **Answer: b**
   The nurse will warn against putting the child to bed with a bottle of milk or juice because this allows the sugar content of these fluids to pool around the child's teeth at night. Not cleaning a neonate's gums when he is done eating will have minimal impact on the development of dental caries, as will using a cloth instead of a brush for cleaning teeth when they erupt. Failure to clean the teeth with fluoridated toothpaste is not a problem if the water supply is fluoridated.

5. **Answer: b**
   If the parents are keeping the child up until she falls asleep, they are not creating a bedtime routine for her. Infants need a transition to sleep at this age. If the parents are singing to her before she goes to bed, if she has a regular, scheduled bedtime, and if they check on her safety when she wakes at night, then lie her down and leave, they are using good sleep practices.

6. **Answer: c**
   The nurse would advise the mother to watch for increased biting and sucking. Mild fever, vomiting, and diarrhea are signs of infection. The child would more likely seek out hard foods or objects to bite on.

7. **Answer: d**
   When introducing a new food to an infant, it may take multiple attempts before the child will accept it. Parents must demonstrate patience. Letting the child eat only the foods she prefers, forcing her to eat foods she does not want, or actively urging the child to eat new foods can negatively affect eating patterns.

8. **Answer: a**
   The best way to ensure effective feeding is by maintaining a feed-on-demand approach rather than a set schedule. Applying warm compresses to the breast helps engorgement. Encouraging the infant to latch on properly helps prevent sore nipples. Maintaining proper diet and fluid intake for the mother helps ensure an adequate milk supply.

9. **Answer: b**
   If the child's rectal temperature is greater than 100.4° F, the parents should call their care provider. Infants are very susceptible to infection. If the dried umbilical cord stump falls off, or the child wets her diaper 8 times per day, this is

normal. In the first 5 to 10 days of life, it is also normal for the child to eat but still lose weight.

10. **Answer: c**
    At 6 months of age, the child is able to put down one toy to pick up another. He will be able to shift a toy to his left hand to reach for another with his right hand by 7 months. He will pick up an object with his thumb and finger tips at 8 months, and he will enjoy hitting a plastic bowl with a large spoon at 9 months.

11. **Answer: b**
    The average infant's weight doubles at 6 months and will triple at 1 year of life. The rate of increase for the infant's length is an increase of 1 inch per month for the first 6 months.

12. **Answer: b**
    The normal respiratory rate for a 1-month-old infant is 30 to 60 breaths per minute. By 1 year of age the rate will be 20 to 30 breaths per minute. The respiratory patterns of the 1-month-old infant are irregular. There may normally be periodic pauses in the rhythm.

13. **Answer: b**
    Normally infants are not born with teeth. Occasionally there are one or more teeth at birth. These are termed natal teeth and are often associated with anomalies. The first primary teeth typically erupt between the ages of 6 and 8 months.

14. **Answer: c**
    The capacity of the normal newborn's stomach is between one-half and one ounce. The recommended feeding plan is to use a demand schedule. Newborns may eat as often as 1½ to 3 hours. Demand scheduled feedings are not associated with problems sleeping at night.

# CHAPTER 4

## SECTION I: ASSESSING YOUR UNDERSTANDING

### Activity A  FILL IN THE BLANKS

1. Myelinization
2. Drowning
3. Receptive
4. Urethra
5. Preoperational

### Activity B  MATCHING

**Question 1**

| 1. d | 2. f | 3. e | 4. b | 5. a | 6. c |
|------|------|------|------|------|------|

**Question 2**

| 1. c | 2. a | 3. b | 4. e | 5. d |
|------|------|------|------|------|

### Activity C  SEQUENCING

$$4 \rightarrow 3 \rightarrow 1 \rightarrow 2$$

## Activity D  SHORT ANSWERS

*Briefly answer the following.*

1. Prevention is best concerning temper tantrums. Fatigue or hunger may limit the toddler's coping abilities, so adhering to reasonable food and sleep schedules help prevent tantrums. When parents note the beginnings of frustrations during activities, friendly warnings, distractions, refocusing or removal from the situation may prevent the tantrum.

2. Toddler discipline should focus on clear limits, consistency, not involve spanking, and be balanced with a caring and nurturing environment along with frequent praise for appropriate behavior.

3. At the age of 1, every child should have an initial dental visit. To prevent the development of dental caries children should be weaned by 15 months of age. In addition, the use of sippy cups should be limited. Cleaning of the toddler's teeth should progress from brushing simply with water to using a very small pea-sized amount of fluoridated toothpaste with brushing beginning at age 2.

4. Changes in the anatomy of the toddler's genitourinary system make toilet training possible. The kidney functions reach adult levels between 16 and 24 months of age. The bladder is able to hold urine for increased periods of time.

5. The abdominal musculature is weak in the young toddler. This causes a pot-bellied appearance. In addition the child appears sway backed. As the muscles mature this resolves.

## SECTION II: APPLYING YOUR KNOWLEDGE

### Activity E  CASE STUDY

The potentially bilingual child may blend two languages, that is, parts of the word in both languages are blended into one word or may language mix within a sentence; he will combine languages or grammar within a sentence. The assessment of adequate language development is more complicated in bilingual children. Due to the possible language mixing the bilingual child may be more difficult to assess for speech delay.

The bilingual child should have command of 20 words (between both languages) by 20 months of age and be making word combinations; if this is not the case, then further investigation may be warranted.

1. Talking and singing to the toddler during routine activities such as feeding and dressing provides an environment that encourages conversation. Frequent, repetitive naming helps the toddler learn appropriate words for objects. Be attentive to what the toddler is saying as well as to his moods. Listen to and answer the toddler's questions. Encouragement and elaboration convey confidence and interest to the toddler. Give the toddler time to complete his or her thoughts without interrupting or rushing. Remember that the toddler is just starting to be able to make the connections necessary to transfer thoughts and feelings into language.

Do not over-react to the child's use of the word "no." Give the toddler opportunities to appropriately use the word "no" with silly questions such as "Can a cat drive a car?" Teach the toddler appropriate words for body parts and objects. Help the toddler choose appropriate words to label feelings and emotions. Toddlers' receptive language and interpretation of body language and subtle signs far surpasses their expressive language especially at a younger age.

Encourage the use of both English and Spanish in the home.

Reading to the toddler everyday is one of the best ways to promote language and cognitive development. Toddlers particularly enjoy books about feelings, family, friends, everyday life, animals and nature, and fun and fantasy. Board books have thick pages that are easier for young toddlers to turn. The toddler may also enjoy "reading" the story to the parent.

2. Erikson defines the toddler period as a time of autonomy versus shame and doubt. It is a time of exerting independence. Exertion of independence often results in the toddler's favorite response, "No." The toddler will often answer "no" even when he or she really means "yes." Always saying "no," referred to as negativism, is a normal part of healthy development.

If there is no option of avoiding an action, do not ask toddlers if they want to do something. Avoid closed ended yes–no questions, as the toddler's usual response is "No," whether he means it or not. Offer the child simple choices such as "Do you want to use the red cup or the blue cup." This helps give the toddler a sense of control. When getting ready to leave, do not ask the child if he wants to put his shoes on. Simply state in a matter of fact tone that shoes must be worn outside and give the toddler a choice on type of shoe or color of socks. If the child continues with negative answers, then the parent should remain calm and make the decision for the child.

3. Does not use 2-word sentences, does not imitate actions, does not follow basic instructions, and cannot push a toy with wheels.

## SECTION III: PRACTICING FOR NCLEX

### Activity F  NCLEX-STYLE QUESTIONS

*Answer the following questions.*

1. **Answer: c**
   Suggesting that the parents transition the child to a healthier diet by serving him more healthy

choices along with smaller portions of junk food will reassure them that they are not starving their child. The parents would have less success with an abrupt change to healthy foods. Explaining calorie requirements and the time line for acceptance of a new food do not offer a practical reason for making a change in diet.

2. **Answer: a**
This child has most recently acquired the ability to undress himself. Pushing a toy lawnmower and kicking a ball are things he learned at about 24 months. He was able to pull a toy while walking at about 18 months.

3. **Answer: d**
Stopping the child when she is misbehaving and describing proper behavior sets limits and models good behavior and will be the most helpful advice to the parents. The child is too young to use time out or extinction as discipline. Slapping her hand, even done carefully with two fingers, is corporal punishment, which has been found to have negative effects on child development.

4. **Answer: b**
Because they are curious and mobile, toddlers require direct observation and cannot be trusted to be left alone. The priority guidance is to never let the child be out of sight. Gating stairways, locking up chemicals, and not smoking around the child are excellent, but specific, safety interventions.

5. **Answer: b**
The nurse would be concerned if the child is babbling to herself rather than using real words. By this age, she should be using simple sentences with a vocabulary of 150 to 300 words. Being unwilling to share toys, playing parallel with other children, and moving to different toys frequently are typical toddler behaviors.

6. **Answer: c**
The fact that the child does not respond when the mother waves to him suggests he may have a vision problem. The toddler's sense of smell is still developing, so he may not be affected by odors. Their sense of taste is not well developed either, and this allows him to eat or drink poisons without concern. The child's crying at a sudden noise assures the nurse that his hearing is adequate.

7. **Answer: c**
If the child is still speaking telegraphically in only 2- to 3-word sentences, it suggests there is a language development problem. If the child makes simple conversation, tells about something that happened in the past, or tells the nurse her name she is meeting developmental milestones for language.

8. **Answer: a**
Separation anxiety should have disappeared or be subsiding by 3 years of age. The fact that it is persistent suggests there might an emotional problem. Emotional lability, self soothing by thumb sucking, or the inability to share are common for this age.

9. **Answer: b**
The nurse would be sure to tell the mother to feed her child iron-fortified cereal and other iron-rich foods when she weans her child off the breast or formula. Weaning from the breast is dependent upon the mother's need and desires with no set time. Weaning from the bottle is recommended at 1 year of age in order to prevent dental caries. Use of a no-spill sippy cup is not recommended because it too is associated with dental caries.

10. **Answer: d**
The nurse would recommend a preschool where the staff is trained in early childhood development and cardiopulmonary resuscitation. Cleanliness and a loving staff are not enough without competence. Good hygiene procedures require that a sick child not be allowed to attend. It is also important that parents are allowed to visit any time without an appointment.

11. **Answer: b**
The Erickson stage of development for the toddler is autonomy versus shame and doubt. During this period of time the child works to establish independence. Trust versus mistrust is the stage of infancy. Initiative versus guilt is the stage for the preschooler. Industry versus inferiority is the stage for school-aged children.

12. **Answer: a**
The ability to have object permanence is consistent with the phase of tertiary circular reactions.

13. **Answer: d**
The 20-month-old toddler should have a vocabulary greater than 75 to 100 words. A toddler at this age should comprehend approximately 200 words. The ability to point to named body points, discuss past events, and point to pictures in a book when asked are communication skills associated with an older child.

14. **Answer: a**
The social skills of the toddler at this age include parallel play. During parallel play children will play alongside each other not cooperatively. There is no indication that the aggression levels of the child need to be investigated. There is no indication the child needs increased socialization with other children.

# CHAPTER 5

## SECTION I: ASSESSING YOUR UNDERSTANDING

### Activity A FILL IN THE BLANKS

1. Iron
2. Concrete
3. Urethra
4. Terror
5. Dense

### Activity B MATCHING

**Question 1**

1. d    2. a    3. b    4. f    5. c    6. e

### Activity C SEQUENCING

*Place the following motor skills in the order of acquisition:*

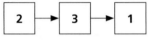

### Activity D SHORT ANSWERS

1. The child in the intuitive phase can count 10 or more objects, correctly name at least 4 colors, can understand the concept of time, and knows about things that are used in everyday life such as appliances, money, and food.
2. A nightmare is a scary or bad dream. After a nightmare, the child is aroused and interactive. Night terrors are different. A short time after falling asleep, the child seems to awaken and is screaming. The child usually does not respond much to the parent's soothing, eventually stops screaming, and goes back to sleep. Night terrors are often frightening for parents, because the child does not seem to be responding to them.
3. The preschooler should have his or her teeth brushed and flossed daily with a pea-sized amount of toothpaste. Cariogenic foods should continue to be avoided. If sugary foods are consumed, the mouth should be rinsed with water if it is not possible to brush the teeth directly after their consumption. The preschool-age child should visit the dentist every 6 months.
4. The parent should ascertain the reason for the lie before punishing the child. If the child has broken a rule and fears punishment, then the parent must determine the truth. The child needs to learn that lying is usually far worse than the misbehavior itself. The punishment for the misbehavior should be lessened if the child admits the truth. The parent should remain calm and serve as a role model of an even temper.
5. The primary psychosocial task of the preschool period is developing a sense of initiative.

## SECTION II: APPLYING YOUR KNOWLEDGE

### Activity E CASE STUDY

1. Magical thinking and playing make believe are a normal part of preschool development. The preschool age child believes her thoughts to be all-powerful. The fantasy experienced through magical thinking and make believe allows the preschooler to make room in his world for the actual or the real and to satisfy her curiosity about differences in the world around her. Encouraging pretend play and providing props for dress-up stimulate and develop curiosity and creativity. Fantasy play is usually cooperative in nature and encourages the preschooler to develop social skills like turn-taking, communication, paying attention, and responding to one another's words and actions. Fantasy play also allows preschoolers to explore complex social ideas such as power, compassion, and cruelty.
2. Kindergarten may be a significant change for some children. The hours are usually longer than preschool and it is usually held 5 days per week. The setting and personnel are new and rules and expectations are often very different. When talking about starting kindergarten with Nila do so using an enthusiastic approach. Keep the conversation light and positive. Meet with Nila's teacher prior to the start of school and discuss any specific needs or concerns you may have. A tour of the school and attending the school's open house can help ease the transition also. Incorporate and practice the new daily routine prior to school starting. This can help the child adjust to the changes that are occurring.
3. The discussion should include the following points:
   - Cannot jump in place or ride a tricycle
   - Cannot stack four blocks
   - Cannot throw ball overhand
   - Does not grasp crayon with thumb and fingers
   - Difficulty with scribbling
   - Cannot copy a circle
   - Does not use sentences with three or more words
   - Cannot use the words "me" and "you" appropriately
   - Ignores other children or does not show interest in interactive games
   - Will not respond to people outside the family, still clings or cries if parents leave

## SECTION III: PRACTICING FOR NCLEX

### Activity F NCLEX-STYLE QUESTIONS

1. **Answer: b**
   The presence of only 10 deciduous teeth would warrant further investigation. The preschooler should have 20 deciduous teeth present. The absence of dental caries or presence of 19 teeth does not warrant further investigation.

2. **Answer: b**
The nurse should encourage the mother to schedule a meeting with the teacher prior to school's start date and set up a time to tour the classroom and school so the boy knows what to expect. The other statements are not helpful and do not address the mother's or boy's concerns.

3. **Answer: c**
The average preschool child will grow 2½ to 3 inches per year. The nurse would expect that the child's height would have increased 2½ to 3 inches since last year's well child examination.

4. **Answer: b**
By the age of 5, persons outside of the family should be able to understand most of the child's speech without the parents "translation." The other statements would not warrant additional referral or follow-up. A child of 5 years should be able to count to at least 10, know his or her address, and participate in long detailed conversations.

5. **Answer: a**
During a night terror, a child is typically unaware of the parent's presence and may scream and thrash more if restrained. During a nightmare, a child is responsive to the parent's soothing and reassurances. The other statements are indicative of a nightmare.

6. **Answer: d**
The preschooler is not mature enough to ride a bicycle in the street even if riding with adults, so the nurse should emphasize that the girl should always ride on the sidewalk even if the mother is riding with her daughter. The other statements are correct.

7. **Answer: c**
The nurse needs to emphasize that there are number of reasons that a parent should not choose a preschool that utilizes corporal punishment. It may negatively affect a child's self-esteem as well as ability to achieve in school. It may also lead to disruptive and violent behavior in the classroom and should be discouraged. The other statements would not warrant further discussion or intervention.

8. **Answer: b**
The nurse should explain to the parents that attributing life-like qualities to inanimate objects is quite normal. Telling the parents that their daughter is demonstrating animism is correct, but it would be better to explain what animism is and then remind them that it is developmentally appropriate. Asking whether they think their daughter is hallucinating or whether there is a family history of mental history is inappropriate and does not teach.

9. **Answer: a**
The nurse needs to remind the parents that the girl should use a helmet when riding any wheeled toy, not just her bicycle. The other statements are correct.

10. **Answer: c**
It is important to remind the parents that they should perform flossing in the preschool period because the child is unable to perform this task. The other statements are correct.

11. **Answer: d**
The average 4-year-old child is 40.5 inches. The average rate of growth per year is between 2.5 and 3 inches. The child in the scenario demonstrates normal stature and growth patterns.

12. **Answer: c**
Preschool-aged children may become occupied with activities around them and not remember to void. Reminding them to void is helpful. Discipline should not be applied to infrequent episodes of incontinence. There is no indication the child has an infection.

13. **Answer: d**
Preschool-aged children often interact with imaginary friends. The nurse should recognize this as normal for the age group. No special actions are needed.

14. **Answer: c**
Sexual curiosity is normal in the preschool-aged child. The parents should be encouraged to provide brief, honest answers to the child. The parents must also determine the type of curiosity the child has. Explanations should be within the level of understanding of the child.

15. **Answer: a**
Fears are normal in the preschool-aged child. Some children are afraid of the dark. The parents should be advised to show patience with their child as he works through this fear. Refusing a night light will further increase the stress of the child. Turning out the light may have the child waking up in darkness and becoming further afraid.

# CHAPTER 6

## SECTION I: ASSESSING YOUR UNDERSTANDING

### Activity A FILL IN THE BLANKS

1. 8
2. 2
3. 10th
4. Energy
5. Injury
6. Stress
7. Industry
8. Peers
9. Lower
10. 12

### Activity B MATCHING

**Question 1**

1. c     2. a     3. e     4. b     5. f     6. d

**Question 2**

1. c     2. b     3. a

**Question 3**

1. b     2. c     3. d     4. a

## Activity C SEQUENCING

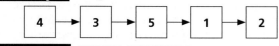

$$4 \rightarrow 3 \rightarrow 5 \rightarrow 1 \rightarrow 2$$

## Activity D SHORT ANSWERS

1. Children aged 6 to 8 enjoy bicycling, skating, and swimming. Children between 8 and 10 years of age have greater rhythm and gracefulness of muscular movements; they enjoy activities such as sports. Those aged 10 to 12 years, especially girls, are more controlled and focused, similar to adults.

2. The child typically feels discomfort in new situations, requires additional time to adjust, and exhibits frustration with tears or somatic complaints. Also described as irritable and moody, the child could benefit from patience, firmness, and understanding when faced with new situations.

3. The nurse's role includes promotion of healthy growth and development through anticipatory guidance, goal attainment, playing, learning, education, and reading. The nurse's role also includes addressing common developmental concerns, assessing the individual child, and recommending intervention or referral where needed.

4. Children between ages 6 and 8 years require approximately 12 hours of sleep per night; those between 8 and 10 years of age require 10 to 12 hours of sleep per night. Children between 10 and 12 years of age require 9 to 10 hours of sleep per night. Some children, regardless of their age group, may need an occasional nap.

5. Body image refers to the perception of one's body. During the school-age period there is a strong interest on the clothing and appearance of others. It is important not to be teased or ridiculed.

## SECTION II: APPLYING YOUR KNOWLEDGE

## Activity E CASE STUDY

1. The discussion should include the following points:
   The role of the family in promoting healthy growth and development is critical. Respectful interchange of communication between the parent and child will foster self-esteem and self-confidence. This respect will give the child confidence in achieving personal, educational, and social goals appropriate for his or her age. During your exam, model appropriate behaviors by listening to the child and making appropriate responses. Serve as a resource for parents and as an advocate for the child in promoting healthy growth and development. Negative comments to the child concerning her appearance may be counterproductive and harm her self-esteem.

2. The discussion should include the following points:
   The school-age child is able to see how her actions affect others and to realize that her behaviors can have consequences. Therefore, discipline

techniques with consequences often work well. For example, the child refuses to put away his or her toys, so the parent forbids him or her to play with those toys. Parents need to teach children the rules established by the family, values, and social rules of conduct. This will help give the child guidelines to what behaviors are acceptable and unacceptable. Parents need to be role models and demonstrate appropriate expressions of feelings and emotions and allow the child to express emotions and feelings. They should never belittle the child, and they need to preserve the child's self-esteem and dignity. Parents should be encouraged to discipline with praise. This positive acknowledgment can encourage appropriate behavior.

When misbehaviors occur, the type and amount of discipline should be based upon the developmental level of the child and the parents, severity of misbehavior, established roles of the family, temperament of the child, and response of the child to rewards. The child should participate in developing a plan of action for his or her misbehavior. Consistency in discipline, along with providing it in a nurturing environment, is essential.

3. The discussion should include the following points:
   Although some television shows and video games can have positive influences on children, guidelines on the use of television and video games are important. Research has shown that the amount of time watching television or playing video games can lead to aggressive behavior, less physical activity, and altered body image.

   Parents should set limits on how much television the child is allowed to watch. The Academy of Pediatrics recommends 2 hours or less of television viewing per day. The parent should establish guidelines on when the child can watch television, and television watching should not be used as a reward. The parents should monitor what the child is watching, and they should watch the programs together and use that opportunity to discuss the subject matter with the child.

   Parents should also prohibit television or video games with violence. There should be no television during dinner and no television in the child's room. The parents need to set examples for the child and encourage sports, interactive play, and reading. They should encourage their child to read instead of watching television or to do a physical activity together as a family. If the television causes fights or arguments, it should be turned off for a period of time.

## SECTION III: PRACTICING FOR NCLEX

## Activity F NCLEX-STYLE QUESTIONS

1. **Answer: a**
   The child will be able to consider an action and its consequences in Piaget's period of concrete

operational thought. However, she is now able to empathize with others. She is more adept at classifying and dividing things into sets. Defining lying as bad because she gets punished for it is a Kohlberg characteristic.

2. **Answer: b**
   The child with an easy temperament will adapt to school with only minor stresses. The slow-to-warm child will experience frustration. The difficult child will be moody and irritable and may benefit from a preschool visit.

3. **Answer: b**
   It is very important to get a bike of the proper size for the child. Getting a bike that the child can "grow into" is dangerous. Training wheels and grass to fall on are not acceptable substitutes for the proper protective gear. The child should already demonstrate good coordination in other playing skills before attempting to ride a bike.

4. **Answer: c**
   Asking how often the family eats together is an appropriate question for the girl. All the others should be directed to the parents.

5. **Answer: c**
   The nurse would have found that the child still has a leaner body mass than girls at this age. Both boys and girls increase body fat at this age. Food preferences will be highly influenced by those of her parents. Although caloric intake may diminish; appetite will increase.

6. **Answer: d**
   Parents are major influences on school-age children and should discuss the dangers of tobacco and alcohol use with the child. Not smoking in the house and hiding alcohol send mixed messages to the child. Open and honest discussion is the best approach rather than forbidding the child to make friends with kids that use tobacco or alcohol.

7. **Answer: b**
   The girl would need approximately 2,065 calories per day. (65 lbs = 29.5 kg × 70 calories per day per kg = 2,065 calories per day).

8. **Answer: b**
   Because they are role models for their children, parents must first realize the importance of their own behaviors. It is possible that the parents are pressuring the child, but that is not the primary message. Punishment should be appropriate, consistent, and not too severe.

9. **Answer: b**
   Lymphatic tissue growth is complete by age 9 better helping to localize infections and produce antibody–antigen responses. Brain growth will be complete by age 10. Frontal sinuses are developed at age 7. Third molars do not erupt until the teen years.

10. **Answer: d**
    The nurse would recommend that the parents be good role models and quit smoking. Locking up or hiding your cigarettes and going outside to smoke is not as effective as having a tobacco-free environment in the home.

11. **Answer: c**
    Self-esteem is developed early in childhood. The feedback a child receives from those perceived in authority such as parents and educators impact the child's sense of self-worth. As the child ages, the influences of peers and their treatment of the child begin to have an increasing influence on self-esteem.

12. **Answer: b**
    The child can be permanently scarred by negative experiences such a bullying. Activities such as self-defense and sports can promote a sense of accomplishment but are not most import option. There is no indication the child in the scenario will become a bully.

13. **Answer: d**
    School-aged children are often preoccupied with thoughts of death and dying. There is no indication these thoughts will lead to mental health issues or the development of depression.

14. **Answer: b**
    The values of a child are determined largely by the influences of their parents. As the child ages the impact of peers does begin to enter the picture. Children may also begin to test the values with their actions. In most cases the values of the family will prevail.

15. **Answer: a, d**
    During hospitalization the school-aged child may exhibit increased clinging behaviors. The child may also demonstrate regression. It will be helpful to promote the child be able to make some decisions or have some age appropriate sense of control. Ignoring the behaviors may be counterproductive.

# CHAPTER 7

## SECTION I: ASSESSING YOUR UNDERSTANDING

### Activity A FILL IN THE BLANKS

1. Psychosocial
2. Infancy
3. Abstract
4. Positive
5. Hispanic
6. Crisis
7. Identity
8. Ossification
9. Coordination
10. Socioeconomics

## Activity B MATCHING

**Question 1**

**1.** c    **2.** f    **3.** a    **4.** e    **5.** b    **6.** d

**Question 2**

**1.** e    **2.** c    **3.** a    **4.** d    **5.** f    **6.** b

**Question 3**

**1.** c    **2.** a    **3.** d    **4.** b    **5.** e

## Activity C SEQUENCING

6 → 3 → 1 → 4 → 5 → 2

## Activity D SHORT ANSWERS

1. Ambivalence, 10% wanted to become pregnant, 40% did not mind being pregnant, escape from home life, rite of passage to adulthood, peer pressure, confrontation of parental authority, ignorance.

2. The adolescent tries out various roles when interacting with peers, family, community, and society; this strengthens his or her sense of self. Past stages revisited tend to be those of trust (who/what to believe in), autonomy (expression of individuality), initiative (vision for what he or she might become), and industry (choices in school, community, church, and at work).

3. Completing school prepares the adolescent for college and/or employment. Schools that support peer bonds, promote health and fitness, encourage parental involvement, and strengthen community relationships lead to better student outcomes. Teachers, coaches, and counselors provide guidance and support to the adolescent.

4. The nurse should encourage parents and teens to have sexuality discussions. Sexuality discussions increase the teen's knowledge and strengthen his or her ability to make responsible decisions about sexual behavior.

5. Diet, exercise, and hereditary factors influence the height, weight, and body build of the adolescent. Over the past three decades, adolescents have become taller and heavier than their ancestors and the beginning of puberty is earlier. During the early adolescent period, there is an increase in the percentage of body fat and the head, neck, and hands reach adult proportions.

6. According to Piaget, the adolescent progresses from a concrete framework of thinking to an abstract one. It is the formal operational period. During this period, the adolescent develops the ability to think outside of the present; that is, he or she can incorporate into thinking concepts that do exist as well as concepts that might exist. Her thinking becomes logical, organized, and consistent. She is able to think about a problem from all points of view, ranking the possible solutions while solving the problem. Not all adolescents achieve formal operational reasoning at the same time.

## SECTION II: APPLYING YOUR KNOWLEDGE

## Activity E CASE STUDY

1. The discussion should include the following points:

    Today, piercing of the tongue, lip, eyebrow, naval, and nipple are common. Generally, body piercing is harmless, but Cho should be cautioned about receiving these procedures under nonsterile conditions and about the risk of complications. Qualified personnel using sterile needles should perform the procedure, and proper cleansing of the area at least twice a day is important. Although body piercing is common and considered relatively harmless, complications can occur. The complications of body piercing vary by site. Infections from body piercing usually result from unclean tools of the trade. Some of the infections that may occur as a result of unclean tools include hepatitis, tetanus, tuberculosis, and HIV. These complications may not become evident for some time after the piercing has been performed. Also, keloid formation and allergies to metal may occur. The naval is an area prone for infection since it is a moist area that endures friction from clothing. Once a naval infection occurs, it may take up to a year to heal.

2. The discussion should include the following points:

    Be open and respectful of the teen's decision about sexual activity. Discuss contraceptive options and a referral to a teen clinic may be appropriate. Provide education and information on abstinence, contraception, and the reality of caring for an infant. Reinforce that pregnancy and STIs, including HIV, can occur with any sexual encounter without the use of contraception. Stress the importance of the use of contraception.

    Identify if Cho is at risk for STIs and pregnancy based on her sexual practices. Encourage frequent and ongoing follow-ups. Encourage discussion with her parents about sexuality. Reinforce that engaging in sexual relations should be her choice and should not be influenced by peers. It is her right to say no. Reinforce that sexual activity in mature relationships should be respectful to both parties.

3. The discussion should include the following points:

    Families and parents of adolescents experience changes and conflicts that require adjustments and understanding of the development of the adolescent. The adolescent is striving for self-identity and increased independence. Maintaining open lines of communication is essential but often difficult during this time. Parents sense that they have less influence on the adolescent as they spend more time with peers, questions family values, and become more mobile.

    To help improve communication, encourage Cho's mother to set aside an appropriate amount of time to discuss matters without interruptions. Encourage her to talk face-to-face with Cho and to be aware of both her and Cho's body language.

Suggest that she ask questions about what Cho is feeling and offer Cho suggestions and advice. Cho's mother should choose her words carefully and be aware of her tone of voice and body language. Cho's mother should listen to what Cho has to say and should speak to her as an equal. It is important that her mother does not pretend to know all the answers and admits her mistakes. The mother should be reminded to give praise and approval to Cho often and to ensure rules and limits are set fairly and discussed.

---

# SECTION III: PRACTICING FOR NCLEX
## Activity F  NCLEX-STYLE QUESTIONS

1. **Answer: c**
   Asking broad, unanswerable questions, such as what the meaning of life is, is a Kohlberg activity for early adolescence. An example of Piaget activities for middle adolescence is wondering why things can't change (like wishing her parents were more understanding) and assuming everyone shares her interests. Comparing morals with those of peers is a Kohlberg activity for middle adolescence.

2. **Answer: b**
   Since most contraception methods are designed for females, it is important to teach the boy that contraception is a shared responsibility. Statistics about adolescent cases of STIs and warnings about getting the girl pregnant can easily be ignored by the child's sense of invulnerability. The fact that girls are more susceptible to STIs may give the boy a false sense of security.

3. **Answer: d**
   Cheese, yogurt, white beans, milk, and broccoli are good sources of calcium. Strawberries, watermelon, raisins, peanut butter, tomato juice, and whole grain bread are all foods high in iron. Beans, poultry, fish, meats, and dairy products are foods high in protein.

4. **Answer: a**
   Peers serve as role models for social behaviors, so their impact on an adolescent can be negative if the group is using drugs, or the group leader is in trouble. Sharing problems with peers helps the adolescent work through conflicts with parents. The desire to be part of the group teaches the child to negotiate differences and develop loyalties.

5. **Answer: c**
   Amphetamine use manifests as euphoria with rapid talking and dilated pupils. Signs of opiate use are drowsiness and constricted pupils. Barbiturates typically cause a sense of euphoria followed by depression. Marijuana users are typically relaxed and uninhibited.

6. **Answer: b**
   Checking for signs of depression or lack of friends would be most effective for preventing suicide. All other choices are more effective for preventing violence to others.

7. **Answer: a**
   The best approach is to describe the proper care using frequent cleansing with antibacterial soap. This is too late for warnings about the dangers of piercing such as skin- or blood-borne infections, or disease from unclean needles.

8. **Answer: c**
   If the boy has entered adolescence, he would also have frequent mood changes. A growing interest in attracting girls' attention and understanding that actions have consequences are typical of the middle stage of adolescence. Feeling secure with his body image does not occur until late adolescence.

9. **Answer: d**
   Increased blood pressure to adult levels indicates the child is in the early stage of adolescence. Increased shoulder, chest, and hip widths and muscle mass increase occurs in mid-adolescence. Eruption of the last four molars occurs in late adolescence.

10. **Answer: b**
    Whole grain bread contains high amounts of iron and is a type of food the child would not have an aversion to. Milk is a good source of vitamin D. Carrots are high in vitamin A. Orange juice is a good source for vitamin C.

11. **Answer: c**
    Teen age boys can experience growth in height until age 17.5. The nurse should reassure the teen that this may happen for him. Telling the client not to be ashamed, or assuring him it is not as short as his peers fails to provide information or support. Determining the height of the other men in the family may be indicated at a later time but is not the most appropriate initial comment.

12. **Answer: c**
    The dietary intake for active teen females should include be approximately 2,200 calories daily.

13. **Answer: c**
    Piaget's developmental theories focus on the cognitive maturation of the child. The ability to critically think is a sign of successful cognitive maturation. A sense of internal identity is consistent with Erikson's theories of development. Kohlberg's theories development focus on morals and values.

14. **Answer: c**
    The sedentary teen needs to consume approximately 1,600 calories each day. The recommended numbers of servings of fruit needed daily are two. A balanced diet includes a small amount of fat. To avoid all fat could place the child's health at risk. Protein intake is important for the development of tissue. The teen will need about 5 ounces of protein daily.

15. **Answer: b**
    The teenaged male has pubic hair that is beginning to curl. This takes place between ages 11 and 14. Absent or sparse pubic hair is consistent with a younger child. Coarse pubic hair is seen in older teens and adult men.

# CHAPTER 8

## SECTION I: ASSESSING YOUR UNDERSTANDING

### Activity A FILL IN THE BLANKS

1. Atraumatic
2. Therapeutic
3. Nonverbal
4. Child life
5. Verbal
6. Active
7. Interpreter

### Activity B MATCHING

**1.** e      **2.** a         **3.** d         **4.** c         **5.** b

### Activity C SEQUENCING

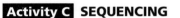
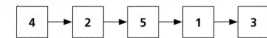

| 4 | → | 2 | → | 5 | → | 1 | → | 3 |

### Activity D SHORT ANSWERS

1. Therapeutic hugging is a method of safely preventing a child from harm during a painful or uncomfortable procedure that decreases fear and anxiety. The parent or caregiver holds the child in a position that promotes close physical contact in a way that restrains the child as necessary for the procedure to be performed successfully. This technique provides atraumatic care during procedures such as injections, venipunctures, and other invasive procedures.
2. The child or family will be able to demonstrate a skill, repeat information in their own words, answer open-ended questions, and act out the proper care procedure.
3. Signs exhibited by families or children that should alert the nurse of problems with health literacy include: difficulty completing registration forms or health care forms that are incomplete; frequently missed appointments; noncompliance with prescribed treatment; history of medication errors; claiming to have forgotten glasses or asking to take forms home to complete in regards to reading material or filling out forms; inability to answer questions about health care or avoiding asking questions regarding health care.
4. Draw pictures or use medical illustrations, use videos, color-code medications or steps of a procedure, record an audio tape, repeat verbal information often and "chunk" it into small bites, and teach a "back-up" family member.
5. The nurse should be an advocate of family-centered care in order to prevent separation, resulting in anxiety of both the family and child during hospitalization. The nurse can provide comfortable accommodations for the family and allow the family to choose if they want to be present for procedures that are uncomfortable for their child.

## SECTION II: APPLYING YOUR KNOWLEDGE

### Activity E CASE STUDY

1. The discussion should include the following:
   The nurse should avoid using terms that Emma may not understand or interpret differently from the intended meaning. The nurse could tell Emma that she will be taken to another room on a "special bed with wheels" rather than on a "stretcher." When describing the CT equipment the nurse could use an explanation such as, "there will be a big machine in the room that works like a camera. It will take pictures of your head since you hurt it when you fell. Your mommy and daddy will be able to go to this room with you and they will stand right outside the room when the camera takes the pictures."
2. The discussion should include the following:
   Therapeutic hugging should be utilized since this will allow Emma's parents to provide a comforting way of safely holding her so that the stitches can be placed with decreased trauma. The nurse should be sure that the parents understand how to hold Emma properly so that the procedure can be performed successfully while maintaining safety and security.

## SECTION III: PRACTICING FOR NCLEX

### Activity F NCLEX-STYLE QUESTIONS

1. **Answer: c**
   Nodding the head while the other person speaks indicates interest in what they are saying. When children and parents feel they are being heard, it builds trust. Sitting straight with feet flat on the floor, looking away from the speaker, and keeping distance from the family may send a message of disinterest.
2. **Answer: a**
   Having a child life specialist play with the child would provide the greatest support for the child and make the greatest contribution to atraumatic care. It is important to explain the procedure to the child and parents, let the child have a favorite toy and keep the parents calm, but these interventions are not as effective for atraumatic care.
3. **Answer: c**
   Since the child has just been diagnosed, concerns about postoperative home care would be least important. Arranging an additional meeting with the specialist and discussing treatment options may be necessary at some point, but involving the child and family in decision making is always a goal and is a part of family-centered care.
4. **Answer: b**
   Asking questions is a valid way to evaluate learning. However, it is far more effective to ask open-ended questions because they will better expose missing or incorrect information. As with teaching, evaluation of learning that involves active

participation is more effective. This includes the child and family demonstrating skills, teaching skills to each other, and acting out scenarios.

5. **Answer: d**
Recognizing the parents' and child's desire regarding treatment options is part of family-centered care. Presenting options for treatment is vague. Informing the child in terms that she can understand is the best example of therapeutic communication, which is goal, focused, purposeful communication.

6. **Answer: c**
The nurse is responsible for determining that the parents or legal guardians understand teaching that has been provided, as well as what they are signing, by asking pertinent questions of them. The physician or advanced practitioner is responsible for informing the child and family about the treatment, the potential risks and benefits, and alternative methods available; simply presenting this information does not ensure understanding. Witnessing the signing of the consent form should not occur until the nurse is sure the family understands teaching.

7. **Answer: c**
While it is important that the nurse recognizes and show respect for the parents' beliefs, and communicates in appropriate terms that they will understand, educating them carefully about the procedure and prognosis is vitally important in ensuring the child receives appropriate care. Assuring the competency of the surgeon is not therapeutic.

8. **Answer: a**
Missing appointments is one of the red flags to health literacy problems as the parents may not have understood the importance of the appointment or may not have been able to read or understand appointment reminders. Being bi-lingual does not indicate health literacy issues. Taking notes or one-parent being the primary leader of the child's health care are not unusual practices.

9. **Answer: a, c, d**
School age children better understand about and participate in their own care than preschoolers and toddlers. They need time to prepare themselves mentally for the procedure and should be given 3 to 7 days. Plays and puppets are more appropriate for preschoolers. Active involvement in self care will help them adjust and learn. Giving them choices to make allows them control and involvement in the process.

10. **Answer: c**
Asking questions or having private conversations with the interpreter may make the family uncomfortable and destroy the child/nurse relationship. Translation takes longer than a same-language appointment, and must be considered so that the family is not rushed. Using a nonprofessional runs the risk that they won't be able to adequately

translate medical terminology. Using an older sibling can upset the family relationships or cause legal problems.

11. **Answer: a, d, e**
RATIONALE: The child life specialist commonly assists with nonmedical preparation for diagnostic testing, provides tours, assists in play therapy, and is the child's advocate. The child's nurse gives medication, vaccines, and starts intravenous lines.

12. **Answer: a, c, d, e**
RATIONALE: Taking notes is an indicator that the mother is literate. All of the other options are "red flags" that indicate the mother may not be literate.

13. **Answers: a, c, d**
RATIONALE: The nurse should position himself or herself at the child's level. The nurse should speak in an unhurried manner. The nurse should ensure that the child's parents are present during education. It is appropriate to use words that the child will understand. It is appropriate to show patience during the interaction and look for nonverbal cues that indicate understanding or confusion.

14. **Answers: a, d, e**
RATIONALE: It is appropriate to use the word "tube" and not a "catheter." It is appropriate to call a "gurney" a "rolling bed." It is better to call "dye" special medicine. Terms used in the other options may be misunderstood by the child.

15. **Answers: b, c, d, e**
RATIONALE: When following the principles of atraumatic care, it is appropriate to apply numbing cream prior to starting the child's intravenous line. It is appropriate to empower the child with choices about care, if possible. It is appropriate for the child to have a security item present in the hospital. It is helpful for the family if the parent is able to stay with the child because it helps make the environment less stressful. The nurse should avoid using the phrase "holding the child down" and replace this with "therapeutic hugging."

# CHAPTER 9

## SECTION I: ASSESSING YOUR UNDERSTANDING

### Activity A FILL IN THE BLANKS

1. Development
2. In-utero
3. Community
4. Prevention
5. When
6. Coronary
7. Bone
8. Immunosuppression
9. Fixate
10. Active

## Activity B MATCHING

**Question 1**

**1.** b      **2.** e      **3.** c      **4.** f      **5.** d      **6.** a

**Question 2**

**1.** c      **2.** a      **3.** b      **4.** e      **5.** d

**Question 3**

**1.** b      **2.** d      **3.** a      **4.** e      **5.** c

## Activity C SEQUENCING

| 4 | → | 1 | → | 6 | → | 2 | → | 3 | → | 5 |

## Activity D SHORT ANSWERS

1. Place a vibrating tuning fork in the middle of the top of the head. Ask if the sound is in one ear or both ears. The sound should be heard in both ears.

2. Conditions in parents or grandparents what would suggest screening for hyperlipidemia in children includes coronary atherosclerosis, myocardial infarction, angina pectoris, peripheral vascular disease, cerebrovascular disease, and sudden cardiac death.

3. If problems are noted in the provided history, objective audiometry should be performed. When the child is capable of following simple commands, the nurse can perform basic procedures to screen for hearing loss. The "whisper," Weber, and Rinne tests can be used to screen for sensorineural or conductive hearing loss.

4. Iron deficiency is the leading nutritional deficiency in the United States. Iron deficiency can cause cognitive and motor deficits resulting in developmental delays and behavioral disturbances. The increased incidence of iron deficiency anemia is directly associated with periods of diminished iron stores, rapid growth, and high metabolic demands. At 6 months of age, the in utero iron stores of a full-term infant are almost depleted. The adolescent growth spurt warrants constant iron replacement. Pregnant adolescents are at even higher risk for iron deficiency due to the demands of the mother's growth spurt and the needs of the developing fetus.

5. Universal hypertension screening for children beginning at 3 years of age is recommended. If the child has risk factors for systemic hypertension, such as preterm birth, very low birth weight, renal disease, organ transplant, congenital heart disease or other illnesses associated with hypertension, then screening begins when the risk factor becomes apparent.

## SECTION II: APPLYING YOUR KNOWLEDGE

### Activity E CASE STUDY

**Case Study 1**

1. The discussion should include the following points:
   Nutritional history should be collected directly from Jasmine. There must be a discussion of her activity levels. Her height and weight should be plotted on a growth chart to observe trends.

2. The discussion should include the following points:
   Screening for iron deficiency is warranted for Jasmine. Iron deficiency is the leading nutritional deficiency in the United States. The increased incidence of iron deficiency anemia is directly associated with periods of rapid growth and high metabolic demands. The adolescent growth spurt warrants constant iron replacement. The Centers for Disease Control and Prevention recommends universal screening of high-risk children at various age intervals. Jasmine demonstrates risk factors for iron deficiency anemia, including the rapid growth spurt of adolescence, meal skipping and dieting, and low intake of fish, meat, and poultry. The American Academy of Pediatrics (AAP) recommends universal screening of all adolescent females during all routine physical examinations, therefore placing Jasmine in this category.

3. The discussion should include the following points:
   Your focus of healthy weight promotions should be health-centered, not weight-centered. Emphasize the benefits of health through an active lifestyle and nutritious eating pattern. Gear the education to focus on Jasmine's growing autonomy in making self-care decisions. Encourage healthy eating habits and healthy activity. Limit sedentary activities such as television viewing, computer usage, and video games.

**Case Study 2**

1. The discussion should include the following points:
   Children with chronic illnesses require repeated assessments to determine their health maintenance needs. How their illnesses impact their functional health patterns determines if standard health supervision visits need to be augmented to meet the individual child's situation.

   Nurses need to ensure comprehensive health supervision with frequent repeated assessments that include psychosocial assessments. The assessments should cover issues such as health insurance coverage, availability of transportation, financial stressors, family coping, and school personnel response to the child's chronic illness. The nurse needs to help develop an effective partnership between the child's medical home, family, and community.

   Coordination of care and access to resources is vital and enhances the quality of life for children with chronic illnesses. Nurses need to assist families in finding support groups and community-based resources, as well as financial and medical assistance programs. The nurse can also educate school personnel about the child's illness and assist them in maximizing the child's potential for academic success.

## SECTION III: PRACTICING FOR NCLEX

**Activity F** NCLEX-STYLE QUESTIONS

1. **Answer: d**
Congenital facial malformations are developmental warning signs. Neonatal conjunctivitis, when properly treated, has no long-term effects on development. Parents who are college students are not risk factors as would be high school dropouts. A 36-week birth is not a warning sign, but 33 weeks or less is.

2. **Answer: b**
Asking what activities that promote exercise for the child is best for several reasons. It provides assessment of the child's activity preferences, whether health-centered (positive) or weight centered (negative), and it offers variety. If on option doesn't work, others might. Emphasizing appropriate weight or dietary shortcomings can lead to eating disorders or body hatred. Suggesting only softball limits the success of the healthy weight promotion.

3. **Answer: c**
The most compelling argument for vaccinating for Varicella is that children not immunized are at risk if exposed to the disease. The mother needs to know about the chance of her child contracting the illness if not immunized. The contagious nature of the disease, low risk of the vaccine, or the low incidence of reactions is not appropriate explanations for why the child should have the vaccine.

4. **Answer: c**
Iron deficiency anemia could be present because the iron stores in the boy's body may have diminished by the adolescent's growth spurt. This would be checked for by blood work. Developmental problems are not caused by the adolescent's growth spurt. Hyperlipidemia could be possible if the child's diet included an excessive amount of fat. Hypertension might be a problem if a family member had the condition in early adulthood or if many family members had this condition.

5. **Answer: d**
The nurse will provide information to prevent injury or disease such as discussing the hazards of putting the baby to sleep with a bottle. Assessing for an infection and taking a health history for an injury are not part of a health supervision visit. Administering a vaccination for Varicella would not occur until 12 months of age.

6. **Answer: a**
The nurse will advise the mother that poor oral health can have significant negative effects on systemic health. Discussing fluoridation and community health may have little interest to the mother. Placing the hands in the mouth exposes the child to pathogens and is appropriate for personal hygiene promotion. Soft drink consumption is better covered during healthy diet promotion.

7. **Answer: b**
Maintaining proper therapy for eczema can be exhausting both physically and mentally. Therefore it is essential that the nurse assess parents' ability to cope with this stress. Changing a bandage is not part of a health supervision visit. Skin hydration is important for a child with eczema; however, fluid volume is not a concern. Systemic corticosteroid therapy is very rarely used and the success of the current therapy needs to be assessed first.

8. **Answer: c**
The Ishihara chart is best for the 6-year-old because the child will know numbers. CVTME charts are designed to assess color vision discrimination for preschoolers. The Allen figures chart and the Snellen charts are for assessing visual acuity.

9. **Answer: d**
Neighborhoods with high crime, high poverty, and lack of resources may contribute to poor health care and illness. If the aged grandparents have healthy lifestyles, they would be positive partners. Developmentally appropriate chores and responsibilities could be positive signs of parental guidance. The doting mother could make a strong health supervision partner.

10. **Answer: a**
The Rinne test compares air conduction of sound with bone conduction of sound and can be performed in the office. The Whisper test requires a quiet room with no distractions. Auditory Brainstem Response (ABR) and the Evoked Otoacoustic Emissions (EOAE) are indicated for newborns and are usually done by an audiologist.

11. **Answer: c**
A 3-year-old child should have the ability to copy a circle. Stacking five blocks, grasping a crayon, and throwing a ball overhand are not reasonable accomplishments for a 3-year-old child.

12. **Answer: a, c, d**
The Denver II screening test is used on children from birth to age 6 months. It is used to assess personal–social, fine motor–adaptive, language, and gross motor skills. The test employs props. These include dolls, crayons, and balls.

13. **Answer: c**
In the absence of risk factors vision screening should begin in children once they reach the age of 3.

14. **Answer: b**
Passive immunity results when immunoglobulins are passed from one person to another. This immunity is temporary. This is the type of immunity that takes place when a mother breastfeeds her child. Active immunity results when an individual's own immunity generates an immune response.

15. **Answer: d**
Populations at an increased risk for elevated blood lead levels include immigrants, refugees, or international adoptees.

# CHAPTER 10

## SECTION I: ASSESSING YOUR UNDERSTANDING

### Activity A FILL IN THE BLANKS

1. PERRLA
2. BMI
3. Fontanel
4. Stethoscope
5. Stridor
6. Milia
7. Auscultation

### Activity B LABELING

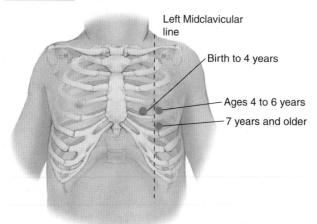

Left Midclavicular line

Birth to 4 years

Ages 4 to 6 years

7 years and older

### Activity C MATCHING

1. c    2. e        3. a        4. d        5. b

### Activity D SEQUENCING

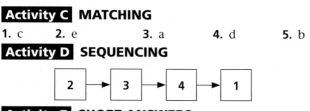

### Activity E SHORT ANSWERS

1. Grade one is barely audible, sometimes heard, sometimes not. Grade two is quiet, yet heard each time the chest is auscultated. Grade three and four are audible with grade three having an intermediate intensity and grade four having a palpable thrill. Grade five is loud and is audible with the edge of stethoscope lifted off the chest. Grade six is very loud and audible with the stethoscope placed near but not touching the chest.

2. Ecchymosis is a purplish discoloration (bruise) that changes from blue, to brown to black. It is common on the lower extremities in young children.

   Petechiae are pinpoint reddish purple macules that do not blanch when pressed. They are broken tiny blood vessels that occur with coughing, bleeding disorders and meningococcemia.

   Purpura is purple larger macules caused by bleeding under the skin and occurs with bleeding disorders and meningococcemia.

3. The canal should be pink, have tiny hairs, and be free from scratches, drainage, foreign bodies, and edema. The tympanic membrane should appear pearly pink or gray and be translucent allowing visualization of the bony landmarks.

4. The heart rate of the child gradually decreases from infancy to adolescence. The infant's normal heart rate ranges from 80 to 150 beats per minute, with the toddlers heart rate decreasing slightly to 70 to 120 beats per minute. The preschooler and school-age child have similar normal heart rates at 65 to 110 and 60 to 100, respectively. The adolescent's normal heart rate drops to 55 to 95 beats per minute.

5. Inaccurate pulse oximetry readings may result from the child having a low hemoglobin value, hypotension, hypothermia, hypovolemia, skin breakdown, carbon monoxide poisoning, interference with the ambient light, and movement of the extremity.

6. Possible risk factors that indicate the need for BP measurement of children under the age of 3 years include: history of prematurity, very low birth weight, or other neonatal complications; congenital heart disease; recurrent urinary tract infections or any other renal complication; any malignancy or transplant; any treatment that causes the BP to increase; systemic illnesses that affect the BP; and increased intracranial pressure.

## SECTION II: APPLYING YOUR KNOWLEDGE

### Activity F CASE STUDY

*The discussion should include the following points:*

**FIRST PRIORITY:** A 7-month-old hospitalized with pneumonia. Vital signs are heart rate of 165 with brief episodes of dropping into the 60's during the previous shift, respiratory rate of 78, blood pressure 112/72, and axillary temperature of 99.5 F.

**RATIONALE:** This child is the most unstable. The tachypnea, tachycardia with bradycardic episodes can be indicative of a potentially unstable airway. The increased blood pressure may also indicate acute distress.

**SECOND PRIORITY:** A 3-month-old hospitalized for rule out sepsis secondary to fever. Vital signs are heart rate of 165, respiratory rate of 34, blood pressure 108/64, rectal temperature of 102.5 F taken immediately before report. No intervention was initiated.

**RATIONALE:** This child is potentially unstable. The tachycardia and increased blood pressure are most likely due to fever and stress. The increased temperature (without intervention) is a concern but overall this child's vital signs are less life-threatening than the tachypnea and bradycardia present in the first priority child.

**THIRD PRIORITY:** A 5-year-old hospitalized with an acute asthma attack. Vital signs are heart rate 124, respiratory rate 28 to 30, blood pressure 93/48, and axillary temperature of 98.6F.

**RATIONALE:** This child has an acute illness and may be potentially unstable due to slightly increased respiratory rate and mild tachycardia. This child warrants close monitoring but at this time is more stable than either of the other two children.

## SECTION III: PRACTICING FOR NCLEX

**Activity G** NCLEX-STYLE QUESTIONS

1. **Answer: a**
   **RATIONALE:** The newborn's labia minora is typically swollen from the effects of maternal estrogen. The minora will decrease in size and be hidden by the labia majora within the first weeks. Lesions on the external genitalia are indicative of sexually transmitted infection. Labial adhesions are not a normal finding for a healthy newborn. Swollen labia majora is not a normal finding.

2. **Answer: c**
   **RATIONALE:** The nurse should first begin with open-ended questions regarding work, hobbies, activities, and friendship in order to make the teen feel comfortable. Once a trusting rapport has been established, the nurse should move on to the more emotionally charged questions. While it is important to assure confidentiality, the nurse should first establish rapport.

3. **Answer: c**
   **RATIONALE:** A good health history includes open-ended questions that allow the child to narrate their experience. The other questions would most likely elicit a yes or no response.

4. **Answer: c**
   **RATIONALE:** It is best to approach a shy 4-year-old by introducing the equipment slowly and demonstrating the process on the girl's doll first. Toddlers are egocentric; referring to how another child performed probably will not be helpful in gaining the child's cooperation. The other questions would most likely elicit a "no" response.

5. **Answer: b**
   **RATIONALE:** Asking "What can I help you with?" is very welcoming and allows for a variety of responses that may include functional problems, developmental concerns, or disease. Asking about the chief complaint may not be clear to all parents. Asking if the child feels sick will most likely elicit a yes or no answer and no other helpful details. Asking whether the child has been exposed to infectious agents is unclear and would not open a dialogue.

6. **Answer: c**
   **RATIONALE:** Preschoolers like to play games. To encourage deep breathing, the nurse should elicit the child's cooperation by engaging the child in a game to blow out the light bulb on the penlight. Telling the child that he or she may not leave or must breathe deeply would not engage the child. Asking whether the child would allow his or her caregiver to listen would most likely elicit a no.

7. **Answer: a**
   **RATIONALE:** The physical examination of children, just as for adults always begins with a systematic inspection, followed by palpation or percussion, then by auscultation.

8. **Answer: b**
   **RATIONALE:** Touching the thumb to the ball of the infant's foot would elicit the plantar grasp reflex. The other reflexes are not elicited by this method.

9. **Answer: c**
   **RATIONALE:** The nurse knows that some of the history must be delayed until after the child is stabilized. After the child is stabilized the nurse can take a detailed history. The child who has received routine health care and presents with a mild illness would need only a problem-focused history. The nurse should be sensitive to repetitive interviews in hospital situations but should not assume that the child's history can be obtained from other providers. A complete and detailed history would be in order if physicians rarely see the child or if the child is critically ill.

10. **Answer: b**
    **RATIONALE:** This indicates a positive Romberg test which warrants further testing for possible cerebellar dysfunction.

11. **Answer: 21**
    **RATIONALE:** Using the metric method, the formula is:
    weight in kilograms divided by height in meters squared
    weight (kg)/height (m)$^2$
    42 kg/1.42$^2$
    42/2.0164 = 20.8292 = 21

12. **Answer: b, c, a, d**
    **RATIONALE:** The proper order of the assessment of the thorax is to inspect, palpate, percuss, and auscultate.

## CHAPTER 11

### SECTION I: ASSESSING YOUR UNDERSTANDING

**Activity A** FILL IN THE BLANKS

1. Hugging
2. 15
3. Bath
4. Eat
5. Therapeutic
6. Individualized Health Plans (IHPs)
7. Health department

**Activity B** MATCHING

1. b    2. e         3. a         4. c         5. d

**Activity C** SEQUENCING

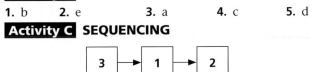

## Activity D  SHORT ANSWERS

1. The nurse can address and minimize separation anxiety by:

   Understanding the stages of separation anxiety and be able to recognize them in children; realizing that behaviors demonstrated during the first stage do not indicate that the child is "bad"; encouraging the family to stay with the child when appropriate; helping the family deal with various reactions and intervene before the behaviors of detachment occur; using guided imagery based on the use of the child's imagination and enjoyment of play in order to help the child relax.

2. Discharge planning actually begins upon admission. The nurse should assess the family's resources and knowledge level upon admission to determine the need for education and possible referrals.

3. Some common coping behaviors/methods include: stoicism, ignoring or negating problem, acting out, anger, withdrawal, rejection, and intellectualizing.

4. Under the age of 5 years, children are most commonly admitted to the hospital for respiratory issues. Older children are typically hospitalized for issues such as diseases of the respiratory system, mental health problems, injuries, and gastrointestinal disorders. In regards to adolescents, problems related to pregnancy, childbearing, mental health, and injury account for the majority of hospitalizations.

5. The home care nurse should be sure to include the child in the conversation; address the caregivers formally unless asked to address them otherwise; be friendly and respectful, and use a soft, calm voice; use good listening skills; and be sure to schedule the first visit when the primary caregiver is present.

## SECTION II: APPLYING YOUR KNOWLEDGE

## Activity E  CASE STUDY

*The discussion should include the following points:*

1. **INTERVENTIONS:** Assess if irritability is related to surgical intervention, including pain.

   **RATIONALE:** The irritability could be related to the surgery, especially pain, resulting from the procedure. Once this is ruled out address the infant's basic needs (trust versus mistrust).

   **INTERVENTIONS:** Encourage and facilitate family presence at the bedside and rooming-in. Provide consistent nursing staff. Arrange to have a volunteer hold and rock the baby when family is not present at bedside. Place the baby in a room near the nurse's station.

   **RATIONALE:** Infants gain a sense of trust in the world through reciprocal patterns of contact. Crying without comfort and lack of stimulation can lead to distress in the infant. By 5 to 6 months infants are acutely aware of the absence of their primary caregiver and may be fearful of unfamiliar persons. Providing caregivers who will address the comfort and care needs of the infant consistently is important for the developing infant. Response time to crying may be reduced by placing the infant near the nurse's station.

2. **INTERVENTIONS:** Address discomfort or pain that may be associated with disease process. Promote home routine related to bedtime and naptime. Provide a quiet, darkened room. Allow the parent to lie in bed or crib next to toddler if possible. Group care activities and allow undisturbed periods of rest during designated nap/sleep times.

   **RATIONALE:** Pain and discomfort could be contributing to lack of rest. Once ruled out, address the toddler's developmental needs. The change in routine caused by the hospitalization could be contributing to the lack of rest. Maintaining home rituals can help to normalize naptime and bedtime. Toddlers have a need of familiarity and the closeness of a primary caregiver. Providing parental comfort can help to minimize the toddler's distress. Allowing undisturbed times for naps can also help promote adequate rest.

3. **INTERVENTIONS:** Address pain management needs. Explain procedures honestly, using concrete terms. Encourage expression of feelings using therapeutic play. Consult child life  physician if available. Encourage family member to room in. Leave a small light on at night.

   **RATIONALES:** Fantasy and magical thinking may be heightened when pain and discomfort are experienced. Once ruled out address the preschoolers developmental needs. Preschoolers fear mutilation and are afraid of intrusive procedures. They interpret words literally and have an active imagination. Explaining procedures in terms the child can understand can help allay fears. Therapeutic play can help the child express and work through fears. Child life physician are excellent resources to encourage medical play and assist with preparation of the child. Presence of family provides comfort and security. Simply having a small amount of light in the room can help prevent fantasies and fears related to darkness leading to nightmares.

4. **INTERVENTIONS:** Talk to the child about the reasons for his lack of eating. Provide the child's favorite foods and allow the child to choose his meals (allow foods from home, if possible allow child to go to cafeteria to pick out food).

   **RATIONALE:** The refusal to eat may be related to a lack of appetite due to disease process. Once ruled out, focus on the school-age child's developmental needs. Lack of eating may be a reaction to the hospitalization or a dislike of the foods provided. Offering favorite foods and asking the child the reasons he is not eating may help determine the cause of the lack of appetite. School-age children are accustomed to controlling self-care and they like being involved. They are used to making decisions about their meals and activities. By allowing them to pick their food you give them the opportunity to maintain independence, retain self-control, enhance self-esteem, and continue to work toward achieving a sense of industry.

5. **INTERVENTIONS:** Establish rapport with the adolescent. Encourage her to discuss her feelings. Provide a phone at her bedside. Encourage her to call her friends and family. Encourage her friends to visit. Encourage use of a journal. Collaborate with a psychologist if appropriate.

**RATIONALE:** Adolescents typically do not experience separation anxiety from being away from their parents; instead, their anxiety comes from separation from their friends. They typically do not like to be different than their peers and appearance is an important factor for them. Adolescents with a chronic illness may become depressed due to prolonged separation from peers, altered body image, lack of self-esteem, and feeling different. Loss of control may lead to behaviors of anger, withdrawing, and general uncooperativeness. Developing rapport with the adolescent and encouraging discussion and expression of her feelings can help the adolescent cope. Also connecting the adolescent with her peers can be an important factor in improving coping. Collaboration with a psychologist may be appropriate if depression seems severe.

# SECTION III: PRACTICING FOR NCLEX
## Activity F NCLEX-STYLE QUESTIONS

1. **Answer: a**
   **RATIONALE:** Children in the first phase, protest, react aggressively to this separation, and reject others who attempt to comfort the child. The other behaviors are indicators of the second phase, despair.

2. **Answer: d**
   **RATIONALE:** It is best to include the families whenever possible so they can assist the child in coping with their fears. Preschoolers fear mutilation and are afraid of intrusive procedures. Their magical thinking limits their ability to understand everything, requiring communication and intervention to be on their level. Telling the child that we need to put a little hole in their arm might scare the child. Talking about taking or removing blood might be interpreted literally.

3. **Answer: a**
   **RATIONALE:** Previous experience with hospitalization can either add to the positive aspects of preparation or distract if the experiences were perceived as negative. If the child associates the hospital with the death of a relative, the experience is likely viewed as negative. The other statements would most likely indicate that the child's previous experiences were viewed as positive.

4. **Answer: c**
   **RATIONALE:** Distraction with books or games would be the best remedy to provide an outlet to distract him from his restricted activity. The other

responses would be unlikely to affect a change in the behavior of a 6-year-old.

5. **Answer: a**
   **RATIONALE:** Parents who do not tell children the truth or do not answer their questions confuse, frighten, and may weaken the children's trust in the parent. The other statements are effective forms of communication.

6. **Answer: d**
   **RATIONALE:** The nurse should start the initial contact with children and their families as a foundation for developing a trusting relationship. Asking about a favorite toy would be a good starting point. The nurse should allow the child to participate in the conversation without the pressure of having to comply with a request or undergo any procedures.

7. **Answer: c**
   **RATIONALE:** The nurse needs to describe the procedure and equipment in terms the child can understand. For a 4-year-old, a simple explanation along with the chance to touch and feel the tiny tubes would be best. Using the term tympanostomy tubes is not age-appropriate and does not teach. Telling the child that he or she will be asleep the whole time might increase their fears. Showing the child the operating room might increase fear with all of the strange and imposing equipment.

8. **Answer: b**
   **RATIONALE:** The nurse understands that a toddler is most likely to develop anxiety and fears due to separation from the parents. Separation from friends, loss of control, and loss of independence are fears typically experienced by an adolescent.

9. **Answer: c**
   **RATIONALE:** It is important to be honest and encourage the child to ask questions rather than wait for the child to speak up. The other statements are correct.

10. **Answer: c**
    **RATIONALE:** The best approach would be to write the name of his nurse on a small board and then identify all staff members working with the child (each shift and each day). Reminding the boy he will be going home soon or telling him not to worry does not address his concerns or provide solutions. Encouraging the boy's parents to stay with him at all times may be unrealistic and may place undue stress on the family.

11. **Answer: d, a, c, b**
    **RATIONALE:** Nursing care for a hospitalized child typically occurs in four phases: introduction, building a trusting relationship, decision-making phase, and providing comfort and reassurance.

12. **Answer: a, b, d**
    **RATIONALE:** It is important to assess the child's peripheral vascular circulation especially when the child has a restraint placed on an extremity. Capillary refill, color, temperature, and pulses are appropriate to assess to ensure that the child's peripheral vascular circulation has not been compromised.

13. **Answers: b, c, d**
    **RATIONALE:** Even minor nursing interventions should not be performed in the playroom. The playroom should be referred to as the "activity room" or "social room" instead of "playroom" when speaking with adolescent children. It is inappropriate to perform procedures in the child's crib. It is better to perform procedures in the treatment room. It is important to give anti-emetics prior to mealtimes. Parents can be encouraged to bring in security items to help reduce the child's level of stress.

14. **Answer: 2 cups of fluid**
    **RATIONALE:** Ice is approximately equivalent to half the same amount of water.

# CHAPTER 12

## SECTION I: ASSESSING YOUR UNDERSTANDING

### Activity A FILL IN THE BLANKS

1. 3
2. Respite
3. Family
4. Cancer
5. Written
6. Palliative
7. Hospice

### Activity B MATCHING

1. e    2. a    3. b    4. c    5. d

### Activity C SEQUENCING

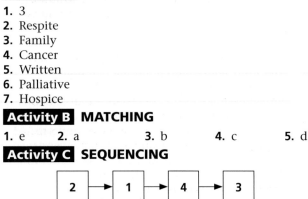

### Activity D SHORT ANSWERS

1. Answers may include homeopathic and herbal medicine, pet therapy, hippotherapy, massage or music. Discharge planning actually begins upon admission. The nurse should assess the family's resources and knowledge level upon admission to determine the need for education and possible referrals.

2. Formerly premature infants need extra calories for growth. They also need extra calcium and phosphorus for adequate bone mineralization. Their diet consists of breast milk fortified with additional nutrients or a commercially prepared formula specific for premature infants.

3. The nurse should explain that DNR (do not resuscitate) refers to withholding cardiopulmonary resuscitation should the child's heart stop beating. It is important to ensure that this does not mean they are giving up on their child. Nurses must educate families that resuscitation may be inappropriate and lead to more suffering than if death were allowed to occur naturally. Families may wish to specify a certain extent of resuscitation that they feel more comfortable with (e.g., allowing supplemental oxygen but not providing chest compressions). Some institutions are now replacing the DNR terminology with "allow natural death" (AND), which may be more acceptable to families facing the decision to withhold resuscitation.

4. Respecting the child and family's goals, preferences, and choices; comprehensive caring; using the strengths of interdisciplinary resources; acknowledging and addressing caregivers' concerns; building systems and mechanisms of support (Association of Pediatric Oncology Nurses, 2003).

5. Do not excessively try to get the child to eat or drink; offer small frequent meals or snacks, such as soups or shakes; provide the child with foods they request; administer anti-emetics as needed; provide good mouth care; ensure environment is free of odors and is conducive to eating.

## SECTION II: APPLYING YOUR KNOWLEDGE

### Activity E

*The discussion should include the following points:*

Children with special health care needs require comprehensive and coordinated care from multiple health care professionals. The nurse can facilitate communication and help to ensure collaboration to address the child's health, educational, psychological, and social service needs. The nurse needs to promote family-centered care and work with the parents as a team. Include both parents and other caregivers in learning skills needed to care for this child. The nurse can assist the family to incorporate the child's medical needs into daily life and to minimize the child's self perception of being different. Developing a trusting and permanent relationship with the family will allow the nurse to identify the family's changing needs and will allow better two-way communication. The nurse should support and empower the family and assist parents and families to find support systems and resources.

The nurse needs to be attuned to the entire family's needs and emotions and be fully present with the child and family. Listen to the child and family and foster respect for the whole child. Respect the parents and help them to honor the commitments they have made to their child. Work collaboratively with the family and health care team. Acknowledge that the parents have diverse needs for information and encourage participation in decision making. The school-age child has a concrete understanding of death. Give Georgia specific honest details when they are requested. Encourage participation in decision making and help the child to establish a sense of control.

## SECTION III: PRACTICING FOR NCLEX

### Activity F NCLEX-STYLE QUESTIONS

1. **Answer: c**
   **RATIONALE:** A good therapeutic relationship is built on trust and communication. It is strengthened by

listening to the parents, acknowledging their triumphs, and supporting them when they fail. Continuing to educate them, helping them access resources, and helping them to save money on medications are good interventions, but not as effective at building a trusting relationship.

2. **Answer: a**
RATIONALE: Providing full participation in decision making gives the adolescent a sense of worth and builds his self-esteem. The adolescent may have difficulty initiating conversation, but wants and needs to voice his fears and concerns. He also requires direct, honest answers to his questions. However, these needs are not as effective in meeting his need for sense of self-worth or self-esteem.

3. **Answer: d**
RATIONALE: School-age children need specific details about procedures related to dying. Explaining how a morphine drip keeps her sister comfortable would best minimize the child's anxiety. Saying her sister won't need food any more when she dies is more appropriate for a younger child. School-age children are curious about death and may deny that it is impending. These behaviors should be handled with understanding and patience.

4. **Answer: b**
RATIONALE: Serving on his individualized education plan committee will be most beneficial to his education because this plan is designed to meet his individual educational needs. Collaborating with the school nurse and assessing the health effects of attending school, and getting a motorized wheel chair do not address his educational needs.

5. **Answer: b**
RATIONALE: Watching the interaction between mother and child to see if the child maintains eye contact may indicate that the child is being neglected which is an inorganic cause for failure to thrive. Refusing the nipple is a sign of organic cause for failure to thrive. Prematurity is a risk factor for failure to thrive. Checking the health history may disclose other organic causes for failure to thrive.

6. **Answer: c**
RATIONALE: Communication can best be improved if the nurse uses reflective listening techniques to show the parents that their input is heard and valued. Giving direct, understandable answers and saying the same thing different ways helps ensure effective communication with the parents but does nothing to build communication between the nurse and family. Sharing cell phone numbers only allows the nurse and family to talk to each other.

7. **Answer: d**
RATIONALE: A good way to involve the father and gain his input regarding in the child's care is to schedule education sessions in the evening when he can get away from the office. Leaving voice mails and sending email reports leave him isolated from care group. Lunchtime visits are not long enough for him to focus on the situation.

8. **Answer: a**
RATIONALE: Nurses can help parents build on their strengths and empower them to care for their child by educating them about the course of treatment and the child's expected outcome. Evaluating emotional strength, assessing the home, and preparing a list of supplies do not empower the parents for the task ahead of them.

9. **Answer: b**
RATIONALE: Young adolescents require time with their peers. Encouraging her to have visitors would best meet this need. Assuring her illness is not her fault and acting as her personal confidant are interventions suited to school-age children. Explaining her condition in detail meets the needs of an older adolescent.

10. **Answer: c**
RATIONALE: The child may be struggling to fit in with his peers by avoiding his treatment regimen in an effort to hide his illness. Monitoring his compliance would disclose this risky behavior. Assessing for depression, encouraging participation in activities, and joining a support group would not address risky behavior.

11. **Answers: b, c**
RATIONALE: Hearing deficits and strabismus are associated with prematurity.

12. **Answer: 7-month-old**
RATIONALE: When assessing growth and development of the infant or child who was born prematurely, determine the child's adjusted or corrected age so that you can perform an accurate assessment. 40 weeks–32 weeks is 8 weeks or 2 months. The child was born 2 months early.

13. **Answer: 2,784 kilocalories**
RATIONALE: 23.2 kilograms × 120 kilocalories/ 1 kilogram = 2,784 kilocalories

14. **Answer: d, b, a, c**
RATIONALE: The proper order of occurrence is trust, autonomy, initiative, and industry.

15. **Answer: c, d, e**
RATIONALE: Risk factors for the development of vulnerable child syndrome include newborn jaundice, an illness that the child was not expected to recover from, and congenital anomalies.

# CHAPTER 13

## SECTION I: ASSESSING YOUR UNDERSTANDING

### Activity A FILL IN THE BLANKS

1. Implanted
2. Pharmacodynamics
3. Distraction
4. Fifth
5. Hypoglycemia
6. Nasogastric
7. Opthalmic

## Activity B LABELING

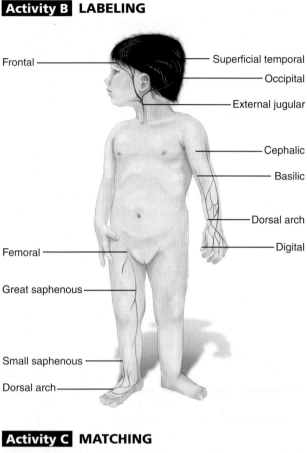

Frontal — Superficial temporal
— Occipital
— External jugular
— Cephalic
— Basilic
— Dorsal arch
— Digital
Femoral —
Great saphenous —
Small saphenous —
Dorsal arch —

## Activity C MATCHING

**1.** e **2.** a **3.** b **4.** c **5.** d

## Activity D SEQUENCING

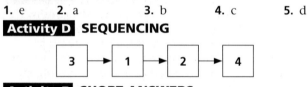

## Activity E SHORT ANSWERS

1. The child's room should remain a safe and secure area. In the hospital, all invasive procedures should be performed in the treatment room.
2. Check identification since children may deny their identity in attempt to avoid unpleasant situations, play in another child's bed, or remove ID bracelet; confirm identity each time medication is given; verify the child's name with the caregiver to provide additional assurance of identification.
3. Monitor the child's vital signs closely for changes; adhere to strict aseptic technique when caring for the catheter and administering TPN; ensure that the system remains a closed system at all times, including securing all connections, using occlusive dressings, and clamping catheter or having child perform the Valsalva maneuver during tubing and cap changes; follow agency policy for flushing of catheter and maintaining catheter patency; assess intake and output frequently; monitor blood glucose levels and obtain laboratory tests as ordered to evaluate for changes in fluid and electrolytes.

4. The eight rights of medication administration for children are the right: medication, patient, time, route of administration, dose, documentation, to be educated, and to refuse.
5. A feeding tube can be checked for placement by checking the pH (results vary between gastric and intestinal tubes); observing the appearance of the fluid removed from the tube upon aspiration; instilling air and performing gastric auscultation; checking external markings on tube and external tube length; assessing for signs indicative of feeding tube misplacement; and reviewing any chest or abdominal X-rays for placement.

## SECTION II: APPLYING YOUR KNOWLEDGE

## Activity F CASE STUDY

*The discussion should include the following points:*

1. **a.** Identify the need for the PRN medication based on the order. Rationale: Identification of the child's condition that warrants the medication is the first step in administering a PRN medication. Jennifer's rectal temperature of 102.5 F demonstrates a need for acetaminophen for fever (per the order).
   **b.** Verify medication order. Rationale: To ensure appropriate medication will be administered.
   **c.** Calculate the correct dose. Rationale: To ensure that the amount of medication is appropriate for the child based on weight.
   **d.** Calculate amount to be drawn up from the bottle of acetaminophen. Rationale: To ensure the appropriate amount of medication is given based on the available medication concentration.
   **e.** Wash hands. Rationale: To prevent infection
   **f.** Verify correct medication and expiration date of medication. Verify time of last dose given and ensure at least 4 hours ago. Verify oral route is the ordered route of administration. Draw up acetaminophen from the bottle using an oral syringe. Rationale: Right medication, right time, and right route of administration are three of the 8 right parts of medication administration. A syringe is the best way to accurately measure the liquid medication. It is also the best way to administer medicine to an infant.
   **g.** Prepare a bottle of juice, formula, or breastmilk. Rationale: It is recommended to have a "chaser" for the infant to drink immediately after the medication is given.
   **h.** Educate Jennifer's parents at the bedside regarding why the medicine is needed, what the child will experience and the desired effect of the medication, what is expected of the child and how the parents can participate and support their child. Rationale: Parent teaching is an important part of medication administration. Involvement of parents in medication administration can reduce stress for the infant.

i. Invite the parents to assist and/or give suggestions for techniques. Rationale: The parents may have helpful suggestions for how their child best takes medications. Involvement of parents in medication administration can reduce stress for the infant, validates their roles as caregivers, and may increase the likelihood of successful medication administration.

j. Check identification of the child. Rationale: To ensure medicine is given to correct child.

k. Administer the medication into the back of the infant's mouth between the teeth and gums. Give small amounts and allow the child to swallow before more medicine is placed in the mouth. Have the child upright or at least 45 degree angle. Rationale: Allows infant to swallow the medication and decreases the likelihood of spitting, coughing up, or aspirating the medication.

l. Offer the infant a sip from the prepared bottle. Rationale: The juice can help rinse the medication taste from the mouth and sucking on the bottle often will help soothe and calm the infant.

m. Document the medication administration and within 30 to 60 minutes document the child's response (recheck temperature). Rationale: Documentation should be done after the medication is administered. Since this is a PRN medication the infant's response should be noted.

2. Dosing for acetaminophen is 10 to 15 mg/kg every 4 to 6 hours. Convert 15 lbs to kg (1 kg = 2.2 lbs)

   Therefore 15 lb equals 6.8 kg multiplied by 10 = 68 mg; 6.8 multiplied by 15 = 102 mg. The range of acetaminophen Jennifer can receive is 68 mg to 102 mg every 4 to 6 hours; therefore 70 mg every 4 hours po is a safe and therapeutic dose.

3. Ratio method:

   70 mg:x = 80 mg:0.8 mL-multiply means and extremes and get 56 = 80x, solve for x

   x = 0.7 mL

   Proportion method:

   $\dfrac{70\text{ mg}}{x} = \dfrac{80\text{ mg}}{0.8\text{ mL}}$ (cross multiply) = 56 = 80x solve for x, x = 0.7 mL

## SECTION III: PRACTICING FOR NCLEX

### Activity G NCLEX-STYLE QUESTIONS

1. **Answer: a**
   **RATIONALE:** The nurse should provide a description of and reason for the procedure in age-appropriate language. The nurse should avoid the use of terms such as culture or strep throat as it is not age appropriate for a 4-year-old. The nurse should also avoid confusing terms like "take your blood" that might be interpreted literally.

2. **Answer: b**
   **RATIONALE:** Signs of infiltration included cool, puffy, or blanched skin. Warmth, redness, induration, and tender skin are signs of inflammation.

3. **Answer: b**
   **RATIONALE:** The priority nursing action is to verify the medication ordered. The first step in the eight rights of pediatric medication administration is to ensure that the child is receiving the right medication. After verifying the order, the nurse would then gather the medication, the necessary equipment and supplies, wash hands and put on gloves.

4. **Answer: c**
   **RATIONALE:** The nurse should emphasize that the parents should never threaten the child in order to make him take his medication. It is more appropriate to develop a cooperative approach that will elicit the child's cooperation since he needs ongoing, daily medication. The other statements are correct.

5. **Answer: d**
   **RATIONALE:** The preferred injection site for infants is the vastus lateralis muscle. An alternative site is the rectus femoris muscle. The dorsogluteal is not a recommended site for the infant. The deltoid muscle, which is a small muscle mass, is used as an IM injection site in children after the age of 4 to 5 years of age due to the small muscle mass.

6. **Answer: b**
   **RATIONALE:** The nurse should explain what is to occur and enlist the child's help in the removal of the tape or dressing. This provides the child with a sense of control over the situation and also encourages his or her cooperation. The nurse should avoid using scissors to remove the tape or dressing and the comment regarding cutting may be perceived as threatening and/or frightening. Telling the child to be a big girl is inappropriate and does not teach. Telling the child the procedure will not hurt and using the terms tug and pinch could increase the child's fear and lead to misunderstanding.

7. **Answer: a**
   **RATIONALE:** A good way to involve the father and gain his input regarding in the child's care is to schedule education sessions in the evening when he can get away from the office. Leaving voice mails and sending email reports leave him isolated from care group. Lunchtime visits are not long enough for him to focus on the situation.

8. **Answer: c**
   **RATIONALE:** The child's daily intravenous fluid maintenance is 1700 mL. The child requires 100 mL/kg for the first 10 kg plus 50 mL/kg for the next 10 kg plus 20 mL/kg for each kg more than 20 kg equals the number of kg required for 24 hours. (10 × 100) + (10 × 50) + (10 × 20) = 1,700.

9. **Answer: b**
   RATIONALE: Yellow or bile-stained aspirate indicates intestinal placement. Clean, tan, or green aspirate indicates gastric placement.

10. **Answer: a**
    RATIONALE: The nurse should convert the child's weight in pounds to kilograms by dividing the child's weight in pounds by 2.2 (70 pounds divided by 2.2 = 32 kg). The nurse would then multiply the child's weight in kilograms by 3 mg (32 kg × 3 mg = 96 mg) for the low end and then by 4 mg for the high end (32 pounds × 4 mg = 128 mg).

11. **Answer: 21.4 kg**
    RATIONALE: There are 2.2 pounds per kg

    47 pounds × 1 kg/2.2 pounds = 21.363636 kg

    When rounded to the tenth place, the answer is 21.4 kg.

12. **Answer: 1,640 mL**
    RATIONALE:

    (First 10 kg) 10 kg × 100 mL/kg = 1,000 mL
    (Second 10 kg) 10 kg × 50 mL/kg = 500 mL
    (remaining kilograms of body weight) 7 kg × 20 mL/kg = 140 mL
    1,000 + 500+ 140 = 1,640 mL.

13. **Answer: 411 mL**
    RATIONALE: The child weighs 113 pounds. 113 pounds × 1 kg/2.2 pounds = 51.363636 kg

    51.363636 kg × 1 mL/1 kg = 51.363636 mL/hour
    51.363636 × 8 hours = 410.90908

    when rounded to the nearest whole number = 411 mL

14. **Answer: 35 mL**
    RATIONALE: The diaper must be weighed before being placed on the infant and after removal to determine urinary output. For each 1 gram of increased weight, this is the equivalent of 1 mL of fluid.

    75 grams − 40 grams = 35 grams = 35 mL

15. **Answers: a, e**
    RATIONALE: It is true that infants and young children have an increased percentage of water in their bodies. Infants and young children have immature livers.

# CHAPTER 14

## SECTION I: ASSESSING YOUR UNDERSTANDING

### Activity A FILL IN THE BLANKS

1. Midazolam
2. 60
3. Depressed
4. Morphine
5. Seven
6. Pain threshold
7. Oucher

### Activity B MATCHING
**Question 1**
1. d    2. a    3. b    4. e    5. c

**Question 2**
1. b    2. d    3. a    4. d

### Activity C SEQUENCING

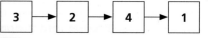

### Activity D SHORT ANSWERS

*Briefly answer the following.*

1. Somatic pain refers to pain that develops in the tissues. Superficial somatic pain is also called cutaneous pain. It involves stimulation of nociceptors in the skin, subcutaneous tissue, or mucous membranes. It is typically well localized and described as sharp, pricking, or burning sensation. Tenderness is common. Deep somatic pain typically involves the muscles tendons, joints, fascia, and bones. It can be localized or diffuse and is usually described as dull, aching, or cramping.

2. The three principles that guide pain management in children are:
   - Individualize interventions based on the amount of pain experiences during procedure and the child's personality
   - Use nonpharmacologic approaches to ease or eliminate the pain
   - Use aggressive pharmacologic treatment with the first procedure

3. The situation factors can be changed. They include behavioral, cognitive, and emotional aspects.

4. Conscious sedation utilizes medications to place the child in a depressed state. This is used to allow the physician to perform procedures. Conscious sedation enables the child to retain protective reflexes. The child is then able to maintain a patent airway and respond to verbal and physical stimuli. Medications used to achieve conscious sedation may include morphine, fentanyl, midazolam, chloral hydrate, or diazepam.

5. Epidural anesthesia is administered after the placement of a catheter in the epidural space. The locations used are L 1–2, L 3–4, or L 4–5. Medications used include fentanyl or morphine. The medications enter the cerebrospinal fluid and cross the dura mater to the spinal cord.

## SECTION II: APPLYING YOUR KNOWLEDGE

### Activity E CASE STUDY

1. The discussion should include the following:
   Recent research supports that infants do feel pain and short- and long-term consequences of inadequately treating their pain do occur. Infants cannot tell us in words that they feel pain like older children or adults but they do give cues with

their behaviors, expressions, and vital signs. Infants will act differently when they are in pain than when they are comfortable. Typically, infants respond to pain with irritability, crying, withdrawal, pushing away, restless sleeping, and poor feeding. They may indicate pain by their facial expressions. A facial expression with brows lowered and drawn together, eyes tightly closed, and mouth opened can be a sign of pain. They are preverbal so this facial expression, diffuse body movements and other signs, as indicated above, provide feedback that the infant is in pain. As parents you play an important role in helping us assess Owen's pain and informing us of changes in his behavior that may indicate pain.

2. The discussion should include the following:

The FLACC scale is an appropriate pain assessment tool for an infant. Based on the scale (refer to Table 14-6 in Essentials of Pediatric Nursing textbook) Owen's pain level is a three at this time.

Owen's vital signs including oxygen saturation as well as how well Owen is feeding may be helpful. (Children in acute pain will often have an increased heart rate, respiratory rate, or elevated blood pressure. Decreased oxygen saturation may be seen secondary to pain. Also, infants in pain will often demonstrate poor feeding.)

3. The discussion should include the following:

Parents are important components in both pain assessment and intervention. Many of the nonpharmacologic techniques can be done by parents and are often received better from the parents. Holding the child with as much skin to skin contact as possible, repositioning, rocking, and massaging the child can help decrease pain. Nonnutritive sucking, breastfeeding, or sucrose or other sweet tasting solutions such as glucose water can decrease discomfort. Distracting the infant with a soothing voice, music, stories, and songs can also be helpful.

# SECTION III: PRACTICING FOR NCLEX

## Activity F NCLEX-STYLE QUESTIONS

1. **Answer: a**
   A preschooler may have difficulty distinguishing between the types of pain such as if the pain is sharp or dull. It also limits the information being obtained by the nurse. They can, however, tell someone where it hurts and can use various tools such as the FACES scale (cartoon faces) or the OUCHER scale (photograph and corresponding numbers) to rate their pain.

2. **Answer: a**
   When administering parenteral or epidural opioids, the nurse should always have naloxone readily available in order to reverse the opioids effects, should respiratory distress occur. Premedication with acetaminophen is not required with opioids. After administration, the nurse should continually

assess for adverse reaction. The nurse should assess bowel sounds for decreased peristalsis after administration.

3. **Answer: d**
   Respiratory depression, although rare when epidural analgesia is used, is always a possibility. However, when it does occur it usually occurs gradually over a period of several hours after the medication is initiated. This allows adequate time for early detection and prompt intervention. The nurse should also monitor for pruritus, urinary retention, and nausea and vomiting but the priority is to monitor for respiratory depression.

4. **Answer: c**
   EMLA is contraindicated in children less than 12 months who are receiving methemoglobin-inducing agents, such as sulfonamides, phenytoin, phenobarbital, and acetaminophen. Children with darker skin may require longer application times to ensure effectiveness. EMLA is not contraindicated for children less than 6 weeks of age or those undergoing venous cannulation or intramuscular injections.

5. **Answer: b**
   When a child is manifesting extreme anxiety and behavioral upset, the priority nursing intervention is to serve as an advocate for the family and ensure that the appropriate pharmacologic agents are chosen to alleviate the child's distress. Ensuring emergency equipment is readily available and lighting is adequate for the procedure is also part of nursing function, but secondary interventions. Conducting an initial assessment of pain is important but would likely be difficult if the child was crying inconsolably or extremely anxious.

6. **Answer: a**
   Just because the girl is sleeping does not mean she is not in pain. Sleep may be a coping strategy or reflect excessive exhaustion due to coping with pain. An easy going temperament and the ability to articulate how she feels will be helpful for the nurse to establish a baseline assessment. If the girl had never had surgery before, she is less likely to have previous memories or episodes of prolonged or severe pain.

7. **Answer: b**
   The parents must understand that they should begin the technique or method chosen before the child experiences pain or when he first indicates he is anxious about or beginning to experience pain. The other statements are accurate.

8. **Answer: b**
   Decreased heart rate is not a physiologic response to pain. Instead, infants demonstrate an increased heart rate, usually averaging approximately 10 beats per minute with possible bradycardia in preterm newborns. Decreased oxygen saturation and palmar and plantar sweating are common physiologic responses to pain in the infant.

**9. Answer: b**

The FLACC behavioral scale is a behavioral assessment tool that is useful in assessing a child's pain when the child is unable to report accurately his or her level of pain or discomfort and is reliable for children from age 2 months to 7 years. The preferred base age for the visual analog and numerical scales is 7 years. The FACES pain rating scale and Oucher pain rating scale are appropriate for children as young as 3; however, in this situation the FLACC is required due to the child's inability to report his level of pain.

**10. Answer: a**

The nurse should select the pain assessment tool that is appropriate for the child's cognitive abilities. The FACES pain rating scale is designed for use with children ages 3 and up. A child with limited reading skills or vocabulary may have difficulty with some of the words listed to describe pain on the word graphic scale. Some of the concepts might be too difficult on the visual analog and numerical scales for a developmentally disabled child. The base age for the Adolescent pediatric pain tool is 8 years, but would likely be inappropriate for an 8-year-old with cognitive delays.

**11. Answer: d**

The nervous system structures needed for pain impulse transmission and perception are present by the 23rd week of gestation. Therefore, children of any age, including preterm newborns, are capable of experiencing pain.

**12. Answer: d**

The epidural is placed at the level of L 1–2, L 3–4, or L 4–5. This is below the area of the spinal cord. Advising the child and family that paralysis is not a serious concern trivializes the concerns and does little to promote therapeutic communication. Nurses have the responsibility to provide education to the child and caregivers. Simply telling them that the cord ends above the area of the epidural does not provide the needed information to promote reassurance. Assuring the child and family that their physician has skills does not meet the needed education.

**13. Answer: c**

Responsible nursing care requires the nurse administer pain medication as needed. The nurse has the authority to discuss the child's pain control needs with the parents. There is no need to discuss the reduction of medications with the physician. Family history of drug abuse is not a factor in the care of this child. Young children can become addicted to analgesics. There is, however, no indication that addiction is a valid concern with this child.

**14. Answer: c**

Children may underreport feelings of pain. They may assume that adults know how they are feeling or they may feel worried about spearing to lose

control. The nurse should assess for the presence of behavioral cues that might be consistent with pain. The nurse should not simply administer analgesics without cause.

**15. Answer: c**

Toradol (ketorolac) is an NSAID medication. It is associated with gastrointestinal upset. To reduce this side effect the nurse may administer the medication with food.

# CHAPTER 15

## SECTION I: ASSESSING YOUR UNDERSTANDING

### Activity A FILL IN THE BLANKS

1. Pyrogens
2. Phagocytosis
3. Antibodies
4. Neutrophils
5. Ibuprofen

### Activity B MATCHING

**Question 1**

1. b  2. e  3. f  4. c  5. d  6. a

**Question 2**

1. b  2. c  3. a  4. e  5. d

### Activity C SEQUENCING

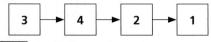

3 → 4 → 2 → 1

### Activity D SHORT ANSWERS

1. Risk factors for sepsis associated with pregnancy include:
   - premature or prolonged rupture of membranes
   - difficult delivery
   - maternal infection or fever, including sexually transmitted infections
   - resuscitation and other invasive procedures
   - positive maternal group beta streptococcal vaginosis

2. The nurse primarily manages the patient's symptoms. Acetaminophen may be given for fever management. Narcotic analgesics may be required for pain management. Oral fluids prevent dehydration. If orchitis is present, ice packs and gentle support for the testicles may be necessitated. Hospitalized children should be confined to respiratory isolation. Children are considered to no longer be contagious after 9 days following the onset of parotid swelling.

3. Concurrent use of passive and active immunoprophylaxis is recommended. It consists of a regimen of one dose of immune globulin and five doses of human rabies vaccine over a 28-day period. Rabies immune globulin and the first dose of rabies vaccine should be given as soon as possible after

exposure, ideally within 24 hours. Additional doses of rabies vaccine should be given on days 3, 7, 14, and 28 after the first vaccination. Rabies immune globulin is infiltrated into and around the wound with any remaining volume administered intramuscularly at a site distant from the vaccine inoculation. Human rabies vaccine is administered intramuscularly into the anterolateral thigh or deltoid depending on the age and size of the child.

4. Fever is a protective mechanism the body uses to fight infection. Evidence exists that an elevated body temperature actually enhances various components of the immune response. Fever can slow the growth of bacteria and viruses and increase neutrophil production and T-cell proliferation (Crocetti & Serwint, 2005). Studies have shown that the use of antipyretics may prolong illness. Another concern is that reducing fever may hide signs of serious bacterial illness.

5. Sepsis is a systemic over response to infection resulting from bacteria (most common), fungi, viruses, or parasites. It can lead to septic shock, which results in hypotension, low blood flow, and multi-system organ failure. Septic shock is a medical emergency and children are usually admitted to an intensive care unit. The cause of sepsis may not be known, but common causative organisms in children include *Neisseria meningitidis, Streptococcus pneumoniae*, and *Haemophilus influenzae*. Sepsis can affect any age group but is more common in neonates and young infants. Neonates and young infants have a higher susceptibility due to their immature immune system, inability to localize infections, and lack of IgM immunoglobulin, which is necessary to protect against bacterial infections.

## SECTION II: APPLYING YOUR KNOWLEDGE
**Activity E** CASE STUDY

1. The discussion should include the following points:
   Continue attempting to open dialogue with Jennifer. Make sure your style, content, and message are appropriate to her developmental level. Do not talk down to her and approach her in a direct and nonjudgmental manner. Work on identifying risk factors and risk behaviors.
2. The discussion should include the following points:
   Encourage completion of antibiotic prescription. Encourage sexual partners to get an evaluation, testing, and treatment.
   Once risk factors and risk behaviors have been identified, guide Jennifer to develop specific individualized actions of prevention. You can encourage abstinence at this point along with encouraging Jennifer to minimize her lifetime number of sexual partners, to use barrier methods consistently and correctly, and to be aware of the connection between drug and alcohol use and the incorrect use of barrier methods.

3. The discussion should include the following points:
   Reinforce the risk she is putting herself at and continue to guide her to develop individualized actions of prevention. For possible discussion about other STI's common in adolescents refer to Table 15.9). Discuss barriers to condom use and ways to overcome them (refer Table 15.10).
   To address specific concerns – condoms are uncomfortable and sex with condoms is not as exciting or as good.
   Encourage Jennifer and her boyfriend to try condoms and provide suggestions such as trying smaller or larger condom sizes, placing a drop of water based lubricant or salvia inside the tip of the condom or on the glans of the penis prior to putting on the condom. Try a thinner latex condom or a different brand or more lubrication. Encourage the incorporation of condom use during foreplay. Remind Jennifer that peace of mind may enhance pleasure for herself and her partner.
   Instruct Jennifer on proper condom use (refer to teaching guideline 15.3).
   The discussion should include the following points:
   - Use latex condoms
   - Use a new condom with each sexual act of intercourse and never reuse a condom
   - Handle condoms with care to prevent damage from sharp objects such as nails and teeth
   - Ensure condom has been stored in a cool, dry place away from direct sunlight. Do not store condoms in wallet or automobile or any place where they are exposed to extreme temperatures
   - Do not use a condom if it appears brittle, sticky, or discolored. These are signs of aging.
   - Place condom on before any genital contact
   - Place condom on when penis is erect and ensure it is placed so it will readily unroll.
   - Hold the tip of the condom while unrolling. Ensure there is a space at the tip for semen to collect but make sure no air is trapped in the tip
   - Ensure adequate lubrication during intercourse. If external lubricants are used only use water-based lubricants such as KY jelly with latex condoms. Oil-based or petroleum-based lubricants, such as body lotion, massage oil, or cooking oil, can weaken latex condoms
   - Withdraw while penis is still erect and hold condom firmly against base of pen

## SECTION III: PRACTICING FOR NCLEX
**Activity F** NCLEX-STYLE QUESTIONS

1. **Answer: c**
   If the family had been camping or in a wooded area, the girl could have been bitten by a tick which would not be easy to discover because of her long hair. Ticks like dark, hair-covered areas

and the signs and symptoms presented are neurological, with a rapid onset, which can be characteristic of a tick bite. The other questions are important but are not focusing on the causative agent.

2. **Answer: b**
Recurrent arthritis in large joints, such as the knees, is an indication of late-stage Lyme disease. The appearance of erythema migrans would suggest early-localized stage of the disease. Facial palsy or conjunctivitis would suggest the child is in the early disseminated stage of the disease.

3. **Answer: c**
It is very important to ensure that the proper dose is given at the proper interval because an overdose can be toxic to the child. Concerns with allergies and taking the entire, prescribed dose are precaution when administering antibiotics and all medications. Drowsiness is not a side effect of antipyretics.

4. **Answer: d**
In order to ensure a successful culture, the nurse must determine if the child is taking antibiotics. Throat cultures require specimens taken from the pharyngeal or tonsilar area. Stool cultures may require three specimens, each on a different day. The nurse would use aseptic technique when getting a blood specimen as well as the urine, but antibiotics cannot be received by the child prior to the test being done.

5. **Answer: a**
The usual sites for obtaining blood specimens are veins on the dorsal side of the hand or the antecubital fossa. Administration of sucrose prior to beginning helps control pain for young infants. Accessing an indwelling venous access device may be appropriate if the child is in an acute care setting. An automatic lancet device is used for capillary puncture of an infant's heel.

6. **Answer: a**
The presence of petechiae can indicate serious infection in an infant. Grunting is abnormal, indicating respiratory difficulty. The behavior of the 2-month-old is normal after immunizations. The 4-month-old needs to be watched but is adequately hydrated and the 8-month-old also needs to be watched. What the 8-month-old is experiencing is common in infants who are teething and is not indicative of illness.

7. **Answer: a**
Varicella zoster results in a life-long latent infection. It can reactivate later in life resulting in shingles. The American Academy of Pediatrics recommends consideration of Vitamin A supplementation in children 6 months to 2 years hospitalized for measles. Dehydration caused by mouth lesions is a concern with foot and mouth disease. Avoiding exposure to pregnant women is a concern with Rubella, Rubeola, and erythema infectiosum.

8. **Answer: a**
Infants and young children are more susceptible to infection due to the immature responses of their immune systems. Cellular immunity is generally functional at birth; humoral immunity develops after the child is born. Newborns have a decreased inflammatory response. Young infants lose the passive immunity from their mothers, but disease protection from immunizations is not complete.

9. **Answer: b**
The use of immunosuppression drugs is a risk factor for the hospitalized child. Maternal infection or fever and resuscitation or invasive procedures are sepsis risk factors related to pregnancy and labor. Lack of juvenile immunizations is a risk factor affecting the overall health of the child but does not impact the chance of sepsis.

10. **Answer: d**
Penicillin V or erythromycin is the preferred antibiotic for treatment of scarlet fever. Scarlet fever transmission is airborne, not via droplet. Lymphadenopathy occurs with cat scratch disease and diphtheria. Close monitoring of airway status is critical with diphtheria because the upper airway becomes swollen.

11. **Answer: c**
Pruritis may be managed by pressing on the area instead of scratching. Increases in temperature will result in vasodilation and increase the pruritis. Warm baths and hot compresses should be avoided. Rubbing may result in increased itching.

12. **Answer: a**
When treating a child suspected of having an infection the blood cultures must be obtained first. The administration of antibiotics may impact the culture's results. A urine specimen may be obtained but is not the priority action. Intravenous fluids will likely be included in the plan of care but are not the priority action.

13. **Answer: d**
Sepsis may be associated with lethargy, irritability, or changes in level of consciousness. The septic child will likely not be anxious to have a high activity level and would prefer to remain in bed. The temperature elevation of 98.8 °F is not significant and does not confirm the presence of sepsis. Hypotension is a late manifestation of sepsis.

14. **Answer: b**
Pressing the tube against the skin may result in the contamination of the specimen with bacteria from the skin. The remaining options are correct.

15. **Answers: b, c, d**
Aspirin should be avoided in children with fever. It may be associated with Reyes Syndrome. Activities that result in over-cooling or chilling such as using fans and cold baths should be avoided.

# CHAPTER 16

## SECTION I: ASSESSING YOUR UNDERSTANDING

### Activity A FILL IN THE BLANKS

1. Kernig's
2. Painful
3. Circumference
4. Gait
5. Doll's eye
6. Touch
7. Intracranial
8. Bruit

### Activity B LABELING

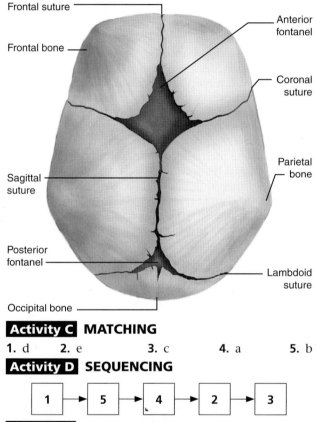

Frontal suture
Frontal bone
Anterior fontanel
Coronal suture
Parietal bone
Sagittal suture
Posterior fontanel
Lambdoid suture
Occipital bone

### Activity C MATCHING

1. d  2. e   3. c   4. a   5. b

### Activity D SEQUENCING

1 → 5 → 4 → 2 → 3

### Activity E SHORT ANSWERS

1. Kernig's sign is tested by flexing the legs at the hip and knee, then extending the knee. A positive report of pain along the vertebral column is a positive sign and indicates irritation of the meninges, or the presence of meningitis.
2. An infant will hyperextend its head and neck assuming an opisthotonic position in order to relieve discomfort due to bacterial meningitis.
3. Proper positioning for newborns is upright with the head flexed forward. An older infant or child is positioned on its side with head flexed forward and knees flexed toward the abdomen.
4. A ventriculoperitoneal (VP) shunt is designed to relieve the build up of CSF in hydrocephalus

children and maintain proper intracranial pressure. Malfunctions may be due to kinking, clogging, or separation of the tubing. The most common malfunction, however, is due to blockage. Signs and symptoms include vomiting, lethargy, headache in the older child, and altered, diminished, or change in the level of consciousness.

5. The Glasgow Coma scale is a tool used to standardize the degree of consciousness in the child. It consists of three parts: eye opening, verbal response, and motor response. A low score indicates a decreased level of consciousness or responsiveness.

## SECTION II: APPLYING YOUR KNOWLEDGE

### Activity F CASE STUDY

*The discussion should include the following points:*

1. The nurse should anticipate the following diagnostic and laboratory tests: Complete blood count (CBC); electrolytes; culture (if febrile); phenobarbital level; toxicology if ingestion of medicine or chemicals is suspected; lumbar puncture (LP) if signs of central nervous system infection are present; and imaging studies, such as CT or MRI, if head injury is suspected.
2. Interventions should include:
   - If child is standing or sitting ease child to the ground if possible, cradle head, place on soft area. Do not attempt to restrain. Place child on one side and open airway if possible.
   - Place blow-by oxygen by child and have suction ready if needed.
   - Remove any sharp or potentially dangerous objects. Tight clothing and jewelry around the neck should be loosened if possible.
   - Observe length of seizure and activity such as movements noted, as well as cyanosis or loss of bladder or bowel control, and any other characteristics about the child's condition during the seizure.
   - If child's condition deteriorates or seizures persist, call for help.
   - Report seizures to physician promptly.
   - Administer anticonvulsants as ordered.
   - Remain with child until fully conscious.
   - Allow postictal behavior without interfering while providing environmental protection.
   - When possible, reorient child.
   - Accurately document information in chart, including preseizure activity.
   - Provide emotional support and education to family.
   - Obtain anticonvulsant levels as ordered.
3. Teaching should include:
   - Discuss seizure warning signs.
   - Teach the family to recognize warning signs and how to care for the child during and after a seizure (refer to Teaching Guidelines 16.1).

- Discuss the disease process and prognosis of condition and life-long need for treatment if indicated.
- Teach parents the need for routine medical care and that it is important for the child to wear a medical bracelet.
- Review medication regimen and the importance of maintaining a therapeutic medication level and administering all prescribed doses.
- Encourage parents to discuss with the child why she does not want to take the medicine.
- Explain to the child in simple terms why the medicine is needed and how it will help her. Encourage participation from physician and parents.
- Discuss alternative ways to administer phenobarbital, such as crushed tablets or elixir, with the physician and family.
- Explain to the family to use an understanding and gentle yet firm approach with medication administration.
- Encourage the family to give medicine at same time and place, which helps create a routine.
- Help the family to identify creative strategies to gain the child's cooperation, such as using a sticker chart and allowing child to do more, such as administering the medication.
- Offer choices when possible, such as "Do you want your medicine before or after your bath, and would you like to have apple or grape juice after your medicine?"
- Praise the child's improvements.

# SECTION III: PRACTICING FOR NCLEX

## Activity G NCLEX-STYLE QUESTIONS

1. **Answer: a**
   RATIONALE: Always start by assessing the family's knowledge. Ask them what they need to know. Knowing when to clamp the drain is important, but they might not be listening if they have another question on their minds. Autoregulation is too technical. Teaching should be based on the parents' level of understanding. Keeping her head elevated is not part of the information which would be taught regarding the drainage system.

2. **Answer: c**
   RATIONALE: Horizontal nystagmus is a symptom of lesions on the brain stem. A sudden increase in head circumference is a symptom of hydrocephalus suggesting that there is a build up of fluid in the brain. An intracranial mass would cause only one eye to be dilated and reactive. A closed posterior fontanel is not unusual at 2 months of age.

3. **Answer: a**
   RATIONALE: The fact that swelling did not cross the midline or suture lines suggests cephalohematoma. Swelling that crosses the midline of the infant's scalp indicates caput succedaneum which

is common. Low birth weight is not an accompanying factor for cephalohematoma. Facial abnormalities may accompany encephalocele, not cephalohematoma.

4. **Answer: a**
   RATIONALE: Signs and symptoms for cerebral contusions include disturbances to vision, strength, and sensation. A child suffering a concussion will be distracted and unable to concentrate. Vomiting is a sign of a subdural hematoma. Bleeding from the ear is a sign of a basilar skull fracture.

5. **Answer: a**
   RATIONALE: Positional plagiocephaly can occur because the infant's head is allowed to stay in one position for too long. Because the bones of the skull are soft and moldable, they can become flattened if the head is allowed to remain in the same position for a long period of time. Massaging the scalp will not affect the skull. Measuring the intake and output is important but has no effect on the skull bones. Small feedings are indicated whenever an infant has increased intracranial pressure, but feeding an infant each time he fusses is inappropriate care.

6. **Answer: d**
   RATIONALE: Fragile capillaries in the periventricular area of the brain put preterm infants at risk for intracranial hemorrhage. Closure of the fontanels has nothing to do with fragile capillaries within the brain. Larger head size gives children a higher center of gravity which causes them to hit their head more readily. Congenital hydrocephalus may be caused by abnormal intrauterine development or infection.

7. **Answer: c**
   RATIONALE: Folic acid supplementation has been found to reduce the incidence of neural tube defects by 50%. The fact that the mother has not used folic acid supplements puts her baby at risk for spina bifida occulta, one type of neural tube defect. Neonatal conjunctivitis can occur in any newborn during birth and is caused by virus, bacteria, or chemicals. Facial deformities are typical of babies of alcoholic mothers. Incomplete myelinization is present in all newborns.

8. **Answer: c**
   RATIONALE: A video electroencephalogram can determine the precise localization of the seizure area in the brain. Cerebral angiography is used to diagnose vessel defects or space-occupying lesions. Lumbar puncture is used to diagnose hemorrhage, infection, or obstruction in the spinal canal. Computed tomography is used to diagnose congenital abnormalities such as neural tube defects.

9. **Answer: c**
   RATIONALE: Brain and spinal cord development occur during the first 3 to 4 weeks of gestation. Infection, trauma, teratogens (any environmental substance that can cause physical defects in the developing embryo and fetus), and malnutrition

during this period can result in malformations in brain and spinal cord development and may affect normal central nervous system (CNS) development. Good health before becoming pregnant is important but must continue into the pregnancy. Hardening of bones occurs during 13 to 16 weeks gestation, and the respiratory system begins maturing around 23 weeks gestation.

10. **Answer: b**
    RATIONALE: Educating parents how to properly give the antibiotics would be the priority intervention because the child's shunt has become infected. Maintaining cerebral perfusion is important for a child with hydrocephalus, but the priority intervention for the parents at this time is in regards to the infection. Establishing seizure precautions is an intervention for a child with a seizure disorder. Encouraging development of motor skills would be appropriate for a microcephalic child.

11. **Answer: a, b, c, e**
    RATIONALE: The child with bacterial meningitis should be placed in droplet isolation until 24 hours following the administration of antibiotics. Close contacts of the child should receive antibiotics to prevent them from developing the infection. The nurse should administer antibiotics and initiate seizure precautions. Children with bacterial meningitis have an increased risk of developing problems associated with an increased intracranial pressure.

12. **Answer: a, b, c, d**
    RATIONALE: The following people have an increased risk of becoming infected with meningococcal meningitis: college freshman living in dormitories, children 11 years old or older, children who travel to high risk areas, and children with chronic health conditions.

13. **Answers: a, b, d**
    RATIONALE: A child with Reye's syndrome may require an anti-emetic for severe vomiting. The nurse should monitor the child's intake and output every shift for the development of fluid imbalance. The child may require an anticonvulsant due an increased intracranial pressure that may induce seizures. A distinctive rash is associated with the development of meningococcal meningitis. The nurse should monitor the Reye's syndrome child's laboratory values for indications that the liver is not functioning well.

14. **Answer: 8**
    RATIONALE: The child would be given a score of 2 for best eye response, 2 for best verbal response, and 4 for best motor response. The total score is 8.

15. **Answers: b, d, e**
    RATIONALE: Late signs of increased intracranial pressure are: decerebrate posturing, bradycardia, and pupils that are fixed and dilated. The other options are early signs of increased intracranial pressure.

# CHAPTER 17

## SECTION I: ASSESSING YOUR UNDERSTANDING

### Activity A FILL IN THE BLANKS
1. 3
2. Horizontal
3. Antibiotics
4. Deterioration
5. Developmental
6. Distance

### Activity B MATCHING
1. b    2. d    3. a    4. e    5. c

### Activity C SEQUENCING

3 → 2 → 1 → 4

### Activity D SHORT ANSWERS
1. Signs and symptoms of children with a hearing loss include:
   a. Infant:
      - Wakes only to touch, not environmental noises
      - Does not startle to loud noises
      - Does not turn to sound by 4 months of age
      - Does not babble at 6 months of age
      - Does not progress with speech development
   b. Young child:
      - Does not speak by 2 years of age
      - Communicates needs through gestures
      - Does not speak distinctly, as appropriate for his or her age
      - Displays developmental (cognitive) delays
      - Prefers solitary play
      - Displays immature emotional behavior
      - Does not respond to ringing of the telephone or doorbell
      - Focuses on facial expressions when communicating
   c. Older child:
      - Often asks for statements to be repeated
      - Is inattentive or daydreams
      - Performs poorly at school
      - Displays monotone or other abnormal speech
      - Gives inappropriate answers to questions except when able to view face of speaker
2. According to the Delta Gamma Center for Children with Visual Impairments, there are several ways to successfully interact with the visually impaired child, including:
   - Use the child's name to gain attention.
   - Identify yourself and let the child know you are there before you touch the child.
   - Encourage the child to be independent while maintaining safety.

- Name and describe people/objects to make the child more aware of what is happening.
- Discuss upcoming activities with the child.
- Explain what other children or individuals are doing.
- Make directions simple and specific.
- Allow the child additional time to think about the response to a question or statement.
- Use touch and tone of voice appropriate to the situation.
- Use parts of the child's body as reference points for the location of items.
- Encourage exploration of objects through touch.
- Describe unfamiliar environments and provide reference points.
- Use the sighted-guide technique when walking with a visually impaired child.

3. Signs and symptoms that would lead the nurse to suspect that a child was visually impaired include:
   a. Infants:
      - Does not fix and follow
      - Does not make eye contact
      - Unaffected by bright light
      - Does not imitate facial expression
   b. Toddlers and older children:
      - Rubs, shuts, covers eyes
      - Squinting
      - Frequent blinking
      - Holds objects close or sits close to television
      - Bumping into objects
      - Head tilt, or forward thrust

4. Possible risk factors for acute otitis media (AOM) in children include any of the following:
   - Eustachian tube dysfunction
   - Recurrent upper respiratory infection
   - First episode of AOM before 3 months of age
   - Day care attendance (increases exposure to viruses causing upper respiratory infections)
   - Previous episodes of AOM
   - Family history
   - Passive smoking
   - Crowding in the home or large family size
   - Native American, Inuit, or Australian aborigine ethnicity
   - Absence of infant breastfeeding
   - Immunocompromise
   - Poor nutrition
   - Craniofacial anomalies
   - Presence of allergies

5. Children with permanent hearing loss, suspected or diagnosed speech and/or language delay, craniofacial disorders, and pervasive developmental disorders are at risk for difficulty with the development of speech or language, or having learning difficulties. Other children at risk include those with genetic disorders or syndromes, cleft palate, and blindness or significant visual impairment.

## SECTION II: APPLYING YOUR KNOWLEDGE

### Activity E  CASE STUDY

*The discussion should include the following points:*

1. The nurse should anticipate the following diagnostic and laboratory tests: Complete blood count (CBC); electrolytes; blood culture (if febrile); phenobarbital level; toxicology if ingestion of medicine or chemicals is suspected; lumbar puncture (LP) if signs of central nervous system infection are present; and imaging studies, such as CT or MRI, if head injury is suspected.

2. Interventions should include:
   - If the child is standing or sitting ease the child to the ground if possible, cradle head, place on soft area. Do not attempt to restrain. Place the child on one side and open airway if possible.
   - Place blow-by oxygen by the child and have suction ready if needed.
   - Remove any sharp or potentially dangerous objects. Tight clothing and jewelry around the neck should be loosened if possible.
   - Observe length of seizure and activity such as movements noted, as well as cyanosis or loss of bladder or bowel control, and any other characteristics about the child's condition during the seizure.
   - If the child's condition deteriorates or seizures persist, call for help.
   - Report seizures to physician promptly.
   - Administer anticonvulsants as ordered.
   - Remain with the child until fully conscious.
   - Allow postictal behavior without interfering while providing environmental protection.
   - When possible, reorient child.
   - Accurately document information in chart, including preseizure activity.
   - Provide emotional support and education to family.
   - Obtain anticonvulsant levels as ordered.

3. Teaching should include:
   - Discuss seizure warning signs.
   - Teach the family to recognize warning signs and how to care for the child during and after a seizure (refer to Teaching Guidelines 16.1).
   - Discuss the disease process and prognosis of condition and life-long need for treatment if indicated.
   - Teach parents the need for routine medical care, and that it is important for the child to wear a medical bracelet.
   - Review medication regimen and the importance of maintaining a therapeutic medication level and administering all prescribed doses.
   - Encourage parents to discuss with the child why she does not want to take the medicine.
   - Explain to the child in simple terms why the medicine is needed and how it will help her. Encourage participation from physician and parents.

- Discuss alternative ways to administer phenobarbital, such as crushed tablets or elixir, with the physician and family.
- Explain to the family to use an understanding and gentle yet firm approach with medication administration.
- Encourage the family to give medicine at same time and place, which helps create a routine.
- Help the family to identify creative strategies to gain the child's cooperation, such as using a sticker chart and allowing child to do more, such as administering the medication.
- Offer choices when possible, such as "Do you want your medicine before or after your bath, and would you like to have apple or grape juice after your medicine?"
- Praise the child's improvements.

# SECTION III: PRACTICING FOR NCLEX
**Activity F** NCLEX-STYLE QUESTIONS

1. **Answer: d**
Reassessing for language acquisition would be most important to the health of the child. There is a risk of otitis media with effusion causing hearing loss, as well as speech, language, and learning problems. Parents should not use over-the-counter drugs to alleviate the child's symptoms, nor should they smoke around her. In addition, proper antibiotic use is important; however, language acquisition is directly related to developmental health.

2. **Answer: c**
The corneal light reflex is extremely helpful in assessment of strabismus. It consists of shining a flashlight into the eyes to see if the light reflects at the same angle in both eyes. Strabismus is present if the reflections are not symmetrical. The visual acuity test measures how well the child sees at various distances. Refractive and ophthalmologic examinations are comprehensive and are performed by optometrists and ophthalmologists.

3. **Answer: b**
Intravenous antibiotics will be the primary therapy for this child, followed by oral antibiotics. Warm compresses will be applied for 20 minutes every 2 to 4 hours. However, narcotic analgesics are not necessary to handle the pain associated with this disorder.

4. **Answer: a**
Assessing for asymmetric corneal light reflex would be the priority intervention as strabismus may develop in the child with regressed retinopathy of prematurity. Observing for signs of visual impairment would not be critical for this child, nor would teaching the parents to check how the glasses fit the child. Referral to Early Intervention would be appropriate if the child was visually impaired.

5. **Answer: c**
Recurrent nasal congestion contributes to the presence of otitis media with effusion. Frequent swimming would put the child at risk for otitis externa. Attendance at school is a risk factor for infective conjunctivitis. Although otitis media is a risk factor for infective conjunctivitis, infective conjunctivitis is not a risk factor for otitis media with effusion.

6. **Answer: d**
Therapeutic management of amblyopia may be achieved by using atropine drops in the better eye. Educating parents on how to use atropine drops would be the most helpful intervention. Explaining postsurgical treatment and discouraging the child from roughhousing would be appropriate only if the amblyopia required surgery. While follow-up visits to the ophthalmologist are important, compliance with treatment is priority.

7. **Answer: d**
Teaching the parents the importance of patching the child's eye as prescribed is most important for the treatment of strabismus. The need for ultraviolet-protective glasses postoperatively is a subject for the treatment of cataracts. The possibility of multiple operations is a teaching subject for infantile glaucoma. Teaching the importance of completing the full course of oral antibiotics is appropriate to periorbital cellulitis.

8. **Answer: c**
Proper hand washing is the single most important factor to reduce the spread of acute infectious conjunctivitis. Proper application of the antibiotic is important for the treatment of the infection, not prevention of transmission; keeping the child home from school until she is no longer infectious and encouraging the child to keep her hands away from her eyes are sound preventative measures, but not as important as frequent hand washing.

9. **Answer: c**
A mixture of ½ rubbing alcohol and ½ vinegar squirted into the canal and then allowed to run out is a good preventative measure, but not when inflammation is present. Cotton swabs should not be placed in the ears to dry them. He can wash his hair as needed. Using a hair dryer on a cool setting to dry the ears works well as long as the vent is clean and free from dust and hair that may have accumulated.

10. **Answer: d**
Encouraging the use of eye protection for sports would be more appropriate if the child was wearing contact lenses that may fall out during athletics. A sport strap would be more appropriate for this child. The child is less likely to wear her glasses if improper fit or incorrect prescription is causing a problem or if the glasses are unattractive. It is important to get scheduled eye examinations on time; watch for signs that the prescription needs changing; and check the condition and fit of glasses monthly.

11. **Answers: a, b**
    **RATIONALE:** Bacterial infections are usually present unilaterally. Drainage from eyes that have been diagnosed with bacterial conjunctivitis is often thick and purulent.

12. **Answers: a, d**
    **RATIONALE:** Visine is not appropriate to use because rebound vasoconstriction may occur and it is not actually treating the infection. The child can go back to school 24 to 48 hours after the mucopurulent drainage is no longer present.

13. **Answers: a, c, e**
    **RATIONALE:** The child with a corneal abrasion may have a normal assessment of the pupils bilaterally. The child may experience photophobia and tearing noted in the eye. The child with a corneal abrasion will typically experience eye pain. The child with a simple contusion of the eye will have bruising and edema around the eye.

14. **Answers: b, c, d, e**
    **RATIONALE:** Children who are 2 years old or younger and have a severe form of acute otitis media with a temperature of 102.2 F or greater (39 °C) will most likely receive antibiotics to treat the infection. Children who are older than 2 years of age with severe otalgia and a fever over 102.2 F (39 °C) typically receive antibiotics. Children who are older than 2 years of age and have mild otalgia and a fever less than 102.2 F have a nonsevere illness. In these cases, the physician may just observe the children to see if their symptoms persist over time or get worse.

# CHAPTER 18

## SECTION I: ASSESSING YOUR UNDERSTANDING

### Activity A FILL IN THE BLANKS

1. Tracheostomy
2. Atopic
3. Coryza
4. Indirect
5. Wheezes
6. Mantoux
7. Decongestant

### Activity B LABELING

### Activity C MATCHING

1. d    2. e    3. b    4. a    5. c

### Activity D SEQUENCING

### Activity E SHORT ANSWERS

1. Signs and symptoms of sinusitis are similar to those found with a cold, with the difference being that sinusitis signs and symptoms are more persistent than with a cold, with nasal discharge lasting more than 7 to 10 days. Common signs and symptoms include cough, fever, halitosis in preschoolers and older children, eyelid edema, irritability, and poor appetite. Facial pain may or may not be present.

2. Laboratory and diagnostic tests typically ordered for the child suspected of having cystic fibrosis and possible findings indicative of cystic fibrosis include the sweat chloride test (above 50mEq/L is considered suspicious levels and above 60mEq is indicative); pulse oximetry (oxygen saturation is usually decreased); chest X-ray (hyperinflation, bronchial wall thickening); and pulmonary function tests (decreased forced vital capacity and forced expiratory volume with increases in residual volume).

3. There is typically no illness that precedes croup or epiglottitis other than possibly mild coryza with croup or a mild upper respiratory infection with epiglottitis. Both have a rapid or sudden onset, with croup frequently occurring at night. Several differences exist between the two illnesses including age groups usually affected (3 months to 3 years with croup and 1 to 8 years for epiglottitis); fever (variable with croup and high with epiglottitis); barking cough and hoarseness with croup; dysphagia and toxic appearance with epiglottitis; lastly, the cause of croup is generally viral whereas the cause of epiglottitis is generally *Haemophilus influenzae* type B.

4. Relief of symptoms is the goal of treatment of the common cold. This may be achieved a number of methods including relief of nasal congestion by providing a humidified environment or using saline nasal sprays or washes. Saline washes are followed by suctioning with a bulb syringe. Over-the-counter cold remedies may reduce the symptoms of the cold, but not the duration and should not be used in children less than 6 years of age due to possible side effects. Additionally, antihistamines should be avoided as they cause excess drying of secretions.

5. Respiratory syncytial virus (RSV) is the most common cause of bronchiolitis, which is an acute inflammation of the bronchioles. The peak incidence of this disorder occurs in the winter and spring seasons. RSV infection is common in all children, with bronchiolitis RSV occurring most often in infants and toddlers. The severity of the infection typically decreases with age.

# SECTION II: APPLYING YOUR KNOWLEDGE

## Activity F CASE STUDY

1. The discussion should include the following points:
   - Is there a family history of atopy?
   - Does James have a history of allergic rhinitis or atopic dermatitis?
   - Has James had recurrent episodes diagnosed as wheezing, bronchiolitis, or bronchitis?
   - Has James had these symptoms before?
   - When did James first develop symptoms?
   - Which symptoms developed first?
   - Are there any factors that could have precipitated the attack?
   - Describe James' home environment (include pets, smokers, type of heating use)
   - Does James have any allergies to food or medication?
   - Does James have a seasonal response to environmental pollen or dust allergies?
   - Is James taking any medication?

2. The discussion should include the following points:
   Ineffective airway clearance related to inflammation and increased secretions as evidenced by dyspnea, coughing and wheezing, pallor, tachypnea, tachycardia and bilateral wheezing on auscultation, and c/o chest tightness.

**RATIONALE:** Inflammation and increased mucous secretions can contribute to the narrowing of air passages and interfere with airflow during an acute asthma attack. This is the highest priority nursing diagnosis.

Ineffective breathing pattern related to inflammatory or infectious process as evidenced by dyspnea, coughing and wheezing, pallor, tachypnea, tachycardia and bilateral wheezing on auscultation, and c/o chest tightness.

**RATIONALE:** Tachypnea and increased work of breathing can lead to inadequate ventilation.

Risk for impaired gas exchange related to dyspnea, coughing and wheezing, pallor, tachypnea, tachycardia and bilateral wheezing on auscultation, and c/o chest tightness.

**RATIONALE:** Unresolved ineffective airway clearance or ineffective breathing pattern may lead to deficits in oxygenation and carbon dioxide retention and hypoxia.

Risk for anxiety related to respiratory distress.

**RATIONALE:** Respiratory distress and related hypoxia may lead to agitation and anxiety as the child struggles to breathe.

Education should include a discussion about the pathophysiology, asthma triggers, and prevention and treatment strategies.

The nurse should explain that asthma is a chronic, inflammatory airway disorder that decreases the size of the airways leading to respiratory distress.

Teaching should include information regarding how attacks of asthma can be prevented by avoiding environmental and emotional triggers (refer to Teaching Guidelines 18.4).

Discussion of appropriate use of medication delivery devices, including the nebulizer and metered-dose inhaler are important. Teaching should include the purposes, functions, and side effects of the prescribed medications. It is essential to require return demonstration of equipment use to ensure that children and families are able to utilize equipment properly. (refer to Teaching Guidelines 18.5).

# SECTION III: PRACTICING FOR NCLEX

## Activity G NCLEX-STYLE QUESTIONS

1. **Answer: c**
   The 4-year-old with pharyngitis has a sore, swollen throat placing the child at risk for dysphagia (difficulty swallowing). Erythematous rash and mild toxic appearance are typical of influenza. Fever and fatigue are symptoms of a common cold. Influenza and the common cold may cause sore throats but would not be the highest risk for dysphagia.

2. **Answer: a**
   Until the family adjusts to the demands of the disease, they can become overwhelmed and exhausted, leading to noncompliance, resulting in worsening of

symptoms. Typical challenges to the family are becoming over vigilant, the child feeling fearful and isolated, and the siblings being jealous or worried.

3. **Answer: d**
Attending day care is a known risk factor for pneumonia. Being a triplet is a factor for bronchiolitis. Prematurity rather than postmaturity is a risk factor for pneumonia. Diabetes is a risk factor for influenza.

4. **Answer: b**
A chest X-ray is usually ordered for the assessment of asthma to check for hyperventilation. A sputum culture is indicated for pneumonia, cystic fibrosis, and tuberculosis; fluoroscopy is used to identify masses or abscesses as with pneumonia; and the sweat chloride test is indicated for cystic fibrosis.

5. **Answer: b**
Oxygen administration is indicated for the treatment of hypoxemia. Suctioning removes excess secretions from the airway caused by colds or flu. Saline lavage loosens mucus that may be blocking the airway so that it may be suctioned out. Saline gargles are indicated for relieving throat pain as with pharyngitis or tonsillitis.

6. **Answer: c**
Infants consume twice as much oxygen (6 to 8 L) as adults (3 to 4 L). This is due to higher metabolic and resting respiratory rates. Term infants are born with about 50 million alveoli, which is only 17% of the adult number of around 300 million. The tongue of the infant, relative to the oropharynx is larger than adults. Infants and children will develop hypoxemia more rapidly than adults when in respiratory distress.

7. **Answer: d**
If the airway becomes completely occluded due to epiglottitis, respiratory distress may lead to respiratory arrest and death. Aseptic meningitis is a complication of infectious mononucleosis, resulting in nuchal rigidity; acute otitis media resulting in ear pain is a complication of influenza; and children with pneumonia are at risk for pneumothorax.

8. **Answer: a**
A flutter valve device is used to assist with mobilization of secretions for older children and adolescents with cystic fibrosis. Teaching regarding the use of metered dose inhalers, nebulizers, and the peak flow meter is typically for asthma therapy.

9. **Answer: b**
Mucus plugging can occur in the neonate placed on a ventilator after surfactant has been administered; therefore, it is important to monitor for adequate lung expansion for early detection of this complication. Promoting adequate gas exchange, maintaining adequate fluid volume, and preventing infection would be interventions for a neonate on a ventilator, but they are not specific to the complication of mucus plugging.

10. **Answer: a**
Using nasal washes to improve air flow will help prevent secondary bacterial infection by preventing the mucus from becoming thick and immobile. Teaching parents how to avoid allergens such as tobacco smoke, dust mites, and molds helps prevent recurrence of allergic rhinitis. Discussing anti-inflammatory nasal sprays and teaching parents about using oral antihistamines would help in prevention and treatment of the disorder.

11. **Answer: 33%**
RATIONALE: Room air is 21%. Each 1 liter of oxygen flow is equal to an additional 4% of oxygen. The child is receiving 3 liters of oxygen. 21% (room air) + 3(4%) = 33% of oxygen.

12. **Answer: b, d, c, a**
RATIONALE: The first step is to administer a short-acting beta 2-agonist as needed. The second step is to administer a low-dose inhaled corticosteroid. The third step is to administer a medium-dose inhaled corticosteroid. The fourth step is to administer a medium-dose inhaled corticosteroid and a long-acting beta 2-agonist.

13. **Answers: c, d**
RATIONALE: Until 4 weeks of age, newborns are obligatory nose breathers and breathe only through their mouths when they are crying. A newborn's respiratory tract makes very little mucus. Children have an increased risk of developing problems associated with airway edema. Children's tongues are proportionally larger than adults. Children under the age of 6 years have a reduced risk of developing sinus infections.

14. **Answer: 157 mg per dose**
RATIONALE: 23 pounds × 1 kg/2.2 pounds = 10.4545 kg

10.4545 kg × 45 g/kg = 470.455 mg
470.455 mg/3 = 156.82 = 157 mg per dose

15. **Answers: b, c, d, e**
RATIONALE: Children with pneumonia may exhibit the following: a chest X-ray with perihilar infiltrates, an elevated leukocyte level, an increased respiratory rate, and a productive cough. The child with pneumonia typically has a fever.

# CHAPTER 19

## SECTION I: ASSESSING YOUR UNDERSTANDING

### Activity A FILL IN THE BLANKS

1. Angiography
2. Electrophysiologic
3. Narrowing
4. Pulmonary
5. 6 months
6. Acquired
7. Rheumatic fever

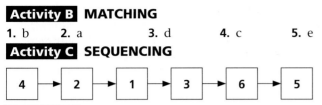

**Activity C  SEQUENCING**

4 → 2 → 1 → 3 → 6 → 5

**Activity D  SHORT ANSWERS**

1. Digoxin is prescribed to increase contractility of the heart muscle by decreasing conduction and increasing force. It is commonly indicated for HF, atrial fibrillation, atrial flutters, and supraventricular tachycardia. Digoxin should be given at regular intervals, every 12 hours, such as 8AM and 8 PM, one hour before or two hours after feeding. If a digoxin dose is missed and more than 4 hours have elapsed, give the missed dose. If the child vomits digoxin, a second dose should not be given. Potassium levels should be carefully monitored as a decrease enhances the effects of digitalis causing toxicity. Digoxin should not be held if the child's heart rate is below or above normal ranges.

2. Heart murmurs must be evaluated on the basis of the following characteristics:
   Location
   Relation to the heart cycle and duration
   Intensity Grades I to VI
   Quality-harsh, musical, or rough in high, medium, or low pitch
   Variation with position (sitting, lying, standing)

3. The three types of ASDs are identified based on the location of the opening:
   Ostium primum (ASD1): the opening is located at the lower portion of the septum.
   Ostium secundum (ASD2): the opening is located near the center of the septum.
   Sinus venosus defect: the opening is located near the junction of the superior vena cava and the right atrium.

4. Ventricular septal defect (VSD) accounts for 30% of all congenital heart defects. By the age of 2 years approximately 50% of small VSD's spontaneously close, and VSD's that require surgical intervention have a high rate of success. Upon assessment, newborns may not exhibit any signs or symptoms. Signs and symptoms of heart failure typically occur at 4 to 6 weeks of age and may include easily tiring and/or color changes and diaphoresis during feeding; lack of thriving; pulmonary infections, tachypnea, or shortness of breath; edema; murmurs; thrill in the chest upon palpation.

5. Risk factors for infective endocarditis include children with:
   Congenital heart defects;
   Prosthetic heart valves;
   Central venous catheters;
   Intravenous drug use.

## SECTION II: APPLYING YOUR KNOWLEDGE

**Activity E  CASE STUDY**

1. The discussion should include:
   Prepare the parents and child for the procedure by discussing what the procedure involves, how long it will take, special instructions from the physician, and what to expect after the procedure is complete. Inform the parents of the possible complications that might occur, such as bleeding, low-grade fever, loss of pulse in the extremity used for the catheterization, and arrhythmias. Explain that the child will have a dressing over the catheter site and the leg may need to remain straight for several hours after the procedure. Discuss that frequent monitoring will be required after the procedure. Use a variety of teaching methods such as videotapes, books, and pamphlets. Discussion with the child should be age appropriate.
   Preprocedure care includes a thorough history and physical examination, including vital signs, to establish a baseline. The nurse should obtain height and weight to assist in determining medication dosages. The child should be assessed for allergies, especially iodine or shellfish, because some contrast material contain iodine as a base. The medication history as well as laboratory testing results should be reviewed. The nurse should keep in mind that some medications, such as anticoagulants, are typically held prior to the procedure to reduce the risk of bleeding. Peripheral pulses, including pedal pulses, should be assessed. The location of the child's pedal pulses should be marked in order to facilitate their assessment after the procedure. Ensure informed consent has been obtained and a signed form is in the chart. Premedications ordered should be administered, and the parents should be allowed to accompany the child to the catheterization area if permitted.

2. Discussion should include:
   Following the procedure, the child should be monitored for complications of bleeding, arrhythmia, hematoma, and thrombus formation and infection. Assessment includes vital signs, neurovascular status of the lower extremities (pulses, color, temperature, and capillary refill), and the pressure dressing over the catheterization site every 15 minutes for the first hour and then every 30 minutes for 1 hour (depending on hospital policy). Monitoring of cardiac rhythm and oxygen saturation levels for the first few hours after the procedure should occur. Maintain bedrest in the immediate post procedure period. The leg might need to be kept straight for approximately 4 to 8 hours, depending on the approach used and facility policy. Reinforcement of the pressure dressing as necessary should be performed, and any evidence of drainage on the dressing should be noted. The infant's intake and output should be monitored closely. The parents should be provided with post-care and follow-up care education prior to discharge.

# SECTION III: PRACTICING FOR NCLEX

## Activity F NCLEX-STYLE QUESTIONS

**1. Answer: b**
Softening of nail beds is the first sign of clubbing due to chronic hypoxia. Rounding of the fingernails is followed by shininess and thickness of nail ends.

**2. Answer: d**
The normal infant heart rate averages 120 to 130 beats per minute (bpm); the toddler's or preschooler's is 80 to 105, the school-age child's is 70 to 80 bpm, and the adolescent's heart rate average 60 to 68 bpm.

**3. Answer: b**
The nurse should pay particular attention to assessing the child's peripheral pulses, including pedal pulses. Using an indelible pen, the nurse should mark the location of the child's pedal pulses as well as document the location and quality in the child's medical records.

**4. Answer: c**
Some medications, like lithium, taken by pregnant women may be linked with the development of congenital heart defects. Reports of nausea during pregnancy and an Apgar score of eight would not trigger further questions. Febrile illness during the first trimester, not the third, may be linked to an increased risk of congenital heart defects.

**5. Answer: a**
Edema of the lower extremities is characteristic of right ventricular heart failure in older children. In infants, peripheral edema occurs first in the face, then the presacral region, and the extremities.

**6. Answer: b**
A bounding pulse is characteristic of patent ductus arteriosis or aortic regurgitation. Narrow or thready pulses may occur in children with heart failure or severe aortic stenosis. A normal pulse would not be expected with aortic regurgitation.

**7. Answer: d**
An accentuated third heart sound is suggestive of sudden ventricular distention. Decreased blood pressure, cool, clammy, and pale extremities, and a heart murmur are all associated with cardiovascular disorders; however, these findings do not specifically indicate sudden ventricular distention.

**8. Answer: d**
A heart murmur characterized as loud with a precordial thrill is classified as Grade IV. Grade II is soft and easily heard. Grade I is soft and hard to hear. Grade III is loud without thrill.

**9. Answer: d**
The normal adolescent's blood pressure averages 100 to 120/50 to 70 mm Hg. The normal infant's blood pressure is about 80/40 mm Hg. The toddler or preschoolers blood pressure averages 80 to 100/64 mm Hg. The normal schoolager's blood pressure averages 94 to 112/56 to 60 mm Hg.

**10. Answer: a**
A mild to late ejection click at the apex is typical of a mitral valve prolapse. Abnormal splitting or intensifying of S2 sounds occurs in children with major heart problems, not mitral valve prolapse. Clicks on the upper left sternal border are related to the pulmonary area.

**11. Answer: 0.7 milligrams**
RATIONALE: The infant weighs 15.2 pounds (2.2 pounds = 1 kg.)

$$15.2 \text{ pounds} \times 1 \text{ kg}/2.2 \text{ pounds} = 6.818 \text{ kg}$$

The infant weighs 6.818 kg. For each kilogram of body weight, the infant should receive 0.1 mg of morphine sulfate.
6.818 kg × 0.1 mg/ 1 kg = 0.6818 mg, when rounded to the tenth place = 0.7 mg
The infant will receive 0.7 mg of morphine sulfate.

**12. Answers: a, b**
RATIONALE: Abrupt cessation of chest tube output and an increased heart rate are indicators that the child may have developed cardiac tamponade. The child's right atrial filling pressure will increase. The child may be anxious and their apical heart rate may be faint and difficult to auscultate.

**13. Answers: c, d, e**
RATIONALE: The nurse should not administer digoxin to children with the following issues: The adolescent with an apical pulse under 60 beats per minute, the child with a digoxin level above 2 ng/mL, and the child who exhibiting signs of digoxin toxicity.

**14. Answers: c, d**
RATIONALE: Subcutaneous nodules and carditis are considered major criteria used in the diagnosing process of acute rheumatic fever. The other options are minor criteria.

**15. Answers: b, c, d**
RATIONALE: The following information should be reported to the physician following a cardiac catheterization because they are indicative of possible complications: Negative changes to the child's peripheral vascular circulatory status (cool foot with poor pulse), a fever over 100.4 °F, and nausea or vomiting.

# CHAPTER 20

## SECTION I: ASSESSING YOUR UNDERSTANDING

### Activity A FILL IN THE BLANKS

**1.** Retching
**2.** Atresia
**3.** 2
**4.** Fungal
**5.** Stones
**6.** Probiotic
**7.** Intussusception

## Activity B  LABELING

*The colostomy is the diagram on the left and the ileostomy is the diagram on the right.*

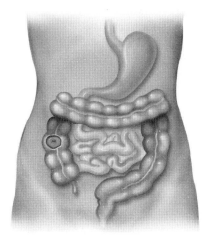 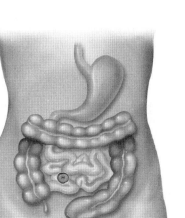

## Activity C  MATCHING

**1.** b   **2.** c   **3.** d   **4.** a   **5.** e

## Activity D  SEQUENCING

2 → 4 → 3 → 1

## Activity E  SHORT ANSWERS

1. (S) set up equipment, (T) take off the pouch, (O) observe the stoma and surrounding skin, (M) measure the stoma and mark the new pouch backing, (A) apply the new pouch.
2. The mouth is highly vascular making it a common entry point for infectious invaders. This increases the infant's and young child's risk for contraction of infectious agents via the mouth.
3. Acute hepatitis is mainly treated with rest, hydration, and nutrition.
4. Complications of a cleft palate that are of most concern during infancy pertain to feeding. The deformity often prevents the infant from being able to form an adequate seal around a nipple, preventing the ability to suction nutrients and cause excessive air intake. Feeding times are greatly extended, which causes insufficient intake and fatigue – both being precursors to problems with normal growth. Cleft palate during infancy also leads to gagging, choking, and nasal regurgitation of milk during feedings.
5. Data collected during the health history that would indicate pyloric stenosis include forceful, nonbilious vomiting that is not related to the feeding position of the infant, with subsequent weight loss, dehydration, and lethargy. These symptoms most commonly occur 2 to 4 weeks after birth. A positive family history of the disorder also increases the risk for pyloric stenosis. Physical assessment findings reveal a hard, movable "olive-like" area palpated in the right upper quadrant of the abdomen.

## SECTION II: APPLYING YOUR KNOWLEDGE

## Activity F  CASE STUDY

1. The discussion should include:
   Weight loss of 6 ounces in 2 weeks, sunken anterior fontanel, sticky mucous membranes, and poor skin turgor.
2. The discussion should include the following:
   The nurse should anticipate interventions that are going to rehydrate and restore Nico's fluid volume. Oral rehydration with pedialyte may be sufficient (refer to Teaching Guidelines 20.2). If dehydration appears to be severe, intravenous fluids may be necessary with a bolus of 20 mL/kg of normal saline or lactated ringers. Blood for electrolytes may need to be drawn to assess the extent of dehydration.
3. To evaluate Nico's hydration status the nurse should assess his fontanels, mucous membranes, skin turgor, urine output, pulses, capillary refill, temperature of extremities, and eyes.
4. Medical management of gastroesophageal reflux disease (GERD) usually begins with appropriate positioning such as elevating the head of the crib 30 degrees and keeping the infant or child upright for 30 to 45 minutes after feeding. Smaller more frequent feedings with a nipple that controls flow well may be helpful. Explain to the family to frequently burp the infant during feeds. Thickening of formula or pumped breast milk with products such as rice cereal can help in keeping the feedings and gastric contents down. Positioning of an infant for sleep with GERD is controversial; infants can be positioned safely on their sides or upright in a car

seat to minimize the risk of aspiration while on their backs. However, always check with the physician to discuss his or her recommendations regarding sleeping positions for infants with GERD.

If reflux does not improve with these measures medications are prescribed to decrease acid production and stabilize the pH of the gastric contents. Also, prokinetic agents may be used to help empty the stomach more quickly, minimizing the amount of gastric contents in the stomach that the child can reflux. If prescribed, thoroughly explain medications and their side effects and or adverse reactions. If the GERD cannot be medically managed effectively or requires long-term medication therapy, surgical intervention may be necessary.

Explain to Nico's parents that reflux is usually limited to the first year of life; though, in some cases, it may persist. Teach Nico's parents and caregivers the signs and symptoms of potential complications. GERD symptoms can often involve the airway. In rare instances, GERD can cause apnea or acute life-threatening events (ALTE). Teach parents how to deal with these episodes, as anxiety is very high. Provide CPR instruction to all parents whose children have had ALTE previously, and use of an apnea or bradycardia monitor may be warranted. The monitor requires a physician's order and can be ordered through a home health company.

# SECTION III: PRACTICING FOR NCLEX
## Activity G  NCLEX-STYLE QUESTIONS

1. **Answer: d**
   Infants are comprised of a high percentage of fluid that can be lost very quickly when vomiting, fever, and diarrhea are all present. This infant needs to be seen by the physician based on her age and symptoms; hospitalization may be necessary for intravenous rehydration depending upon her status when assessed.

2. **Answer: a**
   Anti-nuclear antibodies are one of the diagnostic tests performed to diagnose autoimmune hepatitis. Ultrasound is to assess for liver or spleen abnormalities. Viral studies are performed to screen for viral causes of hepatitis. Ammonia levels may be ordered if hepatic encephalopathy is suspected.

3. **Answer: d**
   If the parent reports that the child passed a meconium plug, the infant should be evaluated for Hirschsprung's disease. Constipation, not diarrhea, is associated with this condition; however, constipation alone would not necessarily warrant further evaluation for Hirschsprung's disease. Passing a meconium stool in the first 24 to 48 hours of life is normal.

4. **Answer: d**
   While most fruits and fruit juices are allowed, the nurse needs to make sure the mother knows that

some fruit pie fillings and dried fruit may contain gluten.

5. **Answer: b**
   It is very important to encourage large amounts of water/fluids after this test to avoid barium-induced constipation. It is also important to tell the parents about a possible change in stool color, but the fluids are most important. This procedure is unlikely to cause an infection. Diarrhea is usually not a problem after this examination.

6. **Answer: c**
   The best response would be to remind the boy that there are lots of other children with Crohn's disease that could be found at the local support group. Teenagers do not like to be told that they "have" to do anything. Telling the boy that he will eventually accept his condition or that the disease has periods of remission does not address his concerns.

7. **Answer: c**
   Tenting of skin is an indicator of severe dehydration. Soft and flat fontanels indicate mild dehydration. Pale and slightly dry mucosa indicates mild or moderate dehydration. Blood pressure of 80/42 is a normal finding for an infant.

8. **Answer: d**
   It is best to ask an open-ended question in very specific terms so that the nurse can assess for proper laxative use based on a recent history of stool patterns. Using the term daily stool patterns might be confusing to the parents. Asking the parents whether the laxatives are working may not elicit any helpful information. Asking whether they are giving him the laxatives properly would likely result in a positive response even if this is not accurate.

9. **Answer: a**
   Ulcerative colitis is usually continuous through the colon while the distribution of Crohn's disease is segmental. Crohn's disease affects the full thickness of the intestine while ulcerative colitis is more superficial. Both conditions share age at onset of 10 to 20 years, with abdominal pain and fever in 40 to 50% of cases.

10. **Answer: a**
    A hard, moveable "olive-like mass" in the right upper quadrant is the hypertrophied pylorus. A sausage-shaped mass in the upper mid abdomen is the hallmark of intussusception. Perianal fissures and skin tags are typical with Crohn's disease. Abdominal pain and irritability is common with pyloric stenosis but are seen with many other conditions.

11. **Answer: 48 milliliters**
    **RATIONALE:** 13.2 pounds $\times$ 1 kg/2.2 pounds = 6 kg
    6 kg $\times$ 1 mL/kg = 6 mL/hour
    6 mL $\times$ 8 hours = 48 mL/8-hour shift

12. **Answers: a, d**
    **RATIONALE:** Hepatitis A virus is transmitted by contaminated food or water. Hepatitis B virus may be

transmitted perinatally from mother to infant, intravenous drug use with contaminated needles, sexual contact with an infected person, and blood transfusions. The mother may have contracted the virus prior to giving birth to the child. Infection with the hepatitis B virus may result in jaundice, fever, and a rash.

13. **Answers: a, b, c**
    **RATIONALE:** Famotidine may cause fatigue. Omeprazole can cause headaches. Prokinetics use may result in side effects involving the central nervous system. Omeprazole use more likely will result in diarrhea, not constipation. Children with GERD should not lie down after meals.

14. **Answer: 289 milliliters per hour**
    **RATIONALE:** The child weighs 63.5 pounds.
    63.5 pounds × 1 kg/2.2 pounds = 577.2727 mL
    577.2727 mL of normal saline/ 2 hours = 288.6364 mL
    When rounded to the nearest whole number = 289 mL/hour

15. **Answers: b, d, e**
    **RATIONALE:** Newborns with esophageal atresia cough during attempts to feed, may have fluid in their lungs, and X-rays will show that nasogastric tubes just coil in the upper part of the esophagus because the esophagus does not extend to the stomach. They have increased salivation in their mouths and their skin may be dusky or cyanotic.

# CHAPTER 21

## SECTION I: ASSESSING YOUR UNDERSTANDING

### Activity A  FILL IN THE BLANKS

1. Suppression
2. Testicular
3. Renal
4. Flow
5. Enuresis
6. 30 mL

### Activity B  LABELING

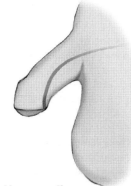 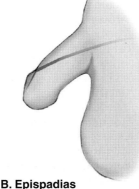

**A. Hypospadias**         **B. Epispadias**

A. Hypospadias: shows the urethral opening located on the ventral side of the penis.
B. Epispadias: shows the urethral opening located on the dorsal side of the penis.

### Activity C  MATCHING

**Question 1**

**1.** f    **2.** d    **3.** a    **4.** b    **5.** c

**Question 2**

**1.** c    **2.** d    **3.** b    **4.** a

### Activity D  SEQUENCING

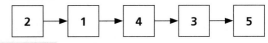

| 2 | 1 | 4 | 3 | 5 |

### Activity E  SHORT ANSWERS

1. After a bladder augmentation the urine may contain mucous.
2. The nurse should encourage fluids and monitor vital signs. The nurse must also be aware that child may feel burning with voiding after the procedure and urine may have a pink tinge because of the irritation of the mucous membrane as a result of the procedure.
3. Medications used in the care and treatment of end-stage renal disease may include:
   - Vitamin D/Calcium to correct hypocalcemia and hyperphosphatemia
   - Ferrous sulfate for anemia
   - Bicitra or sodium bicarbonate tablets to correct acidosis
   - Multivitamins to augment nutrition status
   - Erythropoietin injections to stimulate red blood cell growth
   - Growth hormone injections to stimulate growth in stature
4. A testicle is abnormally attached to the scrotum and twisted. It requires immediate attention because ischemia can result if the torsion is left untreated, leading to infertility. Testicular torsion may occur at any age but most commonly occurs in boys aged 12 to 18 years.
5. Normally both testes are descended at the time of birth. A watch and see approach is taken. If the testes are not descended by 6 months of age surgery is indicated.

## SECTION II: APPLYING YOUR KNOWLEDGE

### Activity F  CASE STUDY

1. The discussion should include the following points:
   Urinary tract infections (UTI) occur most often due to bacteria coming from the urethra and traveling up to the bladder. The most common organism that causes UTI is *Escherichia coli*, which is usually found in the perineal and anal region, close to the urethral opening. UTIs are very common in children, especially infants and young children and after 1 year of age is more common

in females. One explanation for UTI occurring more frequently in females than in males is that the female's shorter urethra allows bacteria to have easier access to the bladder. Additionally, the female urethra is located quite close to the vagina and anus, allowing spread of bacteria such as *Escherichia coli* from those areas.

2. The discussion should include the following points:

   Administer oral antibiotics as prescribed and complete the entire course of antibiotics even if Corey is feeling better and is not showing any signs or symptoms any longer. Push oral fluids, which will help flush the bacteria from the bladder. Administer antipyretics, such as acetaminophen or ibuprofen, in order to reduce fever. A heating pad or warm compress may help relieve abdomen or flank pain. If the child is afraid to urinate due to burning or stinging, encourage voiding in a warm sitz or tub bath.

3. The discussion should include the following points:

   Encourage Corey and her family to follow-up as the physician has ordered for repeat urine culture after completing the course of antibiotics. Ensure Corey drinks adequate fluid to keep urine flushed through the bladder and prevent urine stasis. A decreased fluid intake can contribute to bacterial growth, as the bacteria become more concentrated. Encourage drinking of juices such as cranberry juice that will acidify the urine. If urine is alkaline, bacteria are better able to flourish. Avoid colas and caffeine which irritate the bladder. Encourage Corey to urinate frequently and avoid holding of urine to avoid urinary stasis which allows bacteria to grow. Avoid bubble baths which can contribute to vulvar and perineal irritation. Teach Corey to wipe front to back after using the restroom, to avoid contamination of the urethra with rectal material. Wearing of cotton underwear can decrease the incidence of perineal irritation. Avoid wearing of tight jeans or pants and wash the perineal area daily with soap and water.

## SECTION III: PRACTICING FOR NCLEX

### Activity G  NCLEX-STYLE QUESTIONS

1. **Answer: c**

   Urinalysis is ordered to reveal preliminary information about the urinary tract. The test evaluates color, pH, specific gravity, and odor of urine. Urinalysis also assesses for presence of protein, glucose, ketones, blood, leukocyte esterase, RBCs, WBCs, bacteria, crystals, and casts. Total protein, globulin, albumin, and creatinine clearance would be ordered for suspected renal failure or renal disease. Urine culture and sensitivity is used to determine the presence of bacteria and determine the best choice of antibiotic.

2. **Answer: c**

   Acute glomerulonephritis often follows a group A streptococcal infection. Strep A infections may manifest as an upper respiratory infection. The history of urinary tract infections, renal disorders, or hypotension are not directly associated with the onset of acute glomerulonephritis.

3. **Answer: b**

   The nurse should weigh the old dialysate to determine the amount of fluid removed from the child. The fluid must be weighed prior to emptying it. The nurse should weigh the new fluid prior to starting the next fill phase. Typically, the exchanges are 3 to 6 hours apart so the nurse would not immediately start the next fill phase.

4. **Answer: d**

   The girl cannot eat whatever she wants on dialysis days. She can eat what she wants during the few hours she is actively undergoing treatment in the hemodialysis unit. The other statements regarding a high sodium diet and potassium intake are correct.

5. **Answer: c**

   It is very important to administer in the morning, encourage large amounts of water/fluids and encourage frequent voiding during and after infusion to decrease the risk of hemorrhagic cystitis

6. **Answer: b**

   The best response would be to include the child in plans for nighttime urinary control. This gives the child a sense of hope and reminds him that there are actions he can take to help achieve dryness. Telling him that he will grow out of this does not offer solutions. Providing statistics can be helpful, but does not offer a solution. Reminding him that pull-ups look just like underwear does not address his concerns.

7. **Answer: c**

   Hemolytic uremic syndrome is defined by all three particular features – hemolytic anemia, thrombocytopenia, and acute renal failure. Dirty green colored urine, elevated erythrocyte sedimentation, and depressed serum complement level are indicative of acute glomerulonephritis. Hypertension, not hypotension would be seen and the child would have decreased urinary output which would not cause nocturia.

8. **Answer: c**

   The nurse should withhold routine medications on the morning that hemodialysis is scheduled since they would be filtered out through the dialysis process. His medications should be administered after he returns from the dialysis unit. A Tenckhoff catheter is used for peritoneal dialysis, not hemodialysis. The nurse should avoid blood pressure measurement in the extremity with the AV fistula as it may cause occlusion.

9. **Answer: c**

   The girl's partner should be treated, but she must strongly encourage the girl to require her partner to wear a condom every time they have sex, even after he undergoes antibiotic therapy. The other statements are accurate.

**10. Answer: d**

The nurse should always auscultate the site for presence of a bruit and palpate for presence of a thrill. The nurse should immediately notify the physician if there is an absence of a thrill. Dialysate without fibrin or cloudiness is normal and is used with peritoneal dialysis, not hemodialysis.

**11. Answer: a**

Complications of hydronephrosis include renal insufficiency, hypertension, and eventually renal failure. Hypotension, hypothermia, and tachycardia are not associated with hydronephrosis.

**12. Answer: a, c, e**

A voiding cystourethrogram (VCUG) will be performed to determine the presence of a structural defect that may be causing the hydronephrosis. Other diagnostic tests, such as a renal ultrasound or an intravenous pyelogram, may also be performed to clarify the diagnosis. A urinalysis may be performed to assess the quality and characteristics of the urine but the test will not confirm a diagnosis of hydronephrosis. A complete blood cell count may be used to assess the level of a genitourinary infection but it will not confirm the diagnosis of hydronephritis.

**13. Answer: c**

Normally both testes will descend prior to birth. In the event this does not happen the child will be observed for the first 6 months of life. If the testicle descends without intervention further treatment will not be needed. Surgical intervention is not needed until after 6 months if the testicle has not descended.

**14. Answer: a**

Epididymitis is caused by a bacterial infection. Treatment may include scrotal elevation, bed rest, and ice packs to the scrotum. Pharmacotherapy may include antibiotics, pain medications, and NSAIDs. Warm compresses would result in vasodilation and do little to relieve the pain and swelling of the condition. Corticosteroid therapy is not included in the plan of care for the condition. Voiding is not impacted by epididymitis. Catheterization is not indicated.

**15. Answer: d**

The discharge instructions for the child who has had a circumcision will include a listing of warning signs to report. Redness or swelling of the penile shaft is not a normal finding and must be reported. Petroleum jelly (Vaseline) is often used for the first 24 hours after the procedure but not for a period of 2 weeks. Small amounts of bleeding may be noted. This bleeding if scant in amount does not warrant reporting to the physician. Reduction of water to impact voiding is inappropriate.

# CHAPTER 22

## SECTION I: ASSESSING YOUR UNDERSTANDING

### Activity A  FILL IN THE BLANKS

1. Autoimmune
2. Clonus
3. Decrease
4. Involuntary
5. Hypotonia
6. Neural tube defects
7. Guillain-Barré

### Activity B  LABELING

Figure A shows meningocele
Figure B shows myelomeningocele.
Figure C shows normal spine
Figure D shows spina bifida occulta

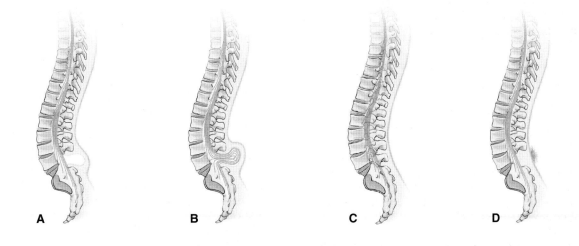

A      B      C      D

**Activity C MATCHING**

**1.** a     **2.** c          **3.** d          **4.** b          **5.** e

**Activity D SHORT ANSWERS**

1. The four classifications are spastic, athetoid (dyskinetic), ataxic, and mixed. Spastic is the most common form and ataxic is the rarest.

2. Nursing management of a child with myelomeningocele focuses on preventing infection, promoting bowel and urinary elimination, promoting adequate nutrition, and preventing latex allergic reaction. The nurse is also concerned with maintaining the child's skin integrity, providing education and support to the family, and recognizing complications such as hydrocephalus or increased intracranial pressure (ICP) associated with the disorder.

3. Pain in the lower extremities is often one of the first symptoms in children. Additional symptoms include fairly symmetrical flaccid weakness or paralysis. Ataxia and sensory disturbances are commonly seen during the course of the illness.

4. Risk factors for neural tube defects include lack of prenatal care; insufficient intake of folic acid preconception and /or prenatally; previous history of a child born with a neural tube defect or a positive family history of neural tube defects; and certain drugs that antagonize folic acid absorption, such as anticonvulsants, that are taken by the mother during pregnancy.

5. There are nine types of muscular dystrophy, with Duchenne muscular dystrophy being the most common childhood type. All types of muscular dystrophy result in progressive skeletal (voluntary) muscle wasting and weakness. The disease is inherited, but there are various patterns of inheritance among the various types of muscular dystrophy.

# SECTION II: APPLYING YOUR KNOWLEDGE
**Activity E CASE STUDY**

1. The discussion should include the following points:
   - Cerebral palsy (CP) is a term used to describe a range of nonspecific clinical symptoms characterized by abnormal motor pattern and postures caused by nonprogressive abnormal brain function. The cause of CP generally occurs before or during delivery and is often associated with brain anoxia. Often no specific cause can be identified. Prolonged, complicated difficult delivery and prematurity are risk factors for CP. CP is the most common movement disorder of childhood and is a life-long, nonprogressive condition. It is one of the most common causes of physical disability in children.
   - There is a large variation in symptoms and disability among those with CP. For some children the disability may be as mild as a slight limp and for others it may result in severe motor and neurologic impairments. However, its primary signs include motor impairment such as spasticity,

muscle weakness, and ataxia. Complications of CP include mental impairment, seizures, growth problems, impaired vision or hearing, abnormal sensation or perception, and hydrocephalus. Most children can survive into adulthood but may endure substantial effects on function and quality of life.

2. The discussion should include the following points:
   - Earliest signs of cerebral palsy include abnormal muscle tone and developmental delay. Primary signs include spasticity, muscle weakness, and ataxia. Children with CP may demonstrate abnormal use of muscle groups such as scooting on their back instead of crawling or walking. Hypertonicity with increased resistance to dorsiflexion and passive hip abduction are common early signs. Sustained clonus may be present after forced dorsiflexion. Children with CP will often demonstrate prolonged standing on their toes when supported in an upright standing position.

3. The discussion should include the following points:
   - Nursing management focuses on promoting growth and development through the promotion of mobility and maintenance of optimal nutritional intake. Treatment modalities to promote mobility include physiotherapy, pharmacological management, and surgery. Physical or occupational therapy as well as medications may be used to address musculoskeletal abnormalities, facilitate range of motion, delay or prevent deformities such as contractures, provide joint stability, and to maximize activity and to encourage the use of adaptive devices. The nurse's role in relation to the various therapies is to ensure compliance with prescribed exercises, positioning, or bracing. Children with CP may experience difficulty eating and swallowing due to poor motor control of the throat, mouth, and tongue. This may lead to poor nutrition and problems with growth. The child with CP may require a longer time to feed because of the poor motor control. Special diets, such as soft or pureed, may make swallowing easier. Proper positioning during feeding is essential to facilitate swallowing and reduce the risk of aspiration. Speech or occupational therapists can assist in working on strengthening swallowing muscles as well as assisting in developing accommodations to facilitate nutritional intake. Consult a dietician to ensure adequate nutrition for children with cerebral palsy. In children with severe swallowing problems or malnutrition, a feeding tube such as a gastrostomy tube may be placed.
   - Providing support and education to the child and family is also an important nursing function. From the time of diagnosis, the family should be involved in the child's care. Refer caregivers to local resources including education services and support groups.

# SECTION III: PRACTICING FOR NCLEX

## Activity F NCLEX-STYLE QUESTIONS

1. **Answer: b**
   The nurse needs to obtain a clear description of weakness. This open-ended question would most likely elicit specific examples of weakness and shed light on whether the boy is simply fatigued. The other questions would most likely elicit a yes or no answer rather than any specific details about his weakness or development.

2. **Answer: d**
   The persistence of a primitive reflex in a 9-month-old would warrant further evaluation. Symmetrical spontaneous movement and absence of the Moro and tonic neck reflex are expected in a normally developing 9-month-old child.

3. **Answer: b**
   Dimpling and skin discoloration in the child's lumbosacral area can be an indication of spina bifida occulta. It would be best to respond that the dimpling and discoloration is possibly a normal variation with no problems and indicate that the doctor will want to take a closer look; this response will not alarm the parent, but it also does not ignore the findings. Spina bifida is a term that is often used to generalize all neural tube disorders that affect the spinal cord. This can be confusing and a cause of concern for parents. It is probably best to avoid the use of the term initially until a diagnosis is confirmed. Nursing care would then focus on educating the family.

4. **Answer: c**
   Symptoms of constipation and bladder dysfunction may result due to an increasing size of the lesion. Increasing ICP and head circumference would point to hydrocephalus. Leaking cerebrospinal fluid would indicate the sac is leaking.

5. **Answer: b**
   It is very important to remind the parents that they must always wash hands very well with soap and water prior to catheterization to help prevent infection. The other statements are correct.

6. **Answer: c**
   The best response would be to remind the boy that there are many children with muscular dystrophy that could be found at the local support group. Teenagers do not like to be told that they "have" to do anything. Telling the boy that he needs to be active or simply suggesting activities does not address his concerns.

7. **Answer: a**
   A sign of Duchenne muscular dystrophy (DMD) is the walking on the toes or balls of the feet with a rolling or waddling gait. Signs of hydrocephalus are not typically associated with DMD. Kyphosis and scoliosis occur more frequently than lordosis. A child with DMD has an enlarged appearance to their calf muscles due to pseudohypertrophy of the calves.

8. **Answer: d**
   The nurse can offer the child a snack and observe if she has any difficulty chewing, swallowing, or feeding herself. Inquiring about a typical day's diet opens up the conversation to discuss the quantity and quality of food the girl eats. Asking about swallowing or whether the girl feeds herself would most likely elicit a yes or no response. Checking her hydration status and respiratory system is important, but does not open a dialogue.

9. **Answer: a**
   The use of ticking is often a successful technique for assessing the level of paralysis in this age of child, either initially or in the recovery phase. Symmetrical flaccid weakness, ataxia, and sensory disturbances are other symptoms seen during the course of the illness.

10. **Answer: b**
    The central nursing priority is to prevent rupture or leaking of cerebrospinal fluid. Keeping infant in prone position will help prevent pressure on lesion. Keeping lesion free from fecal matter or urine is important as well, but the priority is to prevent rupture or leakage. The nurse should consider the lesion first when maintaining the infant's body temperature.

11. **Answers: a, c, d, e**
    RATIONALE: Ditropan is used to increase the child's bladder capacity when they have a spastic bladder. The caregivers and the child should be taught about urinary catheterization techniques to allow the bladder to empty. The child and caregivers should be educated about the clinical manifestations associated with a urinary tract infection so that it can be treated promptly. Sometimes surgical interventions such as vesicostomy and the creation of a continent urinary reservoir are used to treat neurogenic bladders.

12. **Answers: a, b, d**
    RATIONALE: Significant muscle wasting is associated with this diagnosis. Creatine kinase levels increase with muscle wasting. A muscle biopsy will show an absence of dystrophin. Gowers' sign will be positive. An electromygoram will indicate the problem is with the muscles, not the nerves. Genetic testing will reveal the presence of the gene associated with Duchenne muscular dystrophy.

13. **Answers: a, b, d, e**
    RATIONALE: The following are clinical manifestations associated with cholinergic crisis: Sweating, bradycardia, severe muscle weakness, and increased salivation.

14. **Answers: a, b**
    RATIONALE: Corticosteroids should be given with food to minimize gastric upset. Corticosteroids can mask infection. This child should avoid large crowds to prevent exposure to infectious organisms. The other parent responses are correct regarding corticosteroids and dermatomyositis.

15. **Answers: d, b, a, c**
    RATIONALE: Guillain–Barré syndrome paresthesias and muscle weakness. Classically it initially affects the lower extremities and progresses in an

ascending manner to upper extremities and then the facial muscles. Progression is usually complete in 2 to 4 weeks, followed by a stable period leading to the recovery phase.

# CHAPTER 23

## SECTION I: ASSESSING YOUR UNDERSTANDING

### Activity A  FILL IN THE BLANKS

1. Convex
2. Epiphysis
3. Fixator
4. Synovitis
5. Bacterial
6. Ossification
7. Adductus

### Activity B  LABELING

1. Bryant's traction
2. Russell's traction
3. Buck's traction
4. Cervical skin traction
5. Side-arm 90-90
6. Dunlop side-arm 00-90
7. 90-90 traction
8. Cervical skeletal tongs
9. Halo traction
10. Balanced suspension traction

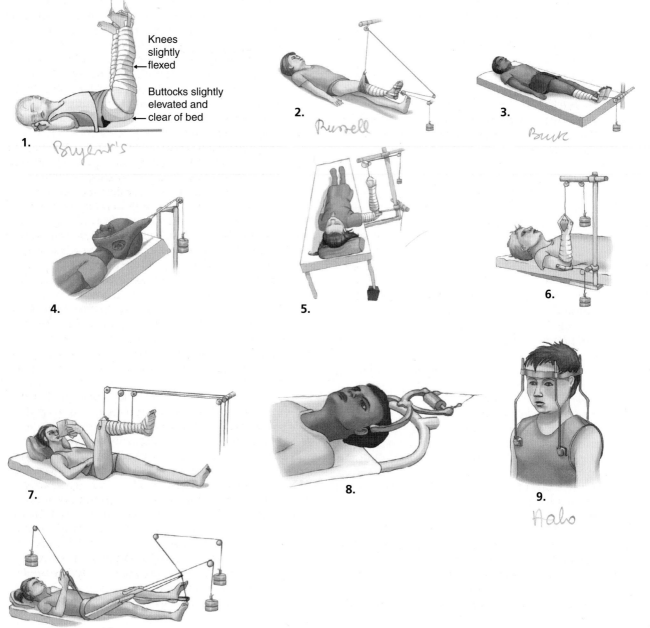

Knees slightly flexed

Buttocks slightly elevated and clear of bed

1. Bryant's

2. Russell

3. Buck

4.

5.

6.

7.

8.

9. Halo

10.

## Activity C MATCHING

**1.** d  **2.** c  **3.** e  **4.** b  **5.** a

## Activity D SEQUENCING

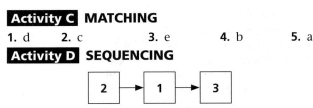

## Activity E SHORT ANSWERS

1. In developmental dysplasia of the hip, the femoral head has an abnormal relationship to the acetabulum. Frank dislocation of the hip is complete dislocation. It may occur in which there is no contact between the femoral head and acetabulum. Subluxation is a partial dislocation, meaning that the acetabulum is not fully seated within the hip joint. Dysplasia refers to an acetabulum that is shallow or sloping instead of cup shaped.

2. A plastic or bowing deformity involves significant bending without breaking of the bone. A buckle fracture is a compression injury; the bone "buckles" rather than breaks. A greenstick fracture is an incomplete fracture of the bone. A complete fracture occurs when the bone breaks into two separate pieces.

3. Osteogenesis imperfecta is a genetic disorder that results in instability of joints and fractures. Parent teaching for care of the child with this disorder should include:
   - Never push or pull on the child's arm or leg
   - Do not bend the child's arm or leg into an awkward position
   - Lift a baby by placing one hand under the legs and buttocks and one hand under the shoulders, head, and neck
   - Do not lift a baby's legs by the ankles to change the diaper
   - Do not lift a baby or small child from under the armpits
   - Provide supported positioning
   - If a fracture is suspected, handle the limb as little as possible

4. Instructions for the child and his parents following removal of the cast should include:
   - Soak the arm in warm water daily to help in removing dead skin and secretions that have accumulated under the cast
   - Advise that new skin may be tender
   - Wash the arm with soapy warm water, but avoid excessive rubbing
   - Apply moisturizing lotion to the arm and avoid scratching dry skin
   - Encourage activity to regain strength and motion of the arm

5. Torticollis is a painless muscular condition that is often seen in infants, and sometimes in children with certain syndromes. Tightness of the sternocleidomastoid muscle causes torticollis, resulting in an infant's or child's head being tilted to one side.

Passive stretching exercises are included in the treatment of the disorder.

## SECTION II: APPLYING YOUR KNOWLEDGE
## Activity F CASE STUDY

1. The discussion should include the following points:
   Perform a baseline neurovascular assessment, including color, movement, sensation, edema, and quality of pulses. Enlist the cooperation of the child, show him the cast materials, discuss colors of the cast materials, and have him help choose the color of his cast. Use an age-appropriate approach to describe the cast application process. Premedicate if ordered and provide distraction throughout cast application.

2. The discussion should include the following points:
   Drying time of the cast will vary depending on type of material used. Help the child keep the cast still and position it on pillows. If a plaster cast has been applied, "petal" the cast with moleskin or other soft material that has adhesive backing in order to prevent skin rubbing. Perform frequent neurovascular checks of the casted extremity. Assess for signs of increased pain, edema, pale or blue discoloration, skin coolness, numbness or tingling, prolonged capillary refill, and decreased pulse strength (if able to assess). Notify physician of changes in neurovascular status, persistent complaints of pain, odor, or drainage from the cast. Elevate casted extremity and apply ice if needed.

3. The discussion should include the following points:
   The child can resume increased levels of activity as the pain subsides. The right arm should be elevated above the level of the heart for the first 48 hours. Ice may be applied for 20 to 30 minutes, then off 1 hour and repeat for the first 24 to 48 hours. Check his right fingers for swelling (have him wiggle his fingers) hourly. Check the skin around the cast for irritation daily. If he complains of itching inside the cast blow cool air in from a hair dryer set on the lowest setting. Never insert anything into the cast for scratching and do not use lotions or powders. Keep the cast dry. Apply a plastic bag around the cast and tape securely for bathing or showering. Do not let the child submerge the cast in a bathtub. Call the physician if the casted extremity is cool to touch; inability to move his fingers; severe pain occurs with movement of his fingers; persistent numbness or tingling; drainage or a foul smell comes from the cast; severe itching inside the cast; temperature above 101.5 °F for longer than 24 hours; skin edges are red, swollen, or exhibit breakdown; or the casts gets wet, cracks, splits, or softens. Educate the family on follow-up needs and medications (including pain medication) if ordered.

# SECTION III: PRACTICING FOR NCLEX

## Activity G NCLEX-STYLE QUESTIONS

1. **Answer: b**
   The baby will most likely wear the harness for 3 months. Telling the parents that the harness does not hurt the baby is appropriate, but stressing the importance of wearing the harness continuously is a higher priority to ensure proper care and effective treatment. Only the physician or nurse practitioner can make adjustments to the harness.

2. **Answer: a**
   Asymmetry of the thigh or gluteal folds is indicative of DDH. Hip and knee joint relationship are not indicative of DDH. The lower extremities of the infant typically have some normal developmental variations due to in utero positioning.

3. **Answer: a**
   It is important to be vigilant in inspecting the child's skin for rashes, redness, and irritation to uncover areas where pressure sores are likely to develop. Applying lotion is part of the routine skin care regimen. Applying lotion, gentle massage, and keeping skin dry and clean are part of the routine skin care regimen.

4. **Answer: c**
   In Type II metatarsus adductus, the forefoot is flexible passively past neutral, but only to midline actively. The forefoot is flexible past neutral actively and passively in Type I. The forefoot is rigid, does not correct to midline even with passive stretching in Type III. An inverted forefoot turned slightly upward is indicative of clubfoot.

5. **Answer: b**
   It is very important to teach parents to identify the signs of neurovascular compromise (pale, cool, or blue skin) and tell them to notify the physician immediately. The other statements are correct.

6. **Answer: c**
   The best response for a 6-year-old is to use distraction throughout the cast application. He is resisting the application of the cast, so the best approach at this point is distraction. Telling him that application will not hurt is not helpful; nor is asking the child whether he wants pain medication. It is helpful to enlist the cooperation of the child by showing the child cast materials before beginning the procedure; but if he is resisting treatment, distraction would be the best approach.

7. **Answer: c**
   The nurse should emphasize that the child should not be allowed to lie on his side for 4 weeks following the surgery to ensure the bar does not shift. The parents should be aware of signs of infection; but the position must be emphasized to protect the bar. The nurse would be expected to monitor the child's vital capacity, not the parents. The prone position is acceptable.

8. **Answer: a**
   The Ilizarov fixator uses wires that are thinner than ordinary pins, so simply cleansing by showering is usually sufficient to keep the pin site clean.

9. **Answer: d**
   Because the mother is crying and experiencing the initial shock of the diagnosis, the nurse's primary concern is to support the mother and assure her that she is not to blame for the DDH. While education is important, let the mother adjust to the diagnosis and assure her that the baby and her family will be supported now and throughout the treatment period.

10. **Answer: d**
    Blue sclera is not diagnostic of osteogenesis imperfecta, but it is a common finding. Foot drawn up and inward (talipes varus) and sole of foot facing backwards (talipes equinus) are associated with clubfoot. Dimpled skin and hair in the lumbar region are common findings with spina bifida occulta.

11. **Answers: a, b**
    RATIONALE: This child has taken a benzodiazepine. Common side effects associated with this medication are dizziness and sedation. The skeletal muscle relaxes and the spasms will diminish. Nausea and upper gastrointestinal pain are not common side effects associated with this medication.

12. **Answers: b, c, e**
    RATIONALE: The parents should call the physician when the following things occur: The child has a temperature greater than 101.5F for more than 24 hours, there is drainage from the casted site, the site distal to the casted extremity is cyanotic, or severe edema is present.

13. **Answer: 1 milliliter**
    RATIONALE: The supplement has 5 mcg of vitamin D in each 0.5 mL. The child is supposed to receive 10 mcg each day of supplemental vitamin D.

    Desired/Have × Quantity = dose
    10 mcg/5 mcg × 0.5 mL = 1 mL

    Ratio/proportion:
    0.5 mL/5 micrograms = x/10 micrograms = 1 mL

14. **Answers: b, c, d, e**
    RATIONALE: Slipped capital femoral epiphysis most often occurs in males between the ages of 12 to 15 years. It more commonly affects African American boys. The femoral plate weakens and becomes less resistant to stressors during periods of growth. Boys are more frequently affected. Obese boys are more likely to develop this condition.

15. **Answer: c**
    RATIONALE: A greenstick fracture (image C) is an incomplete fracture of the bone. Image A shows a plastic or bowing deformity. Image B shows a

buckle fracture (the bone buckles rather than breaks). Image D shows a complete fracture (the bone breaks in two pieces).

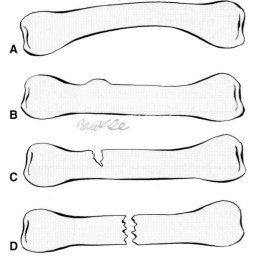

# CHAPTER 24

## SECTION I: ASSESSING YOUR UNDERSTANDING

### Activity A  FILL IN THE BLANKS

1. Decreases
2. IgE
3. Hypersensitivity
4. Cradle cap
5. Androgens

### Activity B  MATCHING

**Question 1**

1. b    2. c        3. d        4. a        5. e

**Question 2**

1. d    2. c        3. a        4. b

### Activity C  SEQUENCING

2 → 5 → 3 → 4 → 1

### Activity D  SHORT ANSWERS

1. Dark-skinned children tend to have more pronounced cutaneous reactions compared to children with lighter skin. Hypopigmentation or hyperpigmentation in the affected area following healing of a dermatologic condition is common.

   Dark-skinned children tend to have more prominent papules, follicular response lichenification, and vesicular or bullous reaction than lighter-skinned children with the same disorder. Additionally, hypertrophic scarring and keloid formation occur more often.

2. Four criteria to describe lesions:
   • Linear refers to lesions in a line
   • Shape: The lesions are round, oval, or annular (ring around central clearing)
   • Morbilliform refers to a rosy, maculopapular rash
   • Target lesions look just like a bull's eye

3. Impetigo is a readily recognizable skin rash. Non-bullous impetigo generally follows some type of skin trauma or may arise as a secondary bacterial infection of another skin disorder, such as atopic dermatitis. Bullous impetigo demonstrates a sporadic occurrence pattern and develops on intact skin resulting from toxin production of *Staphylococcus aureus*.

4. Pressure ulcers develop from a combination of factors, including immobility or decreased activity, decreased sensory perception, increased moisture, impaired nutritional status, inadequate tissue perfusion, and the forces of friction and shear. Common sites of pressure ulcers in hospitalized children include the occipital region and toes, while children who require wheelchairs for mobility have pressure ulcers in the sacral or hip area more frequently.

5. Acne vulgaris affects 50% to 85% of adolescents between the ages of 12 and 16 years. The sebaceous gland produces sebum and is connected by a duct to the follicular canal that opens on the skin's surface. Androgenous hormones stimulate sebaceous gland proliferation and production of sebum. These hormones exhibit increased activity during the pubertal years.

## SECTION II: APPLYING YOUR KNOWLEDGE

### Activity E  CASE STUDY

1. The skin reaction seen in atopic dermatitis is in response to specific allergens (such as food or environmental triggers). So when Eva comes into contact with the triggers it causes her body to respond and her skin starts to feel itchy. This sensation of itchiness comes first and then the rash becomes apparent. Other factors such as high or low temperatures, perspiring, contact with skin irritants (such as fragrance in soaps), scratching, or stress can also trigger the skin to flare up.

2. Management of atopic dermatitis focuses on promoting skin hydration, maintaining skin integrity, and preventing infection. Parents and caregivers need to be instructed to avoid hot water and any skin and hair products that contain perfumes, dyes, or fragrances. Bathing the child twice a day in warm water using a mild soap for sensitive skin is encouraged. Do not rub the child dry but gently pat them and leave the child moist. Apply prescribed ointments or creams to affected areas. Apply fragrance-free moisturizers. Re-moisturize multiple times throughout the day. Avoid clothing made of synthetic fabrics or

wool. Avoid triggers (often food, especially eggs, wheat, milk, and peanut, or environmental triggers such as molds, dust mites, and cat dander) known to exacerbate atopic dermatitis. Cut the child's finger nails short and keep them clean. Avoid tight clothing and heat. Use 100% cotton bed sheets and pajamas. It is very important to stop the child from scratching since this causes the rash to appear and causes trauma to the skin and secondary infection. Antihistamines given at bedtime may sedate the child enough to allow for sleep without awakening because of itching. During the waking hours, behavior modification may help to keep the child from scratching. The parents should keep a diary for 1 week to determine the pattern of scratching. Discuss specific strategies that may raise the child's awareness of scratching such as use of a hand-held clicker or counter to help identify the scratching episode for the child, thus raising awareness. Discuss the use of diversion, imagination, and play to help to detract Eva from scratching. Pressing the skin or fist clenching may replace scratching. Keep the child active and positively reinforce by praising desired behaviors.

## SECTION III: PRACTICING FOR NCLEX

### Activity F  NCLEX-STYLE QUESTIONS

1. **Answer: c**
   Airway injury from burn or smoke inhalation should be suspected if stridor is present. Cervical spine or internal injures would not point to airway injury. Burns on hands would not be indicative of airway injury.

2. **Answer: c**
   Initially, the severely burned child first experiences a decrease in cardiac output with a subsequent hypermetabolic response during which cardiac output increases dramatically. During this heightened metabolic state, the child is a risk for insulin resistance and increased protein catabolism.

3. **Answer: d**
   Staphylococcal scalded skin syndrome results from infection with *S. aureus* that produces a toxin which then causes exfoliation. It is abrupt in onset and results in diffuse erythema and skin tenderness. It is most common in infancy and rare beyond 5 years of age. Bullous impetigo presents with red macules and bullous eruptions on an erythematous base. Nonbullous impetigo presents as papules progressing to vesicles then painless pustules with a narrow erythematous border. Folliculitis presents with red raised hair follicles.

4. **Answer: c**
   The nurse should emphasize that the parents should avoid hot water. The child should be bathed twice a day in warm water. The other statements are correct.

5. **Answer: a**
   Tinea pedis presents with red scaling rash on soles, and between the toes. Tinea capitis presents with patches of scaling in the scalp with central hair loss and the risk of kerion development (inflamed boggy mass filled with pustules). Tinea cruris presents with erythema, scaling, maceration in the inguinal creases and inner thighs.

6. **Answer: b**
   Small round red circles with scaling, symmetrically located on the girls' inner thighs point to nickel dermatitis that may occur from contact with jewelry, eyeglasses, belts, or clothing snaps. The nurse should inquire about any sleepers or clothing with metal snaps. The girl does not have a rash in her diaper area. It is unlikely that an infant this age would have her inner thighs exposed to a highly allergenic plant. Discussing family allergy history is important, but the nurse should first inquire about any clothing with metal that could have come into contact with the girl's skin when she displays a symmetrical rash.

7. **Answer: a**
   Erythema multiforme typically manifests in lesions over the hands and feet, and extensor surfaces of the extremities with spread to the trunk. Thick or flaky/greasy yellow scales are signs of seborrhea. Silvery or yellow-white scale plaques and sharply demarcated borders define psoriasis. Superficial tan or hypopigmented oval-shaped scaly lesions especially on upper back and chest and proximal arms are indicative of tinea versicolor.

8. **Answer: c**
   The nurse should administer diphenhydramine as soon as possible after the sting in an attempt to minimize a reaction. The other actions are important for an insect sting, but the priority intervention is to administer diphenhydramine.

9. **Answer: b**
   Second degree frostbite demonstrates blistering with erythema and edema. First degree frostbite results in superficial white plaques with surrounding erythema. In third degree frostbite, the nurse would note hemorrhagic blisters that would progress to tissue necrosis and sloughing when the fourth degree is reached.

10. **Answer: a**
    It is important to apply moisture multiply times through the day. Petroleum jelly is a recommended moisturizer that is inexpensive and readily available. The other statements are correct.

11. **Answer: a**
    Impetigo is an infectious bacterial infection. The crusts should be removed after soaking prior to applying topical medications. Leaving the lesions open to air is not contraindicated. Children diagnosed with impetigo may attend school during treatment.

12. **Answer: c**
    Tinea pedis is commonly known as athlete's foot. It is a fungal infection. The fungi are able to readily grow in warm, moist conditions such as shower areas.

13. **Answers: a, b, c**
    The treatment of diaper rash may include topical ointments containing vitamins A and D as well as zinc.
14. **Answer: a**
    Atopic dermatitis is commonly associated allergies to food. Common culprits may include peanuts, eggs, orange juice, and wheat-containing products.
15. **Answers: b, c, e**
    When caring for the child with atopic dermatitis the focus of care will be on the prevention of infection, maintenance of skin integrity, and promotion of skin hydration.

# CHAPTER 25

## SECTION I: ASSESSING YOUR UNDERSTANDING

### Activity A FILL IN THE BLANKS

1. Hemogram
2. Volume
3. Kidneys
4. Size
5. Protoporphyrin
6. Mean platelet volume (MPV)
7. Anemia

### Activity B LABELING

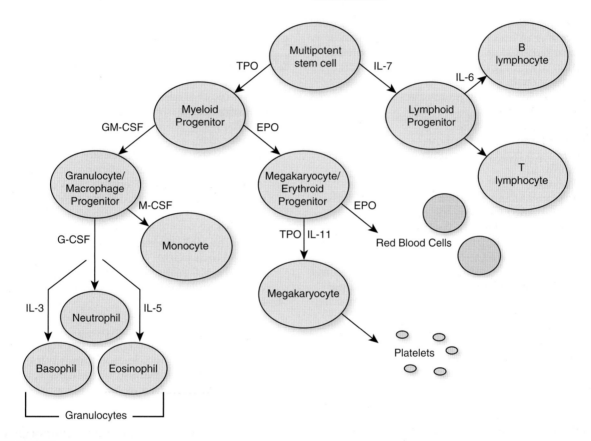

### Activity C MATCHING

**1.** e    **2.** c    **3.** d    **4.** b    **5.** a

### Activity D SHORT ANSWERS

1. Folic acid deficiency is caused by a low dietary intake of green leafy vegetables, liver, and citrus. It can also be caused by malabsorption from medication such as Dilantin or parasitic infections. Pernicious anemia is a deficiency of vitamin B12. Management of folic acid deficiency involves insuring compliance with dietary changes. Pernicious anemia is managed with monthly injections of vitamin B12.
2. The recommended action is to confirm the level with a repeat lab within 1 week, as well as educate the caregivers to decrease lead exposure. Refer the family to the local health department for investigation of the home for lead reduction with referrals for support services.
3. Color changes to the skin such as pallor, bruising, and flushing. Changes in mental status such as lethargy can also indicate a decrease in hemoglobin and decreased oxygenation of the brain.
4. Sickle cell anemia is most commonly seen in persons of African, Mediterranean, Middle Eastern, and Indian decent. In the United States, the number of infants born with sickle cell anemia is approximately 2,000, with 1 in 400 being African American.
5. Iron deficiency anemia occurs when the body does not have enough iron to produce Hgb, often related

to dietary issues. Children between the ages of 6 and 20 months, and those at the age of puberty are the periods when iron deficiency anemia is most prevalent.

## SECTION II: APPLYING YOUR KNOWLEDGE

### Activity E  CASE STUDY

1. The discussion should include:
   - How much milk does Jayda drink per day? (excessive cow's milk consumption, greater than 24 ounces a day, leads to an increased risk for iron deficiency anemia)
   - When did Jayda start on cow's milk? (cow's milk consumption before 12 months of age leads to an increased risk for iron deficiency anemia)
   - Was Jayda formula fed? If so, what type (low iron formula can lead to iron deficiency anemia); or breast fed? If so, did she receive iron supplementation (including eating iron-fortified cereal) after 6 months of age?
   - What are Jayda's food preferences and usual eating patterns?
   - Is she on any restricted diet?
   - Is she taking any medications? (certain medications, such as antacids can interfere with iron absorption)

2. The discussion should include:
   - Oral supplements or multivitamin formulas that have iron are often dark in color as the iron is pigmented. Teaching of Jayda's parents should include to precisely measure the amount of iron to be administered and to be sure to place the liquid behind the teeth since iron in liquid form can stain the teeth. Use of straw and brushing her teeth after administration may help. Another problem that frequently occurs is constipation from the iron. In some cases reduction of the amount of iron can resolve this problem, but stool softeners may be necessary to control painful or difficult to pass stools. Encourage parents to increase their child's fluid intake and maintain adequate consumption of fiber to assist in avoiding the development of constipation. Instruct the parents that stools may appear dark in color due to iron administration. Instruct parents to keep iron supplements and all medications in a safe place to avoid accidental overdose.
   - Providing juice enriched with vitamin C can help aid absorption of iron. Limit cow's milk intake to 24 ounces per day. Limit fast food consumption and encourage iron-rich foods such as red meats, tuna, salmon, eggs, tofu, enriched grains, dried beans and peas, dried fruits, leafy green vegetables, and iron-fortified breakfast cereals (iron from red meat is the easiest for the body to absorb). Encourage parents to provide nutritious snacks and finger foods that are developmentally appropriate for Jayda. Toddlers are often picky eaters. This often becomes a means

of control for the child, and parents should guard against getting involved in a power struggle with their child. Referring parents to a developmental nurse practitioner that can assist them in their approach to diet with their child may prove beneficial.
   - Encourage appropriate follow-up and review signs and symptoms of anemia.

3. The discussion should include:
   - Low socioeconomic status which can lead to a lack of adequate food supply
   - Recent immigration from a developing country
   - Culturally based food influences that lead to dietary imbalances
   - Child abuse or neglect leading to improper nutrition

## SECTION III: PRACTICING FOR NCLEX

### Activity F  NCLEX-STYLE QUESTIONS

1. **Answer: b**
   If neurological deficits are assessed, immediate reporting of the findings is necessary to begin treatment to prevent permanent damage.

2. **Answer: d**
   A convex shape of the fingernails termed 'spooning' can occur with iron deficiency anemia. Capillary refill in less than 2 seconds, pink palms and nail beds, and absence of bruising are normal findings.

3. **Answer: a**
   When the MCV is elevated, the RBCs are larger and referred to as macrocytic. The WBC count does not affect the MCV. The platelet count and Hgb are within normal ranges for a 7-year-old child.

4. **Answer: d**
   If the screening test result indicates the possibility of SCA or sickle cell trait, hemoglobin (Hgb) electrophoresis is performed promptly to confirm the diagnosis. While Hgb electrophoresis is the only definitive test for diagnosis of the disease, other laboratory testing that assists in the assessment of the disease include reticulocyte count (greatly elevated), peripheral blood smears (presence of sickle-shaped cells and target cells), and erythrocyte sedimentation rate (elevated).

5. **Answer: a**
   While iron from red meat is the easiest for the body to absorb, the nurse must limit fast food consumption from the drive thru as they are also high in fat, fillers, and sodium. The other statements are correct.

6. **Answer: b**
   The best response for a 7-year-old is to use distraction and involve him in the infusion process in a developmentally appropriate manner. A 7-year-old is old enough to assist with the dilution and mixing of the factor. Asking for help with the band-aid would be best for a younger child. Teens should be taught to administer their own factor infusions.

Telling him to be brave is not helpful and does not teach.

**7. Answer: a**
The priority is to emphasize to the parents that they precisely measure the amount of iron to be administered in order to avoid overdosing. The other instructions are accurate, but the priority is to emphasize precise measurement.

**8. Answer: c**
Symmetrical swelling of the hands and feet in the infant or toddler is termed dactylitis; aseptic infarction occurs in the metacarpals and metatarsals and is often the first vaso-occlusive event seen with sickle cell disease. Symmetrical swelling of the hands and feet are not typically seen with the other conditions listed.

**9. Answer: b**
This response answers the parent's questions. In the nonsevere form, the granulocyte count remains about 500, the platelets are over 20,000, and the reticulocyte count is over 1%. The other responses do not address what the parents are asking and would block therapeutic communication.

**10. Answer: c**
Laboratory evaluation will reveal decreased hemoglobin and hematocrit, decreased reticulocyte count, microcytosis and hypochromia, decreased serum iron and ferritin levels, and increase FEP level. The other findings do not point to iron deficiency anemia.

**11. Answer: d, c, a, b**
RATIONALE: The bone marrow releases a stem cell. Thrombopoietin acts on the cell to help turn it into a myeloid cell. Erythropoietin acts on the cell and it turns into a megakaryocyte. The megakaryocyte becomes an erythrocyte (red blood cell).

**12. Answers: a, c, d, e**
RATIONALE: This girl's erythrocyte count is below normal, which indicates she is anemic. The mean corpuscular hemoglobin concentration is below normal which indicates that her cells are hypochromic with a diluted amount of hemoglobin available. The mean corpuscular volume of the erythrocytes are decreased which indicates her cells are microcytic or smaller than normal.

**13. Answers: a, c, d, e**
RATIONALE: The caregivers should seek medical treatment promptly for any clinical manifestations associated with an infection. The child should receive prophylactic antibiotics. The child should be provided with immunization against the following organisms: *Streptococcus pneumoniae, Neisseria meningitidis,* and *Haemophilus influenzae* type B. The child should be taught techniques to reduce the transmission of infection. The child should wear his medic alert bracelet all the time.

**14. Answers: b, d**
RATIONALE: Iron supplements should not be mixed in milk because it reduces absorption.

Iron supplements may make the child constipated. All of the other options are correct.

**15. Answer: 36 milligrams**
RATIONALE: 47.3 pounds $\times$ 1 kg/2.2 pounds = 21.5 kg

21.5 kg $\times$ 5 mg/1 kg = 107.5 mg/day
107.5 mg/3 doses = 35.8333 mg/dose

when rounded to the nearest whole number = 36 mg

# CHAPTER 26

## SECTION I: ASSESSING YOUR UNDERSTANDING

### Activity A FILL IN THE BLANKS

1. Self-antigens
2. Chemotaxis
3. Bone marrow
4. Butterfly
5. Peanuts
6. Maculopapular
7. T-helper

### Activity B MATCHING

**1.** e    **2.** d    **3.** b    **4.** a    **5.** c

### Activity C SEQUENCING

$$\boxed{4} \rightarrow \boxed{2} \rightarrow \boxed{3} \rightarrow \boxed{1}$$

### Activity D SHORT ANSWERS

1. The complement system is a series of blood proteins whose action is to augment the work of antibodies by assisting with destruction of bacteria, production of inflammation, and regulation of immune reactions.
2. The enzyme-linked immunosorbant assay (ELISA) method detects only antibodies so results may remain negative for several weeks up to 6 months (false negative). A false-positive result may occur with autoimmune disease.
3. Delayed hypersensitivity reactions are mediated by T-cells rather than antibodies. An infant's skin test response is diminished most likely due to the infant's decreased ability to produce an inflammatory response.
4. If a child acquires HIV infection "vertically" this means the disease was transmitted perinatally, either in utero or through breast milk. Transmission of the disease "horizontally" refers to transmission by nonsterile, HIV-contaminated needles or through unprotected sexual contact; less frequent is contaminated blood product transmission.
5. Avascular necrosis is an adverse effect of long-term use or high dosages of corticosteroids, causing tissue damage to a joint due to lack of blood supply to the joint. Any child receiving long-term or high-dose corticosteroids as treatment, such as a child with

systemic lupus erythematosus (SLE), would be at an increased risk of developing this complication.

## SECTION II: JAI APPLYING YOUR KNOWLEDGE

### Activity E CASE STUDY

1. The discussion should include the following:
   A CBC, which may show a decreased hemoglobin and hematocrit, decreased platelet count, and low white blood cell count.
   Complement levels, C3 and C4, will also be decreased.
   Antinuclear antibody (ANA), though not specific to SLE, is usually positive in children with SLE.

2. The discussion should include the following:
   There is currently no single laboratory test that can confirm whether a person has lupus. In addition, since many of the symptoms with lupus come and go and tend to be vague, lupus can be difficult to diagnose. The physician will look at the entire medical history along with the results from the laboratory tests to determine whether your daughter has lupus.

3. The discussion should include the following:
   Education will focus on the importance of a healthy diet, regular exercise, and adequate sleep and rest. Teach the girl to apply sunscreen (minimum SPF 15) to her skin daily to prevent rashes resulting from photosensitivity. Administer NSAIDs, corticosteroids, and antimalarial agents as ordered. If the girl develops severe SLE or frequent flare-ups of symptoms she may require high-dose (pulse) corticosteroid therapy or medication with immunosuppressive drugs. Teach her to protect against cold weather by layering warm socks and wearing gloves when outdoors in the winter. If she is outside for extended periods during the winter months, educate her about the importance of inspecting her fingers and toes for discoloration. Ensure that yearly vision screening and ophthalmic examinations are performed in order to preserve visual function should any changes occur. Refer the girl and her family to support services such as the Lupus Alliance of America and the Lupus Foundation of America.

## SECTION III: PRACTICING FOR NCLEX

### Activity F NCLEX-STYLE QUESTIONS

1. **Answer: c**
   Children with Wiskott–Aldrich syndrome should not be given rectal suppositories or temperatures since these children are at a high risk for bleeding. Tub baths are not contraindicated. Pacifiers are not contraindicated in Wiskott–Aldrich but should be kept as sanitary as possible to avoid oral infections.

2. **Answer: d**
   Premedication with diphenhydramine or acetaminophen may be indicted in children who have never received intravenous immunoglobulin (IVIG), have not had an infusion in over 8 weeks, have had a recent bacterial infection, or have history of serious infusion-related adverse reactions. The nurse should first premedicate, and then obtain a baseline physical assessment. Once the infusion begins, the nurse should continually assess for adverse reaction.

3. **Answer: c**
   The EpiPen Jr.® should be jabbed into the outer thigh, as this is a larger muscle, at a 90 degree angle, not into the upper arm. The other statements are correct.

4. **Answer: d**
   The ELISA test will be positive in infants of HIV-infected mothers because of transplacentally received antibodies. These antibodies may persist and remain detectable up to 24 months of age, making the ELISA test less accurate in detecting true HIV infection in infants and toddlers than the polymerase chain reaction (PCR). The PCR test is positive in infected infants over the age of 1 month. The erythrocyte sedimentation rate would be ordered for an immune disorder initial workup or ongoing monitoring of autoimmune disease. Immunoglobulin electrophoresis would be ordered to test for immune deficiency and autoimmune disorders.

5. **Answer: a**
   Older children and adolescents with allergic reactions to fish, shellfish, and nuts usually continue to have that concern as a life-long problem. The other statements are correct.

6. **Answer: d**
   Alopecia and the characteristic malar rash (butterfly rash) on the face are common clinical manifestations of SLE. Rhinorrhea, wheezing, and an enlarged spleen are not hallmark manifestations of SLE. Petechiae and purpura are more commonly associated with hematological disorders, not SLE.

7. **Answer: b**
   The parents must understand that their child cannot consume any part of an egg in any form. The other statements are accurate.

8. **Answer: b**
   Lip edema, urticaria, stridor, and tachycardia are common clinical manifestations of anaphylaxis.

9. **Answer: c**
   The nurse should instruct children and their families to avoid foods with a known cross-reactivity to latex, such as bananas.

10. **Answer: a**
    Polyarticular juvenile idiopathic arthritis is defined by the involvement of five or more joints, frequently the small joints, and affects the body symmetrically. Pauciarticular juvenile idiopathic arthritis is defined by the involvement of four or fewer joints. Systemic juvenile idiopathic arthritis presents with fever and rash in addition to join involvement at the time of diagnosis. The child with juvenile idiopathic arthritis is not at greater risk for anaphylaxis.

**11. Answers: b, c, d, e**
RATIONALE: The following are common signs and symptoms of anaphylaxis: tongue edema, urticaria, nausea, vomiting, and syncope. Typically, the child who has developed anaphylaxis will be tachycardic.

**12. Answers: a, e**
RATIONALE: Intravenous immune globulin (IVIG) should be given only intravenously and should not be given as an intramuscular injection. IVIG cannot be mixed with other medications. The nurse should closely monitor the child's vital signs during the infusion of the IVIG. The child may require an antipyretic and/ or an antihistamine during infusion to help with fever and chills.

**13. Answers: b, c, e**
RATIONALE: The following children may have a primary immunodeficiency: a child with a persistent case of oral candidiasis, a child who has been diagnosed with pneumonia at least twice during the previous year, and a child who has taken antibiotics for 2 months or longer with little effect.

**14. Answers: c, d**
RATIONALE: If a child has had a severe reaction to penicillin in the past, then this child should not receive penicillin or cephalosporins. Desensitization involves administration of increasingly larger doses of penicillin in an intensive care setting.

**15. Answers: a, c**
RATIONALE: The child diagnosed with juvenile idiopathic arthritis should not take the oral form of methotrexate with dairy products. The approximate time to benefit from methotrexate is typically 3 to 6 weeks. The child will need blood tests to determine renal and liver function during treatment. Children with juvenile idiopathic arthritis usually find swimming to be a useful exercise for them because it helps maintain joint mobility without placing pressure on the joints. Sleep may be promoted by a warm bath at bedtime.

# CHAPTER 27

## SECTION I: ASSESSING YOUR UNDERSTANDING

### Activity A FILL IN THE BLANKS

1. Langerhans
2. Exophthalmos
3. Polyuria
4. Tetany
5. Kussmaul
6. Deficiency
7. Hyperthyroidism

### Activity B LABELING

Areas on the body corresponding with insulin injection sites.

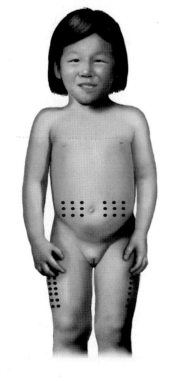 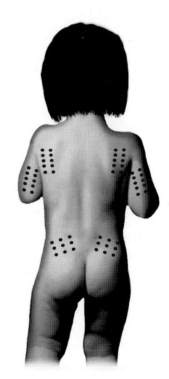

## Activity C MATCHING

**1.** e    **2.** c    **3.** b    **4.** a    **5.** d

## Activity D SEQUENCING

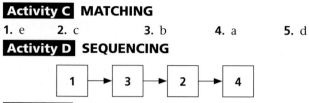

## Activity E SHORT ANSWERS

1. Diet should be low in fats and concentrated carbohydrates. Lists of foods high in carbohydrates, protein, and fat should be provided. The parents need to understand the need to plan for periods of rapid growth, travel, school parties, and holidays. Referring the parents to a nutritionist with diabetes expertise will be helpful. There should be a plan for three meals and two snacks per day in order to maintain blood glucose levels. Regular exercise should be encouraged, as well as participation in age-appropriate sports. The parents should be reminded of the importance of monitoring the insulin dose, food and fluid intake, and hypoglycemic reactions when exercising.

2.

| Hypothyroidism | Hyperthyroidism |
| --- | --- |
| Nervousness/anxiety | Tiredness/fatigue |
| Diarrhea | Constipation |
| Heat intolerance | Cold intolerance |
| Weight loss | Weight gain |
| Smooth, velvet-like skin | Dry, thick skin; edema on the face, eyes, and hands |
| | Decreased growth |

3. Nursing implications when teaching, discussing, and caring for children with diabetes mellitus (DM) are as follows:

    **a.** Infants and toddlers: Attempt to achieve consistent dietary intake. Give the toddler foods to choose from. Help the toddler to find and use a word or phrase to describe feelings when hypoglycemic symptoms occur. Establish rituals/routines with home management.

    **b.** Preschoolers: Use simple explanations and play therapy when instructing or preparing for a procedure or situation related to the disorder.

    **c.** School age: Use concise and concrete terms when instructing. Allow children to proceed at their own rate. Assist the family to incorporate the testing and injections into the school day and plan for field trips. Use the school nurse's assistance and help with the school plan.

    **d.** Adolescents: Care can be slowly turned over to an adolescent with minor supervision from family. Watch for depression in this age group.

4. *Healthy People 2020* recommends screening all children periodically to identify early signs of overweight or obesity based on CDC guidelines. In addition, families should receive education regarding appropriate diet and exercise early during the toddler years in an attempt to prevent obesity, thus decreasing the likelihood of diabetes.

5. The nurse should instruct the family to report headaches, rapid weight gain, increased thirst or urination, or painful hip or knee joints as possible adverse reactions.

## SECTION II: APPLYING YOUR KNOWLEDGE

### Activity F CASE STUDY

1. The discussion should include the following:
    In the past, DM type 2 occurred in adults with only a small percentage of cases seen in childhood. Since the early 1990s, the incidence has increased significantly in children. Many of these children have a relative with type 2 DM or they have other risk factors such as being overweight, African American, Hispanic American, Asian American, or Native American heritage.
    Type 2 DM begins when the pancreas usually produces insulin but the body develops a resistance to insulin or no longer uses the insulin properly. As the need for insulin rises, the pancreas gradually loses its ability to produce sufficient amounts of insulin to regulate blood sugar. Eventually, insulin production decreases with the result similar to type 1 DM.

2. The discussion should include the following:
    Nursing management will focus on regulating glucose control, monitoring for complications, and educating and supporting the child and family. Other important interventions involve nutritional guidelines and exercise protocols.

3. The discussion should include challenges related to educating children with diabetes:
    - Children lack the maturity to understand the long-term consequences of this serious chronic illness.
    - Children do not want to be different from their peers and having to make life style changes may result in anger or depression.
    - Families may demonstrate unhealthy behaviors making it difficult for the child to initiate change because of the lack of supervision or role modeling.
    - Family dynamics are impacted because management of diabetes must occur all day, every day.

## SECTION III: PRACTICING FOR NCLEX

### Activity G NCLEX-STYLE QUESTIONS

1. **Answer: d**
    Administering intravenous calcium gluconate, as ordered, will restore normal calcium and phosphate levels as well as relieve severe tetany. Ensuring patency of the IV site to prevent tissue damage due to extravasation or cardiac arrhythmias is an intervention for any child with an IV, and monitoring fluid intake and urinary calcium output are

secondary interventions. Providing administration of calcium and vitamin D is an intervention for nonacute symptoms.

2. **Answer: b**
Observing pubic hair and hirsutism in a pre-schooler indicates congenital adrenal hyperplasia. Auscultation revealing an irregular heartbeat and palpation eliciting pain due to constipation may be signs of hyperparathyroidism. Observing hyper-pigmentation of the skin would suggest Addison's disease.

3. **Answer: a**
This child may have syndrome of inappropriate antidiuretic hormone (SIADH). Priority interven-tion for this child is to notify the physician of the neurologic findings. Remaining interventions will be to restore fluid balance with IV sodium chloride to correct hyponatremia, set up safety precautions to prevent injury due to altered level of conscious-ness, and monitor fluid intake, urine volume, and specific gravity.

4. **Answer: c**
Monitoring blood glucose levels during this study is the priority task along with observing for signs of hypoglycemia since insulin is given during the test to stimulate release of growth hormone. Pro-viding a wet washcloth would be more appropriate for a child who is on therapeutic fluid restriction, such as with SIADH. Monitoring intake and out-put would not be necessary for this test but would be appropriate for a child with diabetes insipidus. While it is important to educate the family about this test, it is not the priority task.

5. **Answer: b**
Observation of an enlarged tongue along with an enlarged posterior fontanel and feeding difficulties are key findings for congenital hypothyroidism. The mother would report constipation rather than diarrhea. Auscultation would reveal bradycardia rather than tachycardia, and palpation would reveal cool, dry, and scaly skin.

6. **Answer: a**
Observation of acanthosis nigricans in addition to the obesity and amenorrhea is a further indication of polycystic ovary syndrome. Complaint of blurred vision and headaches are signs and symp-toms of DM. Auscultation revealing an increased respiratory rate points to diabetes insipidus. Palpa-tion revealing hypertrophy and weakness is typical of hypothyroidism.

7. **Answer: a**
A history of rapid weight gain and long-term corti-costeroid therapy suggests this child may have Cushing's disease, which could be confirmed using an adrenal suppression test. A round, child-like face is common to both Cushing's and growth hormone deficiency. Observing high weight to height ratio and delayed dentition are findings with growth hormone deficiency.

8. **Answer: c**
The primary nursing diagnosis would be deficient fluid volume related to electrolyte imbalance. It is important to increase the child's hydration to minimize renal calculi formation. Disturbed body image related to hormone dysfunction is a diagno-sis for growth hormone deficiency. Imbalanced nutrition: more than body requirements would be important for a child with DM. Deficient knowl-edge related to treatment of the disease is appro-priate for hyperparathyroidism, but it is not a priority diagnosis.

9. **Answer: b**
Instructing child to rotate injection sites to decrease scar formation is important, but does not focus on managing glucose levels. Teaching the child and family to eat a balanced diet, encourag-ing the child to maintain the proper injection schedule, and promoting a higher level of exercise all focus on regulating glucose control.

10. **Answer: d**
Side effects of hypothyroidism are restlessness, inability to sleep, or irritability and should be reported to the physician. Educating how to recog-nize vitamin D toxicity is necessary for a child with hypoparathyroidism. Teaching parents how to maintain fluid intake regimens is important for a child with diabetes insipidus. Teaching the child and parents to administer methimazole with meals is necessary for hyperthyroidism.

11. **Answer: 393 micrograms**
RATIONALE: The child weighs 72 pounds and 2.2 pounds = 1 kg.
72 pounds × 1 kg/2.2 pounds = 32.727 kg
32.727 kg × 12 µg/1 kg = 392.727 µg
rounded to the nearest whole number = 393 µg

12. **Answers: b, d, a, c**
RATIONALE: Lispro is a rapid-acting insulin. Humu-lin R is a short-acting insulin. Humulin N is an intermediate-acting insulin. Lantus is a long-acting insulin.

13. **Answer: 0.075 milligram per day**
RATIONALE: The child weighs 58 pounds and 2.2 pounds = 1 kg.
58 pounds × 1 kg/2.2 pounds = 26.3636 kg of body weight
26.3636 × 0.2 mg/1 kg = 0.5273 mg of growth hormone per week
0.5273 mg/ week × 1 week/ 7 days = 0.0753 mg/ day

14. **Answers: a, c**
RATIONALE: The child has delayed puberty if any of the following is true: the female has not developed breasts by the age of 13; the male has had no tes-ticular enlargement by the age of 14. In females, pubic hair should appear before the age of 14. In males, pubic hair should appear before the age of 15 and scrotal changes by the age of 14.

**15. Answers: a, b, c**
    RATIONALE: The following are signs and symptoms related to the development of thyroid storm: fever, diaphoresis, and tachycardia. Children who are patients are also typically restless and irritable.

# CHAPTER 28

## SECTION I: ASSESSING YOUR UNDERSTANDING

### Activity A  FILL IN THE BLANKS

1. Mediastinal
2. Leukocoria
3. Sepsis
4. Prevention
5. Limb-salvage
6. Leukemia
7. Clinical trial

### Activity B  LABELING

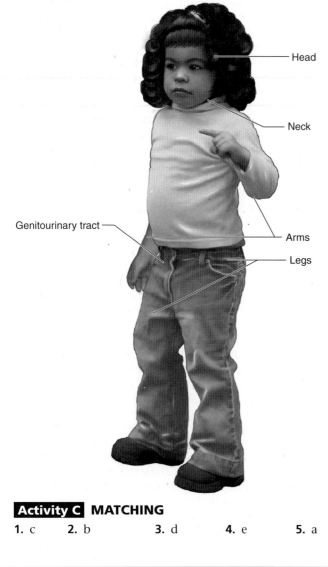

Head

Neck

Genitourinary tract

Arms

Legs

### Activity C  MATCHING

1. c    2. b    3. d    4. e    5. a

### Activity D  SEQUENCING

4 → 1 → 2 → 5 → 3

### Activity E  SHORT ANSWERS

1. Nine locations with presenting signs and symptoms from Table 28.6.
2. Answer can include any of the following types of drugs. Refer to Drug Guide 28.1 for more information on specific drugs, action/indications, and nursing implications.
    Antitumor antibiotics, antimetabolites, antimicrotubulars, mitotic inhibitors, topoisomerase inhibitors, corticosteroids, colony-stimulating factors, interleukins, tumor necrosis factor (protein cytokine), monoclonal anti-bodies, interferons, allopurinol, antibiotics (oral, parenteral), antiemetics, antifungal agents, immunosuppressant drugs, mesna, methotrexate antidote.
3. Chest X-ray, computed tomography (CT), magnetic resonance imaging (MRI), bone scan, and ultrasound. Refer to Common Laboratory and Diagnostic Tests 28.1.
4. There are a number of differences between childhood and adult cancer: Most common sites for childhood cancer are blood, lymph, brain, bone, kidney, and muscle. The most common sites for adult cancer are breast, lung, prostate, bowel, and bladder; Environmental factors have a strong influence on the cause of adult cancers versus minimal influence on childhood cancer; and childhood cancers are typically very responsive to treatment if diagnosed early enough, whereas adult cancers tend to be less responsive to treatment. Additional comparisons of childhood and adult cancer can be found in Comparison Chart 28.1.
5. Chemotherapy drugs are either cell cycle-specific or cell cycle-nonspecific. This is why protocols for chemotherapy treatment often use a combination of drugs to destroy cancer cells during various phases of the cell cycle.

## SECTION II: APPLYING YOUR KNOWLEDGE

### Activity F  CASE STUDY

1. The discussion should include the following:
    The child, who has a low neutrophil count (neutropenia), is at a significant risk for developing a serious infection since neutrophils are the primary infection fighting cells.
    Neutropenia precautions need to be instituted for this child. Precautions related to neutropenia generally include:
    • Maintain hand hygiene prior to and following each child contact
    • Place child in private room
    • Monitor vital signs every 4 hours
    • Assess for signs and symptoms of infection at least every 8 hours

- Avoid rectal suppositories, enemas or examinations, urinary catheterization, and invasive procedures
- Restrict visitors with fever, cough, or other signs/symptoms of infection
- No raw fruits or vegetables, no fresh flowers or live plants in room
- Place mask on the child when transporting outside of room
- Maintain dental care with soft toothbrush if platelet count is adequate

Family and visitors must be educated regarding the need to restrict the child from contact with known infectious exposures and the importance of practicing meticulous hand hygiene. The family should also be educated on the importance of proper nutrition, hydration, and rest for the child.

2. The discussion should include the following:

Teach the family to monitor for fever at home and report temperature elevations to the oncologist immediately (Seek medical care if temperature is 38.3°C (101°F) or greater). Family and visitors must practice meticulous hygiene. The child should avoid any known ill contacts, especially persons with chickenpox. If exposed to chickenpox notify the physician immediately. He should avoid crowded areas, and should not receive live vaccines. The child's temperature should not be taken rectally nor should he be given any medication rectally. Prophylactic antibiotics should be given as ordered by the physician.

3. The discussion should include the following:

Children desire to be normal and in order to maintain appropriate growth and development; parents need to promote this normalization. The child should attend school whenever he is well enough and his white blood cell counts are not dangerously low. Other activities that he enjoys should be promoted if medically appropriate. Encourage him to play with his friends while remembering to avoid ill contacts. Special camps are available for children with cancer and offer the child an opportunity to experience a variety of activities safely and to spend time with many other youngsters who are experiencing the same challenges.

# SECTION III: PRACTICING FOR NCLEX
## Activity G NCLEX-STYLE QUESTIONS

1. **Answer: c**
The parents should seek medical care immediately if the child has a temperature of 101°F or greater. This is because many chemotherapeutic drugs cause bone marrow suppression; the parents must be directed to take action at the first sign of infection in order to prevent overwhelming sepsis. The appearance of earache, stiff neck, sore throat, blisters, ulcers, or rashes, or difficulty or pain when swallowing are reasons to seek medical care, but are not as grave as the risk of infection.

2. **Answers: b, c, d**
Observation revealing a thick, yellow discharge is typical of infectious conjunctivitis, not retinoblastoma. Headaches and hyphema, a collection of blood in the anterior chamber of the eye, are associated with retinoblastoma as is leukocoria, "cat's eye reflex." Most children with retinoblastoma are diagnosed by 3 years of age.

3. **Answer: a**
The priority intervention is to monitor for increases in intracranial pressure because brain tumors may block cerebral fluid flow or cause edema in the brain. A change in the level of consciousness is just one of several subtle changes that can occur indicating a change in intracranial pressure. Lower priority interventions include providing a tour of the ICU to prepare the child and parents for after the surgery, and educating the child and parents about shunts.

4. **Answer: b**
Ewing's sarcoma may result in swelling and erythema at the tumor site. Common sites are chest wall, pelvis, vertebrae, and long bone diaphyses. Dull bone pain in the proximal tibia is indicative of osteosarcoma. Persistent pain after an ankle injury is not indicative of Ewing's sarcoma. An asymptomatic mass on the upper back suggests rhabdomyosarcoma.

5. **Answers: a, c, d, e**
Answer b would not be part of the teaching plan. It would be more accurate and appropriate for the nurse to stress that testicular cancer is one of the most curable cancers if diagnosed early. Self-examination is an excellent way to screen for the disease. Girls should know that they can take responsibility for their own sexual health by getting a Papanicolaou smear. All the children should understand that early intercourse, sexually transmitted disease (STDs), and multiple sex partners are risk factors for reproductive cancer. Information should be provided so the teen girls can discuss the benefits of receiving the human papilloma virus vaccine since many cervical cancers are attributed to human papillomavirus.

6. **Answer: c**
Giving medications as ordered using the least invasive route is a postsurgery intervention focused on providing atraumatic care and is appropriate for this child. Since the child has a stage I tumor, it can be treated by surgical removal, and does not require chemotherapy or radiation therapy. Applying aloe vera lotion is good skin care following radiation therapy. Administering antiemetics and maintaining isolation are interventions used to treat side effects of chemotherapy.

7. **Answer: d**
Increased heart rate, murmur, and respiratory distress are symptoms of hyperleukocytosis (high white blood cell count) which is associated with leukemia. Increased heart rate and blood pressure

are indicative of tumor lysis syndrome, which may occur with acute lymphoblastic leukemia, lymphoma, and neuroblastoma. Wheezing and diminished breath sounds are signs of superior vena cava syndrome related to non-Hodgkin's lymphoma or neuroblastoma. Respiratory distress and poor perfusion are symptoms of massive hepatomegaly which is caused by a neuroblastoma filling a large portion of the abdominal cavity.

**8. Answer: a**
Coupled with the mother's complaints, observation of nystagmus and head tilt would suggest the child may have a brain tumor. Elevated blood pressure of 120/80 might be indicative of Wilm's tumor. Fever and headaches are common symptoms of acute lymphoblastic leukemia. A cough and labored breathing points to rhabdomyosarcoma near the child's airway.

**9. Answer: b**
Along with the symptoms reported by the mother, the fact that the child has Beckwith–Wiedemann syndrome suggests that the child could have a Wilm's tumor. Down syndrome would point to leukemia or brain tumor. Schwachman syndrome would suggest leukemia. A family history of neurofibromatosis is a risk factor for brain tumor, rhabdomyosarcoma, or acute myelogenous leukemia.

**10. Answer: c**
It would not be necessary for the nurse to inform the parents about postoperative care since this is not a treatment method for the disease. The treatment of choice for Hodgkin's disease is chemotherapy, but radiation therapy may be necessary; however, discussing the treatment methods may be overwhelming at this time. Upon first learning the diagnosis, it is most helpful for the nurse to explain that staging refers to the spread of the disease (stages I through IV, see Table 28.3); and that A means the child is asymptomatic, while B means that symptoms are present.

**11. Answers: a, c, d, e**
RATIONALE: Common adverse effects of chemotherapeutic drugs are: immunosuppression, alopecia, hearing changes, and nausea. Another common adverse effect is microdontia, not enlarged teeth.

**12. Answer: 0.99**
RATIONALE: Square root of (height [cm] × weight [kg] divided by 3,600) = BSA
The child is 130 cm tall and weighs 27 kg: $130 \times 27 = 3{,}510$; $3{,}510/3{,}600 = 0.975$; and the square root of 0.975 is 0.9874. The BSA would be 0.987, when rounded to the hundredths place = 0.99.

**13. Answer: d, b, c, a**
RATIONALE: During induction, the child receives oral steroids and IV vincristine. During consolidation, the child receives high doses of methotrexate and mercaptopurine. During maintenance, the child receives low doses of methotrexate and mercaptopurine. During central nervous system prophylaxis, the child receives intrathecal chemotherapy.

**14. Answer: 3,450**
RATIONALE: (Bands + segs/100) × WBC = ANC
$14 + 9 = 23\% = 23/100 = 0.23$
$0.23 \times 15{,}000 = 3{,}450$

**15. Answers: a, b**
RATIONALE: The child in neutropenic precautions should be placed in a private room. Prior to transportation to other areas of the hospital, the nurse should place a mask on the child before she leaves her room. The nurse should monitor the child's vital signs at least every 4 hours. The nurse should carefully assess for signs and symptoms of infection at least every 8 hours. The nurse should perform hand hygiene before and after contact with each child.

# CHAPTER 29

## SECTION I: ASSESSING YOUR UNDERSTANDING

### Activity A  FILL IN THE BLANKS
1. Alleles
2. Consanguinity
3. Phenotype
4. Heterozygous
5. Nondisjunction
6. Genome
7. Chromosome

### Activity B  MATCHING
1. d     2. e          3. a          4. c          5. b

### Activity C  SHORT ANSWERS
1. Complications of Down syndrome include cardiac defects, hearing or vision impairment, developmental delays, mental retardation, gastrointestinal disorders, recurrent infections, atlantoaxial instability, thyroid disease, and sleep apnea.
2. Building a relationship of trust, empathizing with and understanding the family's stresses and emotions, rejecting personal bias, encouraging open discussion.
3. Phenylketonuria excretions exhibit a mousy or musty order caused by a deficiency of the liver enzyme that processes phenylalanine; children with maple syrup urine disease have a maple syrup odor associated with a deficiency of the enzyme that metabolizes leucine, isoleucine, and valine; children with tyrosinemia have excretions with a rancid butter or cabbage like odor as a result of a deficiency of the enzyme that metabolizes tyrosine; and excretions have a rotting fish odor with the disorder trimethylaminuria, resulting from the body's inability to normally produce flavin (which breaks down trimethylamine).
4. Trisomy 21, also known as Down syndrome, occurs in 1 in 800 births across all maternal ages and socioeconomic levels, and 75% of trisomy 21 conceptions result in spontaneous abortion. It is the

most common genetic defect that is linked with intellectual disability. The highest incidence of the disorder occurs in mothers who are over 35 years of age, with the likelihood of having a trisomy 21 baby 1 in 400 at the age of 35, 1 in 100 at the age of 40, 1 in 35 at the age of 45, and 1 in 12 at the age of 49.

5. The infant with trisomy 13 will likely display a microcephalic head with wide sagittal suture and fontanels. Other physical features include malformed ears, small eyes, extra digits, cleft lip and palate, and severe hypotonia. Severe intellectual disability will most likely be exhibited as the child ages.

## SECTION II: APPLYING YOUR KNOWLEDGE
### Activity D CASE STUDY

1. The discussion should include the following:
   Newborn screening is done to detect disorders before symptoms develop. Recent developments in screening techniques allow many metabolic disorders or inborn errors of metabolism to be detected early. Chloe's test results tell us that additional testing is needed to rule out a false positive or confirm the diagnosis. Most inborn errors of metabolism presenting in the neonatal period are lethal or can result in serious complications such as mental retardation if specific treatment is not initiated immediately. This is why it is so important that you came in today for additional testing.

2. The discussion should include the following:
   In fatty acid oxidation disorders (such as medium-chain acyl-CoA dehydrogenase deficiency) the goal is to prevent or avoid prolonged fasts and to provide frequent feedings. Special consideration during illness is very important. If Chloe is unable to tolerate food she needs to be seen by a physician immediately; intravenous dextrose may be required. Supplementation with specific vitamins may also be important in the treatment and a dietician and the physician will work with you. Strict adherence to frequent meals is necessary to prevent complications from arising.
   Nursing management will focus on education and support for the family and caregivers. Ensure they have thorough knowledge about medium chain acyl-CoA dehydrogenase deficiency and its management. Refer the family to a dietician and other appropriate resources, including support groups. Monitor the developmental progress of Chloe and initiate therapies if concern arises.

## SECTION III: PRACTICING FOR NCLEX
### Activity E NCLEX-STYLE QUESTIONS

1. **Answers: b, c, e**
   Numerous café au lait spots on the trunk of the child, a slightly larger head size due to abnormal development of the skull, and abnormal curvature of the spine (especially scoliosis) are clinical signs of this disorder. A first-degree relative rather than a second-degree relative having had neurofibromatosis is clinical sign of the disorder, and freckles in the child's axilla and groin, not the lower extremities, are symptoms of the disorder. Two or more clinical signs and symptoms of the disorder must be present for a diagnosis to be made.

2. **Answers: b, c, d, e**
   Although children with Marfan syndrome have a number of physical problems, respiratory conditions are not one of them, so it would not be appropriate to arrange in home respiratory therapy. The other interventions are needed for children with Marfan syndrome, because they do have ophthalmologic, orthopedic, and cardiac problems.

3. **Answer: d**
   Angelman syndrome is characterized by jerky ataxic movements, similar to a puppet's gait. Hypotonicity is a symptom of Angelman syndrome as well as Prader Willi syndrome, and Cri du chat. Cleft palate is a symptom of velo-cardio-facial/DiGeorge syndrome.

4. **Answer: b**
   This disorder is not X-linked. Either father or mother can pass the gene along regardless of whether their mate has the gene or not. The only way that an autosomal dominant gene is not expressed is if it does not exist. If only one of the parents has the gene, then there is a 50% chance it will be passed on to the child.

5. **Answer: b**
   The priority intervention is to assess the family's ability to learn about the disorder. The family needs time to adjust to the diagnosis and be ready to learn for teaching to be effective. Screening to determine current level of functioning, explaining the care required due to the disorder, and educating the family about available resources are interventions that can be taken once the family is ready.

6. **Answer: c**
   Children with phenylketonuria will have a musty odor to their urine, as well as an eczema-like rash, irritability, and vomiting. Increased reflex action and seizures are typical of maple sugar urine disease. Signs of jaundice, diarrhea, and vomiting are typical of galactosemia. Seizures are a sign of biotinidase deficiency or maple sugar urine disease.

7. **Answer: d**
   The nurse would likely find records of corrective surgery for anal atresia because it is a symptom of VATER association. The nurse may observe that the child has a hearing deficit, underdeveloped labia, and a coloboma, along with heart disease, retarded growth and development, and choanal atresia if the child had CHARGE syndrome. See Table 29.6 for more information.

8. **Answer: a**
   A major anomaly is an anomaly or malformation that creates significant medical problems and

requires surgical or medical management. Café au lait macules are a major anomaly. Polydactyly, or extra digits, syndactyly, or webbed digits, and protruding ears are minor anomalies. Minor anomalies are features that vary from those that are most commonly seen in the general population but do not cause an increase in morbidity in and of themselves.

9. **Answer: b**

Galactosemia is a deficiency in the liver enzyme needed to convert galactose into glucose. This means the child will have to eliminate milk and dairy products from her diet for life. Adhering to a low phenylalanine diet is an intervention for phenylketonuria. Eating frequent meals and never fasting is an intervention for medium-chain acyl-CoA dehydrogenase deficiency. Maple sugar urine disease requires a low-protein diet and supplementation with thiamine.

10. **Answer: c**

Children with Sturge–Weber syndrome will have a facial nevus, or port wine stain, most often seen on the forehead and one eye. While the child may experience seizures, retardation, and behavior problems, they are not definitive findings.

11. **Answers: a, b, d**

RATIONALE: The following are risk factors for genetic disorders: oligohydramnios, paternal age over 50, a family history of genetic disorders, positive alpha-fetoprotein test, and multiple births.

12. **Answers: c, d, e**

RATIONALE: Boys with Klinefelter syndrome may have learning disabilities, underdeveloped testes, and gynecomastia. Typically, they have long legs and short torsos and are taller than their peers.

13. **Answers: c, d, e**

RATIONALE: Babies born with trisomy 18 may have been born with a congenital cardiac defect, webbing between digits and low-set ears. Microcephaly and the development of extra digits are not associated with trisomy 18.

14. **Answers: a, b, c**

RATIONALE: Monogenic disorders (caused by a single gene that is defective) include autosomal dominant, autosomal recessive, X-linked dominant and X-linked recessive disorders. Mitochondrial inheritance and genomic imprinting are considered multifactorial disorders (caused by multiple gene and environmental factors).

15. **Answers: b, c, d, e**

RATIONALE: The following people should receive genetic counseling: paternal age over 50, the presence of consanguinity, parents of African descent, and those parents who have a child at home who was born blind or deaf. A mother-to-be over the age of 35 may also benefit from genetic counseling.

# CHAPTER 30

## SECTION I: ASSESSING YOUR UNDERSTANDING

### Activity A FILL IN THE BLANKS

1. Bowel
2. 6
3. Dyslexia
4. Stocking
5. Neglect
6. Münchausen syndrome by proxy (MSbP)
7. Autism spectrum disorder (ASD)

### Activity B

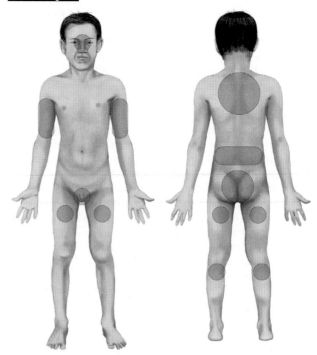

Common nonaccidental injury sites

### Activity C MATCHING

1. b    2. a     3. d     4. e     5. c

### Activity D SHORT ANSWERS

1. Behavior management techniques include the following:
   - Set limits with the child, holding him responsible for his behavior
   - Do not argue, bargain, or negotiate about the limits once established
   - Provide consistent caregivers (unlicensed assistive personnel and nurses for the hospitalized child) and establish the child's daily routine
   - Use a low-pitched voice and remain calm
   - Redirect the child's attention when needed

- Ignore inappropriate behaviors
- Praise the child's self-control efforts and other accomplishments
- Utilize restraints only when absolutely necessary

2. Building a relationship of trust, empathizing with and understanding the family's stresses and emotions, rejecting personal bias, encouraging open discussion.

3. Generalized anxiety disorder (GAD) is characterized by unrealistic concerns over past behavior, future events, and personal competency. Social phobia may result in which the child or teen demonstrates a persistent fear of formal speaking, eating in front of others, using public restrooms, or speaking to authorities.

4. Obtain a health history from the adolescent and his parents separately. Assess for a history of recent changes in behavior, alterations in school, changes in peer relationships, withdrawal from previously enjoyed activities, sleep disturbances, changes in eating behaviors, and an increase in accidents or sexual promiscuity. Ask about potential stressors, conflicts with parents or peers, school concerns, dating issues, and abusive events. If possible utilize a standardized depression screening questionnaire.

   Assess for history of weight loss. Observe for apparent apathy. Inspect the entire body surface for the presence of self-inflicted injuries which may or may not be present.

   Assess for risk factors of suicide including a change in school performance, changes in sleep or appetite, disinterest in former preferred activities, expressing feeling of hopelessness, depression, thoughts of suicide, and any previous attempts at suicide.

5. The most common classifications of medication used for the management of ADHD include psychostimulants, nonstimulant norepinephrine reuptake inhibitors and/or alpha-agonist antihypertensive agents. The goal of treatment with medication is to help increase the child's ability to pay attention and to increase the ability to control impulsive behavior. Medications for ADHD do not cure the disorder.

# SECTION II: APPLYING YOUR KNOWLEDGE
## Activity E  CASE STUDY

1. The discussion should include the following:
   ASD is a developmental disorder that has its onset in infancy or early childhood. Autistic behaviors may be first noted in infancy as developmental delays or between 12 months and 36 months when the child loses previously acquired skills. Children with ASD demonstrate impairments in social interactions and communication. The exact cause of autism is unknown; it is believed to be linked to genetics, brain abnormali-

ties, altered chemistry, a virus, or toxic chemicals. The spectrum of the disorder ranges from mild to severe.

2. The discussion should include the following:
   Warning signs of autism that may be seen with infants and toddlers include: no babbling and no pointing or using gestures by 12 months of age; by 16 months of age the child is not using single words and by 24 months of age is not using any two-word phrases; and the child exhibits loss of language or social skills at any age.

# SECTION III: PRACTICING FOR NCLEX
## Activity F  NCLEX-STYLE QUESTIONS

1. **Answer: b**
   The nurse should pay particular attention to reports of a child spending hours in a repetitive activity, such as lining up cars rather than playing with them. Most 3-year-olds are very busy and would rather play than sit on a parent's lap. The other statements are not outside the range of normal and do not warrant further investigation.

2. **Answer: c**
   The nurse should encourage the family to explore with their physician the option of one of the newer extended-release or once daily attention deficit/hyperactivity disorder medications. The other statements are not helpful and do not address the mother's or boy's concerns.

3. **Answer: b**
   Sudden, rapid, stereotypical sounds are a hallmark finding with Tourette's syndrome. Toe walking and unusual behaviors such as hand-flapping and spinning are indicative of ASD. Lack of eye contact is associated with ASD but is also noted in children without a mental health disorder.

4. **Answer: c**
   The nurse should emphasize the importance of rigid unchanging routines as children with ASD often act out when their routine changes. The other statements would not warrant additional referral or follow-up.

5. **Answer: b**
   An IQ of 35 to 50 is classified as moderate. An IQ of 50 to 70 is classified as mild. An IQ of 20 to 35 is classified as severe, and an IQ less than 20 is considered profound.

6. **Answer: b**
   It is important to continue the usual routine of the hospitalized child, particularly of children with intellectual disability. By asking an open-ended question about a typical day, the nurse can identify the routine activities that can potentially be duplicated in the hospital. Telling the girl she will be going home soon or asking about art supplies does not address her concerns. Asking whether she has talked to her parents is unhelpful at this time.

**7. Answer: a**

The nurse should be aware that rapid nutritional replacement in the severely malnourished can lead to refeeding syndrome. Refeeding syndrome is characterized by cardiovascular, hematologic, and neurologic complications such as cardiac arrhythmias, confusion, and seizures. Orthostatic hypotension, hypertension, and irregular and decreased pulses are complications of anorexia but do not characterize refeeding syndrome.

**8. Answer: a**

The nurse should be sure to carefully assess the mouth and oropharynx for eroded dental enamel, red gums, and inflamed throat from self-induced vomiting. The other findings are typically noted with anorexia nervosa.

**9. Answer: b**

Typical facial features include a low nasal bridge with short upturned nose, flattened midface, and a long filtrum with narrow upper lip. Microcephaly rather than macrocephaly is associated with fetal alcohol syndrome. Clubbing of fingers is associated with chronic hypoxia.

**10. Answer: c**

It is important to remind the parents that medications for the management of ADHD are not a cure but help to increase the child's ability to pay attention and decrease the level of impulsive behavior. The other statements are correct.

**11. Answers: d, e**

RATIONALE: Children diagnosed with dyslexia and dysgraphia experience difficulty with reading, writing, spelling, and producing written words.

**12. Answers: a, b, c**

RATIONALE: An 18-month-old toddler should have babbled by 12 months. He should be using gestures and using single words to communicate. The use of sentences to communicate and the ability to jump rope would be expected later.

**13. Answers: b, d, e**

RATIONALE: Common side effects related to the use of psychostimulants are: headaches, irritability, and abdominal pain. Children typically exhibit a decreased appetite and may have difficulty with insomnia.

**14. Answers: a, b**

RATIONALE: The parents should use a calm, low-pitched voice when communicating with her. They should ignore inappropriate behaviors. The parents should not argue or bargain with the child about set limits. They should praise the child for accomplishments and help the child see the importance of accountability for her own behavior.

**15. Answers: a, b, d**

RATIONALE: Altered sleep patterns, weight loss, and problems at school are commonly found in children with mental health disorders. There also may be alterations in friendships and changes in extracurricular activity participation.

# CHAPTER 31

## SECTION I: ASSESSING YOUR UNDERSTANDING

### Activity A FILL IN THE BLANKS

1. Pediatric
2. "LEAN"
3. Airway
4. Pupil
5. Cyanosis
6. Jaw-thrust
7. Femoral

### Activity B LABELING

A = Sinus tachycardia
B = Supraventricular tachycardia
C = Ventricular tachycardia
D = Coarse ventricular fibrillation

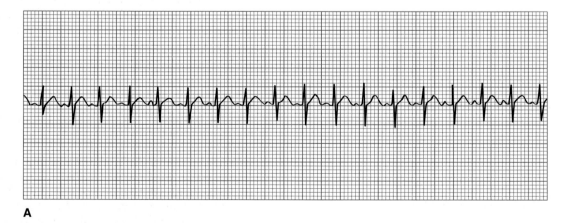

A

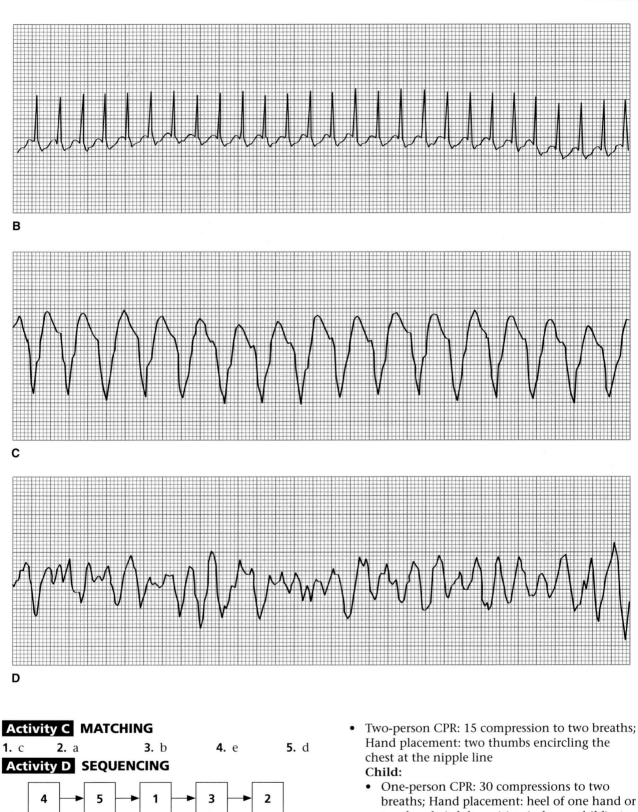

**B**

**C**

**D**

**Activity C** **MATCHING**

**1.** c  **2.** a  **3.** b  **4.** e  **5.** d

**Activity D** **SEQUENCING**

$$4 \rightarrow 5 \rightarrow 1 \rightarrow 3 \rightarrow 2$$

**Activity E** **SHORT ANSWERS**

**1. Infant:**
- One-person CPR: 30 compressions to two breaths; Hand placement: two fingers placed one finger breadth below the nipple line
- Two-person CPR: 15 compression to two breaths; Hand placement: two thumbs encircling the chest at the nipple line

**Child:**
- One-person CPR: 30 compressions to two breaths; Hand placement: heel of one hand or two hands (adult position in larger child) pressing on the sternum at the nipple line
- Two-person CPR: 15 compressions to two breaths; Hand placement: heel of one hand or two hands (adult position in larger child) pressing on the sternum at the nipple line

**2.**

|  | SVT | Sinus Tachycardia |
|---|---|---|
| **Rate (beats/ minute)** | Infants >220, children >180 | Infants <220, children <180 |
| **Rhythm** | Abrupt onset and termination | Beat to beat variability |
| **P-waves** | Flattened | Present and normal |
| **QRS** | Narrow (less than 0.08 seconds) | Normal |
| **History** | Usually none significant | Fever, fluid loss, hypoxia, pain, fear |

3. Choose an appropriate size bag and mask using a Broselow tape or referring to the code reference sheet. Connect the bag valve mask (BVM) via the tubing to the oxygen source and turn on the oxygen. Set the flow rate at approximately 10 L/minute for infants and small children, and 15 L/minute for an adolescent who is adult-sized. Check to make sure that the oxygen is flowing through the tubing to the bag. Open the airway. Place the mask over the child's face. Use the thumb and index finger of one hand to hold the mask on the child's face, and the other hand to squeeze the resuscitator bag. Use upward pressure on the jaw angle while pressing downward on the mask below the child's mouth to keep the mouth open.

4. Cricoid pressure may be used during the ventilation portion of resuscitative efforts to prevent gastric distention, possibly leading to vomiting and aspiration, during ventilation. Pressure is used to occlude the esophagus so that air does not entire the stomach during ventilation.

5. The mnemonic is used to assist in determining a worsening respiratory status of a child who is intubated. Each letter represents possible problems that require further assessment:
D: Displacement of the tracheal intubation tube
O: Obstruction of the tracheal intubation tube from mucus of other sources
P: Pneumothorax
E: Equipment failure

## SECTION II: APPLYING YOUR KNOWLEDGE
### Activity F  CASE STUDY

1. The discussion should include the following:
The use of AEDs on children was not recommended by the AHA until 2005. If the child is over 1 year of age and the emergency is a sudden witnessed collapse, the AHA suggests the use of an AED; this recommendation comes from the result of studies indicating that the AED can be sensitive and specific for detecting and treating arrhythmia by defibrillation in this population.

2. The discussion should include the following:
The chain of survival for children differs from the adult chain of survival due to the common causes of pediatric versus adult cardiopulmonary arrest. These differences affect the priority of steps during an emergency. The pediatric chain of survival begins with prevention of cardiac arrest and injuries, followed by early CPR, then early access to the emergency response system, and ends with early advanced care. The adult chain of survival begins with activation of the EMS, followed by early CPR, then early defibrillation, and ends with early access to advanced care.

## SECTION III: PRACTICING FOR NCLEX
### Activity G  NCLEX-STYLE QUESTIONS

1. **Answer: c**
The AHA emphasizes the importance of cardiac compressions in pulseless clients with arrhythmias, making this the priority intervention in this situation. Current AHA recommendations are for defibrillation to be administered once followed by five cycles of CPR. The AHA now recommends against using multiple doses of epinephrine because they have not been shown to be helpful and may actually cause harm to the child.

2. **Answer: a**
The nurse would be suspicious of a 7-month-old climbing out of his crib, since it is not consistent with his developmental stage. Other areas of concern are if the parents have different accounts of the accident and if the injury is not consistent with the type of accident.

3. **Answer: a**
Due to the potentially devastating effects of drowning-related hypoxia on a child's brain, airway interventions must be initiated immediately. The child's airway should be suctioned to ensure patency. Other interventions such as covering the child with blankets, inserting a nasogastric tube, and assuring that the child remains still during X-ray are interventions that are appropriate once airway patency is achieved and maintained.

4. **Answer: b**
Unilateral absent breath sounds are associated with foreign body aspiration. Dullness on percussion over the lung is indicative of fluid consolidation in the lung as with pneumonia. Auscultating a low-pitched, grating breath sound suggests inflammation of the pleura. Hearing a hyperresonant sound on percussion may indicate pneumothorax or asthma.

5. **Answer: b**
An adolescent, not a 9-year-old, would most likely require an oxygen flow rate of 15 L/minute for effective ventilation. A flow rate of 10 L/minute is appropriate for infants and children. All other options are valid for preparing to ventilate with a bag valve mask.

6. **Answer: c**

Decrease skin turgor is a late sign of shock. Blood pressure is not a reliable method of evaluating for shock in children because they tend to maintain normal or slightly below normal blood pressure in compensated shock. Equal central and distal pulses are not a sign of shock. Delayed capillary refill with cool extremities are signs of shock that occur earlier than changes in skin turgor.

7. **Answer: d**

Once the ABCs have been evaluated, the nurse will move on to "D" and assess for disability by palpating the anterior fontanel for signs of increased intracranial pressure. Observing skin color and perfusion is part of evaluating circulation. Palpating the abdomen for soreness and auscultating for bowel sounds would be part of the full-body examination that follows assessing for disability.

8. **Answer: b**

Inserting a small, folded towel under shoulders best positions the infant's airway in the "sniff" position as is recommended by AHA Basic Cardiac Life Support (BCLS) guidelines. The hand should never be placed under the neck to open the airway. The head tilt chin lift technique and the jaw-thrust maneuver are used with children over the age of 1 year.

9. **Answer: b**

Exhaled $CO_2$ monitoring is recommended when a child has been intubated. It provides quick, visual assurance that the tracheal tube remains in place and that the child is being adequately ventilated. When moving the child, maintaining tube placement would be crucial. The other interventions would also be appropriate but not as essential as monitoring the child's exhaled $CO_2$ level. Unlike the other interventions, exhaled $CO_2$ monitoring can provide an early sign of a problem.

10. **Answer: c**

Attaining central venous access is the priority intervention for a child in shock who is receiving respiratory support. Gaining access via the femoral route will not interfere with CPR efforts. Peripheral venous access may be unattainable in children who have significant vascular compromise. Blood samples and urinary catheter placement can wait until fluid is administered.

11. **Answer: 6 millimeters**

RATIONALE: The following formula should be used to calculate the correct tracheal tube size for a child: Divide the child's age by 4 and add 4 = size in millimeters

$$(8 \text{ years old}/4) + 4 = 6 \text{ mm}$$

12. **Answer: 5,700**

RATIONALE: Cardiac output (CO) is equal to heart rate (HR) times ventricular stroke volume (SV). That is, $CO = HR \times SV$.

$$76 \text{ beats per minute} \times 75 \text{ mL} = 5,700$$

13. **Answer: 25 milliliters per hour**

RATIONALE: 56 pounds $\times$ 1 kg/2.2 pounds = 25.455 kg of body weight.

$$25.455 \text{ kg} \times 1 \text{ mL/kg} = 25.455 \text{ mL/hour}$$

The child must produce 25 mL/hour

14. **Answer: 709 milliliters**

RATIONALE: 78 pounds $\times$ 1 kg/2.2 pounds = 35.455 kg $\times$ 20 mL/kg = 709.1 mL. When rounded to the nearest whole number = 709 mL.

15. **Answer: 84**

RATIONALE: Use the following formula (according to PALS):

$$70 + (2 \text{ times the age in years})$$

Hence, the minimal systolic BP of a 7-year-old is $70 + (2 \times 7) = 84$.